Sustainability and Health

Sustainability and Health

Supporting global ecological integrity in public health

Editors:
Valerie A. Brown, John Grootjans, Jan Ritchie,
Mardie Townsend and Glenda Verrinder

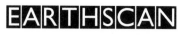

London • Sterling, VA

First published by Earthscan in the UK and USA in 2005

An Innovation Project of the Public Health Education and Research Program, the Australian
Government Department of Health and Ageing. This text represents the views of the authors, and
may not represent the views of the Commonwealth.

For a full list of publications please contact:

Earthscan
8–12 Camden High Street
London, NW1 0JH, UK
Tel: +44 (0)20 7387 8558
Fax: +44 (0)20 7387 8998
Email: earthinfo@earthscan.co.uk
Web: www.earthscan.co.uk

22883 Quicksilver Drive, Sterling, VA 20166-2012, USA

Earthscan is an imprint of James and James (Science Publishers) Ltd and publishes in association
with WWF-UK and the International Institute for Environment and Development

A catalogue record for this book is available from the British Library

Library of Congress Cataloging-in-Publication Data

Sustainability and health : supporting global ecological integrity in public health / Valerie A. Brown
… [et al.].
p. cm.

Includes bibliographical references and index.
ISBN 1-84407-174-X (hbk. : alk. paper)
ISBN 1-84407-173-1 (pbk. : pbk. paper)

1. Public health. 2. Human ecology. 3. Public health–Environmental aspects. I. Brown, Valerie A.

RA425.S876 2004
362.1–dc22
          2004015215

Set in 10.5pt Garamond by Big Island Graphics, Canberra
Printed by South Wind Production, Singapore

Contents

Learning Activities   vii

Boxes and Figures   viii

Acknowledgements   x

Glossary   xiii

Prologue: The way in   xvii

Chapter 1 Living:
Public health and the future of life on the planet   1

1.1   Health and sustainability: a new direction for public health   3

1.2   Defining sustainable development: moving to sustainability   11

1.3   New ideas for new public health: overview of recommended readings   18

1.4   Integrative decision-making about place-based issues (D4P4):
an open learning framework   21

1.5   Sustainability as public health practice: criteria for future-oriented practitioners   28

Chapter 2 Listening:
Co-ordinating ideas on sustainability and health   39

2.1   Sustainability and health   41

2.2   Sustainability and science   43

2.3   Sustainability and economics   48

2.4   Sustainability and environmentalism   59

Chapter 3 Grounding:
Co-ordinating contexts for sustainability and health   81

3.1   Frameworks and tools   83

3.2   Strategic frameworks   84

3.3   Health-based frameworks   93

3.4   Environmental frameworks   106

3.5   Holistic frameworks   121

Chapter 4 Knowing:
Linking the knowledge cultures of sustainability and health   131

4.1   Evidence-based public health   133

4.2   Multiple knowledges   143

4.3   Strategies for synthesis   149

4.4   Tools for synthesis   152

Chapter 5 Scoping:
Designing and monitoring sustainability and health programs   **163**

5.1	Monitoring strategies: what we believe we need to know	165
5.2	The decision-making spiral: what we know we need to know	169
5.3	The file, the grid and the cycle: what we know we don't know	173
5.4	Working with others: what we don't know we don't know	183
5.5	Scoping the program stages: what we now know we need to know	187

Chapter 6 Acting:
Practitioners as actors for sustainability and health   **199**

6.1	Systems thinking	201
6.2	Planning the action	212
6.3	Acting together	226
6.4	Acting individually	235

Chapter 7 Innovating:
Practitioners as innovators for sustainability and health   **243**

7.1	Structural change for sustainability	245
7.2	Capacity building for structural change	251
7.3	Education for sustainability	262
7.4	Research for sustainability	267

Chapter 8 Managing:
Public health leadership and management for sustainability   **273**

8.1	The challenge to public health of managing for sustainability	275
8.2	Analysing issues at multiple levels	277
8.3	Managing complex systems: three organisational forms	278
8.4	Managing hierarchical or formal organisations for sustainability	282
8.5	Managing networks and communities for sustainability	290
8.6	Managing markets for sustainability	296
8.7	Leadership and drivers for sustainability: the role of public health	300

Epilogue: The way forward   **307**

The editors   **315**

Index   **319**

Learning activities

1.1	Value line: clarifying ideas of sustainability and health	6
1.2	Reality check: what holds this planet together?	10
1.3	Decision-making frameworks: how do we put knowledge into action?	27
1.4	Practitioner as change agent: continuum of change	33
2.1	Chinese whispers spiral	43
2.2	Where all the rivers flow: working collaboratively in complex ecological systems	72
3.1	Mind-mapping complex ideas	92
4.1	Assessing the evidence: how do we tell the truth?	140
4.2	Linking the knowledges: case study of decision-making on persistent organic pollutants (POPS)	145
4.3	Using the rules of dialogue: group negotiation exercise	151
4.4	Who do we involve in linking the knowledges?	155
5.1	Synoptic workshop designs	172
5.2	Participatory rapid appraisal (PRA)	183
5.3	Sharing ideas: brainstorming	190
5.4	Scoping and grounding: guided visioning exercise	192
6.1	Systems thinking: the futures wheel	211
6.2	Intersectoral action	220
6.3	Rich pictures or priority-setting: nominal group process	224
6.4	Conflict resolution styles	233
6.5	Acting individually: measure your ecological footprint	239
7.1	Reflection	249
7.2	Diffusion of innovation game	250
7.3	Imagining, settings for innovation	256
7.4	Writing a media release	262
8.1	Building a tower	280

Boxes and Figures

Boxes

1.1	Global indicators of loss of sustainability 1950-95	9
1.2	Sustainable development as principles, issues and processes	12
1.3	Sustainability definitions	13
1.4	Sustainability 2003	16
1.5	Parallels between sustainability, health and environment-based frameworks	18
1.6	Universal competencies and core disciplinary areas in public health education	29
2.1	Indigenous knowledge	71
3.1	Our clients for this chapter	83
3.2	Universal Declaration of Human Rights	86
3.3	Declaration of Alma-Ata	94
3.4	Health for All by the year 2000	98
3.5	Ottawa Charter for Health Promotion	101
3.6	Stockholm Convention on Persistent Organic Pollutants	108
3.7	Montreal Protocol on Substances that Deplete the Ozone Layer	110
3.8	Rio Declaration on Environment and Development	112
3.9	Kyoto Protocol on Greenhouse Gases	118
3.10	Talloires Declaration	119
3.11	Earth Charter Principles	121
4.1	A letter to the editor: being scared of GM	137
4.2	Sustainability in action	146
4.3	Rules for dialogue in a multiple knowledge learning community	150
6.1	Subsystems	205
6.2	The systemic nature of environmental health issues	206
6.3	The Bellagio Principles	215
6.4	Rural City Farm: cultivating a vital urban community	219
6.5	Spectrum of participation	228
6.6	Approaches to participation	229
6.7	Twenty participatory techniques in participatory evaluation	230
6.8	The transformation of Curitiba, Brazil	234
6.9	Ethical guidelines for practice	236
6.10	Climate change: ten solutions for individuals	239
7.1	Overcoming barriers to change	248
7.2	The innovation diffusion game from *Believing Cassandra*	250

7.3	Appreciative inquiry	254
7.4	The shared action story	258
7.5	*Local Heroes*	260
7.6	Seven kinds of intelligence	266
8.1	Three organisational forms co-existing in a complex system	282
8.2	Ideal type characteristics of a bureaucracy	283
8.3	Ideal type characteristics of a network	290
8.4	Ideal type characteristics of a market	296

Figures

1.1	Three eras of public health practice	5
1.2	The Mandala of Health: a systems model of the human ecosystem	17
1.3	Sustainability decision-making framework 1	23
1.4	Change agent continuum	34
4.1	Five paradigms of knowledge	139
4.2	Knowledge cultures within Western decision-making systems	142
4.3	Web of community-based action for sustainability and health	153
5.1	Deductive and inductive problem-solving	167
5.2	A Rose is a rose is a rose	168
5.3	Sustainability decision-making framework 2: decisions-into-practice (D4P4)	171
5.4	Information sources for environment and health reporting	175
5.5	DPSEEA grid for environmental health monitoring	179
5.6	Three-circle diagram of sustainability	179
5.7	Framework for developing environmental health indicators	182
5.8	Extended pressure-state-response framework	183
6.1	Futures wheel using 'no oil' as an example	213
6.2	Windows on environment and health	222
6.3	Grounding the environment for health	222
6.4	A chequerboard model of integrated action for sustainability	223
8.1	Management domains	278
8.2	Three organisational forms for sustainability management	279

Acknowledgements

This resource book is the product of a three-year process, which has involved many people who have generously given their time to move the concept of sustainability and health and this book forward. The project started as a germ of an idea generated by three people, Emeritus Professor Valerie Brown AO, Professor Rod Simpson and Associate Professor Jan Ritchie in 2001.

The project commenced at a point of great debate and relative uncertainty in the field of public health, where public health practitioners were being informed about global environmental events and their potential for significant impact on the wellbeing of populations, and yet were not included in the debate. The question for public health was: what is the role for public health practitioners in the sustainability governance process?

The opportunity to answer this question came with funding from the Public Health Education and Research Program (PHERP) within the Commonwealth Department of Health and Ageing through their Innovation Grants Program. We offer our sincere thanks to Angela McKinnon and Jane Bell, and later Anne Dullow and Brendan Gibson, of that Department, who have guided us throughout. John Grootjans became project manager and Professor Desmond Connell replaced Rod Simpson as the Griffith University representative and administered the project from Griffith University, after Rod took up a senior position at the University of the Sunshine Coast.

Two groups became essential to the success of the project. The first group was invited to act as a steering committee and the second group to act as a set of expert advisors. The steering committee included the project management group and the representatives from PHERP, as well as Michael Sparks, Greg MacAvoy, Adam McEwan, Anne Neller and Kevin Buckett. The expert advisors group was made up of a group of international key thinkers in the area of sustainability and included Alan AtKisson (Sweden), Fran Baum (Australia), Gillian Durham (New Zealand), Trevor Hancock (Canada), Tony McMichael (Australia), Ian Lowe (Australia), Phillip Mills (Torres Strait Islands), Bill Rees (Canada), Colin Soskolne (Canada) and Mathis Wackernagel (USA). This group has contributed to the process in many ways, providing direction in the early stages, giving us permission to use their work extensively, critically reading various reports and participating in web conversations. We thank them most warmly for their commitment to the project.

The editors would like to extend their thanks to the many people who over the last three years have contributed to the iterative and collaborative process which was the heart of the book preparations. Colin Soskolne, through his personal commitment to sustainability and health, made a major contribution, trialling the final draft of the book in a graduate course in the Department of Public Health Sciences at the University of Alberta, Edmonton, Alberta, Canada, with the assistance of Josh J. Marko. The collective suggestions from the group engaged in this course have served to substantially improve the text. The student commentators were: Jody Mackenzie, Geneva Rae, Kim M. Deschamps, Brian Ladd, Vanessa Lam, Jason Klinck and Leila Darwish.

Drawn from the 36 universities teaching public health in Australia, the following people participated in a web-based discussion group which clarified issues surrounding sustainability and health.

Jane Bell, Commonwealth Department of Health and Ageing

Colin Butler, Australian National University

Frank Fisher, Monash University

Ritchie Gun, Flinders University

Elizabeth Hanna, Latrobe University

John Harris, Australian National Biocentre, Inc.

Jane Heyworth, Flinders University

Maggie Hine, University of South Australia

Pierre Horwitz, Edith Cowan University

Bernie Marshall, Deakin University

Rosemary Nicholson, University of Western Sydney

Sharron Pfueller, Monash University

Dino Pisaniello, James Cook University

Helen Ross, University of Queensland

Peter Stephenson, University of Western Sydney

Mardie Townsend, Deakin University

Rae Walker, Latrobe University

And web-site advisors Phil Gang, Mem Gang and Cate Turner-Jamison TIES, Mass.,USA

During this stage of the project, Glenda Verrinder joined the management group. In September 2002 people contributing to linking sustainability and health as individuals, community, specialists and government were invited to attend a writing workshop to prepare the first draft of this book. The following people warrant the editors' special thanks for their contribution to the considerable work and thought that went into the three days of the workshop: Jane Bell, Colin Butler, Barbara Chevalier, Gillian Durham, Frank Fisher, John Harris, Lee Hatcher, Jane Heyworth, Maggie Hine, Pierre Horwitz, Helen Jordan, Angela McKinnon, Tony McMichael, Bernie Marshall, Anne Neller, Rosemary Nicholson, Ron Pickett, Bernard Gilles Rohan, Wendy Rainbird, Michael Sparks, Rae Walker.

Members of our expert advisory group, Gillian Durham, Lee Hatcher (an associate of Alan AtKisson), Tony McMichael and Colin Soskolne attended the writing conference as both expert advisors and full participants. At this stage Mardie Townsend became a full member of the management group. Heather Gardner, Sue Noy and Cesidio Parissi undertook an editorial and critical content review of the book. Regan Field and Tom Chevalier checked the references. Kim Tatnell of Big Islands Graphics worked with us as colleague and editor as well as being responsible for the book's design and production. The editors would particularly like to thank the following people, who assisted the chapter authors by commenting on and helping to finalise each chapter:

Chapter 1   Gillian Durham, Frank Fisher, Maggie Hine and Pierre Horowitz

Chapter 2   Jane Bell, Cecily Maller and Colin Soskolne

Chapter 3   Jane Bell, Colin Soskolne and Joel Townsend

Chapter 4   Gillian Durham, Frank Fisher, Maggie Hine, Pierre Horowitz and Bernard Gilles Rohan. (The foundation material for Chapter 4 was developed during Valerie Brown's residency at the Bellagio Study Centre of the Rockefeller Foundation)

Chapter 5   John Harris, Lee Hatcher, Bernie Marshall, Anne Neller Michael Sparks and Rae Walker

Chapter 6   Barbara Chevalier, Lee Hatcher, Angela McKinnon, Rosemary Nicholson, Ron Pickett, and Wendy Rainbird

Chapter 7   Barbara Chevalier, Lee Hatcher, Angela McKinnon and Wendy Rainbird

Chapter 8   John Harris and Bernie Marshall

Glossary

Access to decision-makers talking to elected representatives; to information, is legislated for and controlled by the privacy act; to services, equality of opportunity

Advocacy presenting a case in favour of meeting the needs of a group or an issue

Agenda 21 United Nations Program of Action for Environment and Development, agreed at Rio de Janeiro in 1992

Airshed volume of air overlying a distinct geographic region

Algal bloom excessive algal growth triggered by sunlight, warm temperatures, still waters and dissolved nutrients

Anthropocentric human-centred view of the world

Biodiversity the number and range of species of plants and animals on the planet

Biological integrity unbroken inter-related biological systems of food webs, energy chains, and photosynthesis

Bio-region a naturally occurring region made up of a comparatively self-contained biological system, such as a valley or a lake

Case studies documentation of a set of events, stories of experiences

Catchment land area drained by a river and its tributaries

Change agent person that acts to change the way things are presently done, often an 'ideas broker' or an innovator

Change management initiatives which lead to immediate and/or strategic change, bringing new skills and new ideas with them and empowering people to change

Civil rights the rights of every citizen, as established in legislation and in the Constitution

Climate change the predicted changes in climate due to accumulation in the atmosphere of carbon dioxide and other gases produced by human activity

Community a group of people living in a common geographical locality or sharing a common interest

Community development working with communities so they have the opportunity of identifying issues of concern and of addressing the issues in their own way

Consultation talking and listening to each other as equals

Corporate plan the forward planning by which organisations coordinate all aspects of their activities, usually for the coming year

Council control statutes legal basis for council's ability to control air, water or soil pollution

D4P4 decisions into practive framework

Data series of observations, measurements, events

Democracy	representative democracy: people entrust others to make decisions on their behalf; participatory democracy: people participate directly in decision-making
Determinants of health development	factors which are known to link statistically to ill-health, such as socio-economic status, diet, physical exercise
Ecocentric	environment-centred view of the world
Ecologically sustainable	the title of an Australian intergovernmental policy with a set of guiding principles
Ecosystem	communities of organisms and their physical environment interacting as a unit
Environment Round Table	national and provincial environmental management committees which include balanced representation from government and community agencies, and from social, economic and environmental interests
Environmental health	refers to the interdependence between the health of individuals and communities and the health of the environment
Environmental Health Impact Assessment	a formal process that answers the question, how will this activity or event affect the environment and human health?
Epidemiology	the study of the determinants and patterns of disease
Equity	equal opportunity to access resources between generations, groups of people, people and the environment
Equity of representation	group made up of equal number of consumers and government members
Evaluation	the process of judging the worth or value of something, usually a periodic assessment of the progress or worth of a program
Facilitation	assisting a person, an event, a change process or a group to meet their goals
Global ecological integrity	refers to the maintenance of the complex relationship between life on the planet and the ecosystems that support this life
Governance	directing and controlling an organisation; establishing and implementing policies that shape activity
Government	direction of the affairs of state, at any scale
Habitat	the type of place where organisms or a community of organisms live (their 'address' in the natural system)
Health	a complete state of physical, mental and social wellbeing and not merely the absence of disease or infirmity (WHO 1948); a resource for everyday life, not the object of living (WHO 1986)

Health and wellbeing	the optimum physical, social, and mental wellbeing (WHO 1948)
Health promotion	the process of enabling people to take control of, and improve, their health
Healthy Cities	a World Health Organisation project based on the idea that a healthy city is the outcome of health-oriented education, transport, economic and housing policies; a supportive environment; a strong community; individual healthy lifestyles and preventive rather than treatment services
Human rights	an ideal that transcends culture, class, language and any other structures or discourses of difference; it assumes that the state has an obligation to ensure that the human rights of citizens are protected and realised; citizens to respect the human rights of others and exercise their own human rights
Indicator	measure or symbol that reflects the status of a system
Indigenous	native to a region
Indigenous values	respect and acknowledgement of local groups' spiritual connections to their land
Knowledge	data applied to a standard becomes information; information absorbed into personal or professional understanding becomes knowledge
Local Agenda 21	a shared management program for a locality which incorporates the goals of all stakeholders in the community and balances social, economic and environmental resources; one of the more powerful programs emerging from the United Nations Conference on Environment and Development held in Brazil in 1992
Multidisciplinary	the combination of several disciplines, can be two (interdisciplinary) or include other modes of knowledge (transdisciplinary)
Negotiating	discussing and settling on terms
Networking	making connections, usually among people
OECD	Office of European Commission for Development
Place management	place-based integration of community and government in the management of place
Point source pollution	point of emission of industrial or other polluted gases (as compared with ambient pollution, which is spread over a wide area)
Policy	principles that guide action
Politics	the science or art of political government; holding the power
Precautionary principle	the absence of scientific certainty should not be used as a reason for failing to avoid risk, or acting to prevent potentially serious harm

Primary health care   delivery of early intervention and preventive health care, by family, community or services

Public health   the art and science of preventing disease, and protecting and promoting the health of the community

Riparian zone   the banks of a waterway (river or creek)

Risk assessment   scientific evaluation of the chances of injury or harm

Risk communication   an interactive process involving exchange among individuals, groups and institutions of information and expert opinion

Risk management   managing the dangers arising from the presence of risks to environment or health

Single bottom line   synthesis of the dimensions of the triple bottom line (economic, social, physical), that is, the whole is greater than the sum of its parts

Social justice   social philosophy that advocates a fair and even distribution of the benefits and burdens in society

Social welfare   government action for those in need

Species   a group of organisms which are biologically capable of breeding and producing fertile offspring with each other but not with members of other species

Stakeholders   those who have a vital or vested interest in the process

Sustainability principles   ensuring continuity for current and future generations; maintaining integrity of ecological life-support systems; practising the precautionary principle; and monitoring social and economic impacts on environmental resources

Sustainable development   the management of environmental resources in such a way that the needs of the present generation are met without reducing the capacity of the next generation to meet their own needs

Systems theory   assumes that real systems are open to, and interact with, their environments, and that they can acquire qualitatively new properties through emergence, resulting in continual evolution

Triple Bottom Line   accounting system that evaluates the status of social, and environmental, as well as financial resources

Wetland   an area of low-lying land that is irregularly, regularly or permanently covered with either fresh or salt water

Wildlife corridor   a passage for migration of free-living populations of native animals

WHO   World Health Organisation

the way in

PROLOGUE

The way in

The challenge

Sustainability and Health: Supporting global ecological integrity in public health addresses a key question in 21st century public health. The cumulative impact of our activities on the self-renewing ecological systems of the planet has been clearly established as unsustainable (McMichael 2001). Governments, social organisations and environmental management agencies have been attempting to address these 'clear and present dangers' for many decades, but public health practitioners have generally been missing from this arena (Brown et al. 2001). They now need to join their colleagues. Our future depends on it.

The generally accepted pathway to a sustainable future is through applying the principles of sustainable development.

The generally accepted pathway to a sustainable future is through applying the principles of sustainable development. The sources and adequacy of the principles need to be critically examined as they apply to public health and re-examined in the light of social priorities, environmental change and the responsibilities of public health practice. The inevitable conclusion is that this will require significant change in perspective and in the acquisition of skills new to public health. This interpretive perspective and these skills make up the content of the book.

The process

The collaborative process which forms a thread throughout this book was also used in the preparation of the book itself. Being fully aware of the gap in public health understanding and practice in this critical arena, the authors applied for an Innovation Grant under the Australian Government's Public Health Education and Research Program. Funding was granted from 2001 to 2003 for a three-year project to support the teaching of sustainability in public health training programs across Australia. A basic discussion paper was compiled and a group of eminent international experts invited to form the project's advisory committee. In 2001 and early 2002 the framework for learning resources was put together in an open learning process through interactive deliberations on a teaching/learning website. Forty academics and policymakers with environmental and public health expertise made up the learning group and most contributed very actively. This process evolved into a writers' workshop where the book chapters and learning activities took further shape; subsequent working groups completed the first drafts. The learning materials were made available for testing as a teaching resource, with volunteers responsible for relevant public health courses in Australia and Canada providing extensive feedback, all of which has contributed to the final content.

The task

This learning resource seeks to address the overall question: Why do we have to worry about health risks from the environment?

The global bodies responsible for informing us about these issues are in strong agreement here as to the answer. A report from the United Nations, the World Bank and the World Resource Institute unequivocally supports the need to address this concern (United Nations Environment Program 2001). The changes we are experiencing in our global air, water, forest and soil life-support systems have already begun to limit the availability of resources that have enabled improvements to human health.

The book also endeavours to offer answers to three questions regularly put to the researchers, teachers and administrators in sustainability and health who prepared this book:

Why do we have to worry about health risks from the environment?

- why is sustainability of key importance for public health?
- why does sustainability require a new approach for public health?
- what difference does sustainability make to my current practice?

While the full answers can be found in the book itself, the short answers are:

- 'sustainability' has become the short-hand expression for the long-term social and economic changes required to re-establish global ecological integrity, the foundation for the planet's life-support systems, thus also of the health of the human population;
- sustainability practices address the unprecedented global scale of simultaneous disruption of population, finance and governance systems, requiring a fresh approach to social support systems including public health; and
- public health practice has now broadened to include matters of:
  - i. living sustainably
  - ii. listening to multiple perspectives
  - iii. grounding in collaborative frameworks
  - iv. acknowledging multiple forms of evidence

v. scoping the global and local context of public health action

vi. acting for global integrity

vii. innovating for global integrity and

viii. managing for the sustainability of health and environment in the long-term future.

These topics are central to the issues, and have therefore been chosen to form the structure and content of the eight chapters in this book.

It can be important to say what a book does not do. This is not a reference file to the latest risks to health from the environment, though it mentions the chief of them frequently as examples. The complementary reading recommended for a briefing on the interactions between health and environment risk is McMichael's *Human Frontiers, Environments and Disease* (2001).

Nor is the book a technical resource, with grids cross-referencing risk factors and responses. Our approach is that health and environment are interactive components of a dynamic system. We offer a range of ways to address changes in that system, including open learning, team-building, strategic frameworks, knowledge synthesis, systems thinking, advocacy and leadership. These are key skills for the public health practitioner in any public health domains, but in *Sustainability and Health* these are related to the need to work in both environment and health fields simultaneously. A comprehensive and far-reaching overview of the contribution of the various specialist fields to our understanding of potential action on environment and health can be found in Soskolne and Bertollini (1999).

Our approach is that health and environment are interactive components of a dynamic system.

Two other relevant and key texts are down-to-earth accounts of sustainability and public health, accessible to individual actors, community members, specialists, industry and government. AtKisson's *Believing Cassandra* (1999) and Baum's *The New Public Health* (2002) make up the other readings complementing our message.

The perspective

During the period we have been developing this resource, we have realised that we are promoting not the mere learning of new knowledge and skills, but much more. We are advocating a major change in mind-set, the taking on of a new world view, the adoption of a whole alternative paradigm. We believe the changes we are recommending for public health practitioners require almost a social revolution for them to be initiated and then accepted—we advocate for an extraordinary change in our manner of working which will lead to sustained action for the benefit of the environment and humans within it.

Our approach is unusual in the more conventional circles of environmental science and public health since we are asking people to leave their bounded intellectual silos and instead reach out towards transdisciplinary and multi-stakeholder consensus. We respect and build on positivist scientific methods, especially as these methods have contributed to the advances in technological understanding. However, we actually take a social constructivist approach in our analysis and synthesis of the issues included here—a kind of approach with which we feel very comfortable, but which may be regarded as radical by those comfortable in their routine manners of working. We hope the perspective we have taken will serve to bring about the change in mind-set we feel must occur for global ecological integrity to be a reality. Our project is now complete. We invite you to read on.

We are advocating a major change in mind-set, the taking on of a new world view, the adoption of a whole alternative paradigm.

The editors:

Valerie A. Brown
John Grootjans
Jan Ritchie
Mardie Townsend
Glenda Verrinder
February 2004

References

AtKisson, A. 1999, *Believing Cassandra: An optimist looks at a pessimist's world*, Scribe Publications, Melbourne

Baum, F. 2002, *The New Public Health*, Oxford University Press, South Melbourne

Brown, V.A., Nicholson, R., Stephenson, P., Bennett, K.-J. and Smith, J. 2001, *Grass Roots and Common Ground: Guidelines for community-based environmental health action*, Hawkesbury Regional Integrated Monitoring Centre, University of Western Sydney, Richmond, New South Wales

McMichael, A.J. 2001, *Human Frontiers, Environments and Disease: Past patterns, uncertain futures*, Cambridge University Press, New York

Soskolne, C.L. and Bertollini, R. 1999, *Global Ecological Integrity and 'Sustainable Development': Cornerstones of Public Health*, WHO European Centre for Environment and Health, Rome, http://www.euro.who.int/document/gch/ecorep5.pdf [22 January 2004]

United Nations Environment Program 2001, *UNEP Annual Report*, UNEP Geneva, http://www.grid.unep.ch/proser/publications/annual/anlrpt2002.pdf [10 February 2004]

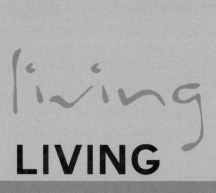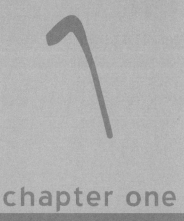

LIVING

Public health and the future of life on the planet

Valerie A. Brown, Jan Ritchie, John Grootjans,
and Bernard G. Rohan

Summary

The task of public health has always been to interpret and respond to the effects on human health of major social and environmental change. This has been true throughout the development of urbanism, industrialisation, globalisation and now planetary environmental change. With global life-support systems at risk, the role of public health has broadened yet again—this time to addressing the integrity of ecological systems so these continue to support the variety of life on Earth. For perhaps the first time it is imperative that the public health practitioner acts as if the sustainability of the environment were of equal importance with the sustainability of our species. In this chapter the work of the 21st century public health practitioner is placed in the context of the global social, economic and ecological changes of our time. We propose an integrative decision-making framework for the public health practitioner or student to use to critically examine the current conditions of global ecological integrity that are affecting the wellbeing of humankind. The framework incorporates an open learning process as the task requires an open, inclusive and innovative perspective—and humility in not assuming that we know all the answers.

Chapter 1 Living

Public health and the future of life on the planet

Valerie A. Brown, Jan Ritchie, John Grootjans and Bernard G. Rohan

Key words

Diversity, equity, globalisation, humility, inclusivity, integrity, learning, localisation, potential, precaution, sustainability, sustainable development

Learning outcomes

Public health practitioners and students will be able to:

- critically evaluate the principles and practices offered for ensuring ecological sustainability as a precondition for safeguarding the future of life on the planet;
- interpret current knowledge and understanding of sustainability principles and practice in the decision-making context and biosocial circumstances in which they operate; and
- use a community learning model of public health practice that will enable them to advance their own and their clients' understanding of the importance of sustainability for health.

Outline

1.1 Health and sustainability: a new direction for public health

1.2 Defining sustainable development: moving to sustainability

1.3 New ideas for new public health: overview of recommended readings

1.4 Integrative decision-making about place-based issues (D4P4): an open learning framework

1.5 Sustainability as public health practice: criteria for future-oriented practitioners

Learning activities

1.1 Value line: clarifying ideas of sustainability and health

1.2 Reality check: what holds this planet together?

1.3 Decision-making frameworks: how do we put knowledge into action?

1.4 Practitioner as change agent: continuum of change

Reading

AtKisson, A. 1999, *Believing Cassandra: An optimist looks at a pessimist's world,* Scribe Publications Pty Ltd, Melbourne, Chapter 1

McMichael, A.J. 2001, *Human Frontiers, Environments and Disease: Past patterns, uncertain futures,* Cambridge University Press, Cambridge, Chapter 1

Soskolne, C.L. and Bertollini, R. 1999, *Global Ecological Integrity and 'Sustainable Development': Cornerstones of Public Health*, WHO European Centre for Environment and Health, Rome, http://www.euro.who.int/document/gch/ecorep5.pdf [22 January 2004]

1.1 Health and sustainability: a new direction for public health

At one of the project management team meetings to discuss the development of this book, a profound question was put to the group: why sustainability? In other words, for what reason were we working so hard? The answer is not as simple as you might imagine. The people at the meeting did not say things such as, 'because our planet is warming', 'our resources are running out', or 'our environments are becoming toxic waste dumps'. Those answers were too simplistic and, as time has shown, there are no simple solutions. After a great deal of discussion, one of the group simply said, 'When in 20 years' time one of my grandchildren asks me why our generation let things go on for so long when everything was telling them time was running out, I want to be able to tell them I did all I could.'

Why sustainability?

As Capra (1983) suggested in *The Turning Point*, we are at a point in history where the essential nature of our relationship to the environment is changing. Like Capra, we believe the next generation will not understand the motivations for our purely growth-driven actions today, just as we found it hard to understand the mid-20th century motivation for tolerating the spread of fascism. We would like readers to begin this book by contemplating answers for the children of 2020.

Baum's *The New Public Health* (2002) puts the argument for a new approach to public health based on the increase in globalisation and decrease in equity in and between populations. This book takes this new direction one step further and argues that if public health is to consider its full responsibility to the health of the public, it has no choice but to give major consideration to global sustainability.

Survey results are indicating most people believe the environment is an important consideration and that the community has good knowledge of environmental issues (Mainieri et al. 1997). If this is so, why is there no corresponding increase in action for the environment, even in simple issues such as waste recycling? This conundrum is also true of the response of public health practice in general: while there is an obvious connection between health and a state of global ecological integrity, there seem to be only isolated reactions on behalf of public health practitioners toward global ecological integrity.

Such a reorientation of public health is nothing new. Public health has always been regarded as a response to changes in the biophysical landscape. Hippocrates of Kos and his school supported the idea that nature—which included the human body—could cure itself, and that the quality of the environment had an important bearing on this process. The beginning of public health as a formal practice was a courageous response by Snow (Ashton and Seymour 1988) to prevent water being pumped from a cholera-infected supply and was carried out in the face of extensive disapproval from the local community. His removing the pump handle, acting on indicative but not final evidence (that is, applying the precautionary principle) halted the epidemic . . . but raised the fury of the water-deprived population. These characteristics—acting for the public good when there is a risk too great not to act on, even if the evidence is not all in and before the public is aware of the risks—are still part of public health practice today.

Public health has always been regarded as a response to changes in the biophysical landscape.

We are now in the third of three phases in public health practice arising from health risks of the industrial revolution, economic development and the current concern about sustainable development (Figure 1.1). Each era has called on different responses from public health practitioners and their colleagues (Brown et al. 1992). In the first phase reducing the risks of infectious disease epidemics lay in the hands of the civic authorities, who made decisions about urban renewal, sewerage and hygiene. Legal action saw the emergence of restraints on public freedom of some to safeguard the health of all, including quarantine, condemned housing and controls on contamination of water sources and waterways.

After major epidemics of infectious diseases had been controlled (at least in developed countries) by changes in public infrastructure, the second phase of public health emerged with the industrial byproducts and wastes of economic development. Technical testing capacities for monitoring air, water and soils became major professional skills of public health practitioners. As the pressures of industrialisation increased, the global changes identified in Figure 1.1 not only arose but also made an increasing and more immediate impact at the local scale.

By the last quarter of the 20th century, public health practice was faced with an even greater change in its application. As well as increases in its existing responsibilities there came the added responsibility of protecting local environmental life-support systems. Moreover, this responsibility is also

Figure 1.1 Three eras of public health practice

Era	Risk	Source	Public health response
1. Industrial revolution	**Infectious disease**		**Technical solutions**
1870-1930	cholera	water	sewerage
	diphtheria	air	domestic hygiene
	tuberculosis	crowding	urban design
2. Economic development	**Ways of living**		**Lifestyle change**
1930-1970	acute toxicity	lead	paint, petrol standards
	lung cancer	asbestos	industry regulation
	chemical overload	wastes	monitoring, reporting
3. Sustainable development	**Global stress**		**Governance solutions**
1970-	melanoma	UV radiation	halogen controls
	disease spread	climate change	limit energy use
	allergies,	environmental	environmental
	toxicity	degradation	management

Source: Adapted from Brown et al. 1992

for the future; not only for the local population but also for that population as a unit of the planetary environment. Long-term protection has always been the concern of public health, but single localities can no longer be protected in isolation from their neighbours. The long shadows of the major cities, the rapid transport of goods and services mean that collaborative regional and national action is required. Local issues still offer the unit of action when dealing with global concerns, leading practitioners to seek to widen their links with a range of professions, expert advisors and community interests at other scales of action. Contamination of city air by transport exhausts, blue-green algae affecting many waterways and the leaching of nitrates into groundwater from crop runoff are examples of unsolved health risks arising from environmental disruption. Maintaining sustainable ecosystems as essential prerequisites for human health is now beginning to be accepted as part of the responsibility of public health. This newly emerging knowledge base for public health utilises knowledge from all three phases in Figure 1.1. This book is designed to stimulate a new generation of public health workers to recognise the connections between the health of the ecosystem and the health of populations. It is the first phase of a continuing dialogue about how public health practitioners can participate in action for sustainability as an essential consideration in promoting the health of populations. It should not be viewed as a new dogma, but rather as the first step in a critical review of the role public health practitioners play currently in sustainability along with actions they can take to improve the situation in the future.

Activity 1.1
Value line: clarifying ideas of sustainability and health

Aim: to help practitioners describe their values in relation to health and sustainability, and to explore ways people with different values can work together.

Description of learning activity

The three-day writing workshop that created this resource book turned out to be a microcosm of the application of the book. The 25 participants crossed two generations and included public health, medicine, education, nursing, environmental management, social research, management, epidemiology and community development professions and more than 15 academic disciplines. They held a range of positions on sustainable development and worked at most points of delivery of public health practice, from epidemiology to community action to national health policy. What they had in common was a combined practitioner and personal interest in linking health and the environment in public health practice. To work together, the workshop needed a way of linking this range of interested parties in a common understanding.

The first activity of the workshop was designed to create such a shared understanding. The group members each took up a position on what is known in education as a 'value line'. Given a notional 10 dollars, participants were asked to position themselves at the point on the line where they would apportion the money, with the limits being 'all for the birds and the bees' (health of the environment) at one end or 'all for the babies' (human health) at the other. As the participants distributed themselves along the line the full range of positions was occupied, though with bunching at each extremity and in the centre.

Feedback

Participants were asked to share their reasons for taking up their positions. The feedback that came from them included:

1. Those at the 'babies' end considered looking after people their primary responsibility, though they acknowledged that to care for people meant the environment must also be considered.

2. Those at the other end had concluded that the environment must take the highest priority for its own sake as the functioning system that underpins the living world and thus as foundation for human life.

3. Where the value line differed from the usual range of positions in public health was in overlapping agreement between the extremes and the reasons given by the group in the centre. In most public health debates such as priorities for treatment or prevention, or addressing the needs of the individual or the population, the middle group would be advocating a mix of both and acting as peacemaker between the extremes.

4. In this exercise those at the poles could agree on the overlap and the central group did not take up a strictly half-and-half-position. On the contrary, it was agreed that a first priority for linking health and environment was a distinctive position in its own right, reflecting a fundamental unity and not merely a combination of the poles.

The 'linking environment and health' group as a whole considered it represented three value positions for incorporating sustainability in public health practice:

- acting as a balancing point between human and environmental interests, ensuring full incorporation of both positions;

- creating a third dimension at right angles to the conventional line, generating and maintaining a fresh perspective on the human/environment relationship; and

- encompassing all the positions along the value line in a circle of a shared knowledge base and collaborative practice.

Source: Brown et al. 2002

Global ecological integrity: the issues for public health

The term global ecological integrity refers to the maintenance of the complex relationship between life on the planet and the ecosystem that supports this life. The concept suggests that for the existing life-support system to remain fully functional, it must be able to regenerate itself in its entirety after addressing any ecological crisis threatening this integrity (Soskolne & Bertollini 1999).

The public health practitioner needs to consider a suite of emerging ecological issues around these threats. These should be viewed as a list of symptoms that result from humanity's poorly considered hunger for rapid growth and unsustainable development, as a result of which ecological symptoms are affecting human wellbeing and resulting in global disintegrity.

> *Human changes to the environment have altered the continuity of global cycles, and the rate of change is expected to increase.*

Human changes to the environment have altered the continuity of global cycles, and the rate of change is expected to increase. Ozone depletion, global warming, urban pollution, non-degradable industrial waste, fresh water contamination and biodiversity depletion are bringing serious and increasing risks to sustainability of the planet's life-support systems and so to human health and wellbeing. Pimentel et al. (1998) claim that 40 per cent of the human disease burden now arises from environmental sources. In a report to the 2002 World Summit, the World Health Organisation (WHO) calculates the figure as closer to 25 per cent—still an amount to be reckoned with (World Summit on Sustainable Development 2002). McMichael (2001) considers structural change is needed in public health practice and in the larger community's cultural and technological processes to recreate a functioning ecosphere that can continue to support biological and social needs.

In 1986 the World Commission on Environment and Development explored ways in which human impact on the environment has endangered the sustainability of global systems (World Commission on Environment and Development 1987). Environmental sustainability was acknowledged as crucial to preserving human health in its own right, not merely as a support system. Despite this recognition the rate of disruption of global air, water, soil and living systems—that is, of the traditional concerns of public health —has increased. The trends recorded in Box 1.1 represent the unprecedented challenges faced by public health practitioners at both global and local scales, and reveal how long these changes have been documented.

Box 1.1 Global indicators of loss of sustainability 1950-95*

Parameter:	1950	1995	
Ozone depletion, Antarctica	110	80	Dobson units
Global warming	14.89	15.39	degrees Celsius
Irrigation	136	248	million hectares
Forests	40%	27%	global cover
Productive land (grain)	0.23	0.12	hectare per person
Population: world total	2.55	5.73	billion people
Annual increase	37	87	million people
Energy use – oil	518	3031	megatonnes
– natural gas	187	2114	megatonnes
– windpower	<10	4880	megawatts

* Measures as agreed by UNDP, Worldwatch and World Resources Institute 1995, confirmed 2002

Source: Brown 1998, p. 270

International conventions have failed to arrest the escalating rates of environmental degradation. The Kyoto Protocol for reducing the production of greenhouse gas emissions causing global warming was not unanimously supported; global temperatures are rising, the ozone hole reappears every year and irrigation and the resulting soil salinisation is increasing. Food production per head is falling, and species are disappearing at the same time that population is rising (although the rate of increase is slowing). Fossil fuel use is increasing, though the proportion of renewable energy use is rising. The unchecked continuation of almost all the trends documented in Box 1.1 has been acknowledged by the major global agencies (World Bank, United Nations Environment Program, World Resources Institute, and the United States National Research Council). The question we need to ask in any teaching/learning program on sustainability and health is: Since all the responsible agencies confirmed those trends in 1995, why is it that those trends continue in 2002? The answer has to lie in re-thinking the solutions we are currently applying. In the context of this book we consider public health practice needs to take these trends into account and act accordingly.

Reports on the state of the global environment suggest that increasing risks from degraded environmental resources of air, water and soil (particularly water) are approaching thresholds beyond which the damage may be irreversible. Thus, risks to the sustainability of environmental systems have become risks to human health in themselves, through:

- directly damaging human systems, for example, through contaminated drinking water;
- degrading small-scale environmental systems on which human systems depend, for example, through forest clearing that reduces local rainfall and so local water supplies;
- disrupting global environmental systems on which all species depend, for example, through contributing to global warming; and
- diminishing biodiversity and indigenous plant knowledge systems, reducing the stock of potential medicines for future generations.

Activity 1.2
Reality check: what holds this planet together?

Aim: this activity aims to illustrate the scope and the interconnectedness of global flows.

Take a globe of any sort, large or small. If you can't find one, take the image of the planet from a geography text. There are at least seven major patterns of global flows:

- information
- people
- air
- fresh water
- food
- finance
- weather

Identify the hubs and patterns of the flows that go around the world. Do they overlap/interact/impede/enhance each other? Are there weak points for a sustainable planet that need watching?

1.2 Defining sustainable development: moving to sustainability

'Sustainable development' has been the generally preferred response to human-generated environmental changes as they affect our wellbeing. The usual working definition is taken from the World Commission on Environment and Development (1987, p. 43) as 'development which meets the needs of the present without compromising the capacity of future generations to meet their own needs'. It is doubtful whether this definition can hold up today, with global systems already significantly changed. The WCED also included global ecological integrity and human collaborative social systems in its recommendations, so perhaps it is time for a new look at this definition. Principles of sustainable development have been adopted by the United Nations and their relevant family of organisations as the basis for policy development, program design, program delivery and monitoring of the outcomes of global and local environmental changes. These principles have also been incorporated in the health, environmental and public health policies of the United Kingdom, Canada and Australia. Sustainable development principles have been translated into action in many different ways. They are referred to in the 27 action groups in Agenda 21 (see Chapter 6). In the Bellagio principles they are set out as modes of action (Chapter 5), and in the Australian Ecologically Sustainable Development Strategy and the Australian National Public Health Strategy and Implementation Plan they are set out as five strategic goals (Chapter 6).

There is much discussion in the literature on whether sustainable development is an oxymoron (a pair of irreconcilable opposites), a paradox (a contradiction in terms), or a newly derived concept in the process of being developed. There are also debates on whether it is a tangible goal, a mode of action or an ideal. We are assuming here that it is a necessary goal, one toward which all professions and practitioners must work, not public health alone. The most generally accepted working definition of sustainable development is that it is a set of principles, issues and processes (Box 1.2).

'Sustainable development' has been the generally preferred response to human-generated environmental changes as they affect our wellbeing.

Box 1.2 Sustainable development as principles, issues and processes

A set of principles:
- equity between generations
- equity within a generation
- conservation of biodiversity
- dealing cautiously with risk
- local/global accountability

Source: Department of Environment Sport and Territories 1992

A set of issues:
- resource depletion and degradation (economic perspective)
- pollution and wastes (ecological perspective)
- society and the human condition (social perspective)

Source: Dovers 1989

A set of actions:
- increased efficiency of resource use and decreased waste production
- management practices that improve the resilience of natural resource systems
- dealing cautiously with risk and irreversibility
- integration of social and environmental considerations into economic decision-making, including proper valuing of environmental resources
- community involvement in decisions

Source: Department of Environment Sport and Territories 1992

While Australia is the only country that has added 'ecologically' to sustainable development, in all other respects the terms are applied internationally in exactly the same way. Publications as various as those of the United States Research Council and the World Bank have moved to use 'sustainability' as a more appropriate concept than sustainable development. This move reflects the progression from working to resolve two conflicting agendas (ecological sustainability and economic development) to that of reconciling both these and social agendas such as health in a co-ordinated long-term solution. Understanding and describing sustainability has been one of the issues of continuing consideration and dialogue for the group engaged in this project. However, at this stage we have settled with a description for sustainability and health proposed by our expert advisors who have agreed that sustainability in public health is about transformational change in environmental governance; it is neither about revolution nor is it about 'business as usual':

> *Sustainability in public health requires both local knowledge and strategic knowledge of environmental change as well as the specialised knowledge of the academic disciplines; and Sustainability and Health teaching programs will need to be different from traditional courses in that they deal with the future as well as the present, and about what to change as well as how to address what to preserve.* (Sustainability and Health Project Expert Advisors 2001)

Box 1.3 Sustainability definitions

Sustainability has been defined by others as:

'Living every day as if we were going to live forever' (Anon)

'Reconciling development goals, social needs and ecological resources' (World Commission for Sustainable Development)

'Supporting a life-sustaining Earth' (USA EPA)

'Valuing a single bottom line' (Australian Local Government Authorities)

'Aspiration, learning, pathway, conceptual, improvement, consideration, equality, caring, being, striving, embracing, changing, thinking, doing, wanting, needing, capacity-building, excellence, will, needed, timely, open-minded, fair play' (Gary Hankinson, Coffs Harbour Council)

'Respecting and sustaining natural and cultural systems and the interplay between them' (Australian National Biocentre)

'Not a problem but a solution' (Human Ecology Forum, ANU)

Source: Keynote addresses at the Indo Pacific Conference on Environment and Health, Perth, Western Australia, November, 2002

The implementation of sustainable development principles has been extremely varied, both in individual countries and worldwide. In Britain, MacDonald (1998) evaluated 45 Agenda 21 projects that had been launched at UNCED 1992 and found only eight still proceeding, all of which were based on local action. In 1999 the United States Institute of Medicine, Research, Engineering and Science reviewed the global situation and, like many similar reviews, found there were structural barriers to the implementation of sustainable development principles in professional education and research (United States National Research Council 1999). Their combined report, Our Common Journey, accepted that a transformation of current research and education frameworks was required if there was to be progress towards sustainable development, and recommended the following changes in direction:

- establish research and education frameworks that integrate global and local perspectives to shape a 'place-based' understanding of the interactions between environment and society;
- ensure that the three key decision-making groups of community, experts and government are fully involved in the research into and the delivery of sustainability programs;
- initiate dedicated research programs on the under-studied questions that are central to a deeper understanding of interactions between society, environment, and the health of all life forms; and
- promote better use of existing tools and processes to link knowledge and action in pursuit of a transition to sustainability.

A place for health will need to be negotiated among the interests of environmental resource management, economic efficiencies, continuity needs of diverse social groups, and organisational territories

These recommendations provide one of the few sets that link education, research and evaluation in the context of global change, and bring together the specialised fields of health, environment and science. They offer useful guidelines for a public health curriculum addressing sustainability and health. One thing is certain: public health initiatives, coming late into the field of sustainability practice, cannot go it alone; the diversity of interests and information means teamwork and multiple alliances will be necessary. Nor can public health practitioners assume that health will be the lead agency in social change, as has often been the case. A place for health will need to be negotiated among the interests of environmental resource management, economic efficiencies, continuity needs of diverse social groups, and organisational territories—no mean task.

One of the early warnings of need for these changes came in the early 1970s. The Club of Rome project headed by Donella and Dennis Meadows (Meadows et al. 1972) developed a thesis titled *The Limits to Growth* using computer modelling to demonstrate the cumulative and interactive effects of growth in population, energy use and polluting byproducts of industry on the self-renewing capacity of the environment. Predictions of ozone depletion, global warming and water depletion date from this time. The warning was partly heeded, with industry and governments of industrialised countries recognising that some controls and re-tooling were necessary. The lessons on social structural change and the need to reinterpret both problems and solutions were lost. The increasing rate of environmental decline has led, by 2003, to recognition that some form of global intervention and reinterpretation of growth and development is required. AtKisson (1999) recalls the impact of the Club of Rome and brings the idea of sustainable development up to date in the light of all we have learnt since then, giving us three necessary conditions for the physical survival of our species:

1. not using up renewable natural resources (air, water, life forms) faster than they can replenish themselves;

2. investing ahead to develop replacements for depleted non-renewable resources (fossil fuels, fertile soils) while we still have the wealth from using up the resources; and

3. not producing wastes faster than natural processes can absorb them.

AtKisson goes on to point out that physical survival is not enough; humanely governed sustainable development is required for the survival to be worthwhile (summarised in Box 1.4). AtKisson's messages, carrying many lessons that echo those of public health practice (making healthy choices the easy choices; turning change into routine behaviour, and moving from treatment of outcomes to prevention of risk), are explored on behalf of public health practice in Chapter 6.

The model known as the Mandala of Health depicts the human ecosystem as a complex web of interrelationships, each component of which has potential to affect human health (Hancock 1985). In the Mandala, the social unit (individual or family) is placed as the centre of concentric circles ever-expanding out to the biosphere. Within the circles are four key factors that determine health. The form the Mandala takes serves first to illustrate that the impacts of changes in one part of the web of relationships are not restricted to that part and instead are likely to make an impact across the entire web. The model especially makes clear that there is a very tight relationship between culture and environment, thus emphasising the risks of this tightening relationship as humans have learned to manipulate the planet. As well as acting to describe the nature of the interrelationships, the Mandala has the potential to serve as a framework for action and in its modified form (Figure 1.2) has been adapted as a guide for practice (Brown et al. 2001).

The increasing rate of environmental decline has led, by 2003, to recognition that some form of global intervention and reinterpretation of growth and development is required.

Box 1.4 Sustainability 2003

Sustainability means yes, not no

While environmentalism has been important in protecting natural resources, we now need more positive initiatives that protect society from the results of the past two centuries of over-use of resources (saying yes to sustainable, healthy futures).

Sustainability is business as very unusual

Redesigning, rebuilding and rethinking our cities, industries, transport systems, educational programs and governance so these remain liveable and workable into the next century require transformational thinking, not business as usual.

Sustainability decouples development and growth

Sustainability is development without growth, decoupling development from production, consumption and pollution and linking it to learning, improving, rebuilding and reorganising. Factor Four is a proposal to halve the growth and double the development.

Sustainability is a way of life

Just as people at the turn of the last century adopted personal hygiene as a way of life that defeated the great plagues and extended lifespans, sustainable practices in living, in business and as a community will allow populations to live well into the future.

Sustainability is the beginning, not the end

As we enter the post-industrial phase of history, the options are endless. The social transformation forecast as inevitable in dealing with the inheritance of degraded systems from the 20th century is also an entry point to a future in which human capabilities are extended in ways we perhaps cannot now imagine.

Source: Summarised from AtKisson 1999

One of the key concepts Hancock advocates as central to the process of the WHO Healthy Cities project is community action (2000):

> . . . *a concern with ecology necessarily becomes part of a social movement because the problem of reversing the present self-destructive treatment of the environment cannot be separated from the right to challenge the authoritarian decision making process invested in corporate and governmental institutions.*

Figure 1.2 The Mandala of Health: a systems model of the human ecosystem

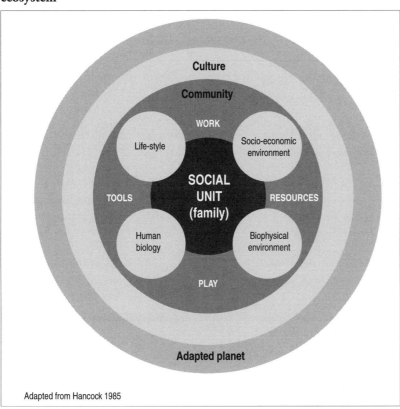

Adapted from Hancock 1985

Hancock states that 'a shared vision can be a powerful force that brings together a community and inspires its members to take action together' (Hancock 2001). Healthy Cities begin their projects by allowing citizens to participate in a process of visualising a common future. The project works with citizens to help them establish indicators of success and participate in a process of evaluation and re-evaluation. In parallel with Healthy Cities, Hancock with others developed the Ottawa Charter for Health Promotion, now known as the blueprint for a new public health (WHO, Health and Welfare Canada and the Canadian Public Health Association 1986). There are clear parallels between the New Public Health, Local Agenda 21 and the principles of sustainable development (Box 1.5).

In *Doing Less Harm*, Hancock takes the medical system's ethical commitment to *primum non nocere*—first, do no harm—to inform the medical profession of its responsibility to make health facilities environmentally healthy (Hancock 2001). This booklet provides simple, commonsense actions for change with case studies of successful stories. Hancock argues that hospitals are significant users of energy and that the health implications of energy use such as carbon dioxide emissions and resource depletion are greater than the health implications of all other aspects of unsustainable hospital buildings put together.

Box 1.5 Parallels between sustainability, health and environment-based frameworks

(Headings 1-5 represent the five core elements of sustainability)

New public health (eg Healthy Cities)	**Sustainable development** (eg Local Agenda 21)
1. Integrated policy and evaluation	
Inter-sectoral collaboration	Valuing social, economic and environmental change
2. Self-supporting ecological systems	
Sustainable environments	Ecological integrity and biodiversity
3. Social equity	
Self-empowered communities	Inter-generational equity
4. Citizens' rights	
Individual skills	Intra-generational equity
5. Precautionary decision-making	
Health promoting services	Precautionary principle

1.3 New ideas for new public health: overview of recommended readings

Baum addresses the strengthening links between environmental issues and the overall health of the public. In *The New Public Health* (Baum 2002), she reviews current public health, especially addressing the translation of the rhetoric into public health practice. She traces the way public health has moved from its basis primarily on bio-medical models to a wider, more holistic and multidisciplinary activity. This more encompassing perspective has been termed the 'New Public Health' (Hancock 1985; Ashton & Seymour 1988; Baum 2002). Baum provides clear evidence of the strong practice links between environmental health practitioners and public health practitioners. An assumption underpinning all her work is that of the primacy of community involvement in decisions and actions that affect members of that community.

In relating the history of public health practice, Baum shows how the values underpinning this recent perspective are developing and are still fragile. She describes how the rather paternalistic collective public health measures of the 19th and early 20th centuries, with their focus on policies and laws across society, gave way late last century to concentration on individual and personal health behaviours, with approaches echoing clinical practice in medicine. Context, situation and locality were not seen to be of importance. Little value was given to proactive or preventive measures, with most effort and funding being directed to reactive responses addressing problems already defined. Although Baum and colleagues have moved to support the principles of the new public health, which they identify as the contemporary view, many in the public health field find any movement away from standard medical practice to be retrogressive and see the work of community-focused public health as of lesser value.

. . . many in the public health field find any movement away from standard medical practice to be retrogressive and see the work of community-focused public health as of lesser value.

The changes in the global environment and its impact on health described by McMichael confirm the need for a further perspective on public health practice, education and research, that we believe could be termed the 'new, new public health'. Soskolne and Bertollini (1999) propose that global ecological integrity, previously taken for granted, is emerging as the cornerstone of public health. They put forward the idea that shifts in current practice and new frameworks are needed to make wise decisions governing the change. Breaches in global environmental integrity are emerging as the biggest challenge in protecting public health, greater even than the move to cities and the great plagues of past centuries, since they threaten the future of the species itself. Soskolne and Bertollini's thesis, which includes contributions by researchers from many disciplines published in the same discussion document, provides an excellent overview of the social, economic and ecological implications of these conclusions.

Soskolne and Bertollini suggest that potential solutions lie in models that focus more on social, information and service-based development than on growth. They argue that knowledge that transcends the barriers of scientific disciplines is necessary for achieving interdisciplinary scientific understanding and consensus, and for reaching agreements among many societal interests to promote appropriate changes in policy and practice. This position is expanded and applied in Chapter 4.

Participants in the Soskolne-Bertollini symposium addressed the 'principle of ecological integrity'. Rees (2000) described humans as a dominant species in the global ecological system, large, adaptable social mammals that live in groups. They have correspondingly large energy and material demands and all resources entering the human economy come from natural systems. Very few unmodified local habitats are productive enough to support even modest groups of people living in permanent settlements for very long. In this respect we are a true 'patch disturbance' species in that we have an impact on the environments we inhabit, a distinction shared with other mammals ranging from beavers to elephants, yet it is evident that the nature of our patch disturbance has a longer lasting if not permanent impact (McMichael 1993; Flannery 1994).

'Accordingly, the appropriate way of approaching nature to learn about her complexity and beauty is not through domination and control, but through respect, cooperation and dialogue'

Capra more recently has revisited this idea by suggesting, 'Accordingly, the appropriate way of approaching nature to learn about her complexity and beauty is not through domination and control, but through respect, cooperation and dialogue' (Capra 1996). Prigogine (1980) describes our society as a 'dissipative structure' drawing resources from external sources to maintain the integrity of society's structures, while all the time increasing the disorder in locations where the resources are drawn. If we accept Prigogine's hypothesis, the nature of our current society can only be maintained through destructively decreasing global ecological integrity (Westra 1998). Not for the first time, public health practice for sustainability and health requires changes in the way we live.

The context of public health education, and particularly the incorporation of sustainability and health into it, reveals a system in the process of change. In responding to this change, continual review and re-evaluation of the application of sustainable development principles in public health is necessary. This will allow these to meet the challenge Soskolne and Bertollini (1999) have described and become a cornerstone of public health and public health practice across the world. Adhering personally to the principles of sustainability can be seen not only as a means of enlarging the focus of public health practice but also as an essential 'role-model' allowing not only more effective distribution of the sustainability 'message' but also encouraging more effective practice in its own right. Personal practice contributes in its own way to closing the gap between sustainability and health in theory and practice.

Hess (in Soskolne & Bertollini 1999), in the same symposium, reviews the significance of impaired ecological integrity for public health. He suggests that unintentionally and unwittingly, public health has contributed to the breaching of the planet's natural systems. The profession of public health has promoted economic development as a means of achieving health. Public health strategies have tended to disregard the ecological consequences of their various interventions. Traditional public health interventions have focused predominantly on humanity as an independent entity and not in the context of the living environment. In both its measures and its interventions, the goal of public health has been to make people impervious to nature by making them immune to disease and by increasing longevity. In such a framework the elements of nature are implicitly reclassified into resources for and threats to human health.

New measures are required to assess health as a balanced system of individuals, communities and the environment. This changing way we view the world around us needs explicit recognition of humankind's niche in the greater environment and of our natural limitations as a species. This new, new public health perspective also requires accepting the public health practitioner as one of a multi-skilled team, a team learning together to support the changing human/environment relationship.

New measures are required to assess health as a balanced system of individuals, communities and the environment.

1.4 Integrative decision-making about place-based issues (D4P4): an open learning framework

Nothing is more certain in our lives than change. Change is all around us; every time we open our front doors to go outside it seems something else is different. Our work here does not involve stopping change, since that would be both impossible and absurd. We do advocate, however, that we become deeply involved in and help to guide a new approach to change. Each of us has ideas—good ideas for improving things—but some of us never get the chance to put those ideas into practice. We suggest throughout this book that change is based on economic, technological, environmental and social considerations, and that somehow all these need to be considered at the same time in the change process. Below we describe a process we believe will lead to sustainable change and development that includes a humane future. The development of this process is necessarily iterative in that it is part of an ongoing dialogue.

Sustainability and health practice is based on the need to respond to and manage change rather than simply follow what has gone before; therefore we need an adaptive, responsive critical learning framework, one that provides the basis for long-term learning. The framework proposed for the design of teaching programs, course materials and field experience in this book is based on a combination of experiential inquiry-based learning principles (Kolb et al. 1974) and place-based cooperation for local sustainability (Brown 1997; Western Sydney Regional Organisation of Councils et al. 2000).

Sustainability and health practice is based on the need to respond to and manage change rather than simply follow what has gone before.

Kolb et al. (1974) argue that all learning is about change, and adult learning is best characterised as a form of personal inquiry into real world problems. This educational approach is well suited to responding to issues of sustainability and health, requiring acceptance of the need for transformational change. Kolb outlines four steps in the experiential learning cycle, linked here with the matching step carrying individual learning into the public sphere: observation and reflection (describing), abstract conceptualisation (designing), active experimentation (doing) and testing the new ideas in fresh situations (developing). This gives us the four Ds described in Figure 1.3.

In his applied research Kolb demonstrated that different professions concentrated on one or more of the steps of the cycle—engineers on concrete observation, scientists on active experimentation, and management on reflection and observation. He argued that an individual or a project team often did not complete the learning/problem-solving cycle; that the learning and/or the inquiry was therefore incomplete and so was unsustainable over the longer term. The learning cycle is in practice a spiral with continual learning throughout an individual's or an organisation's lifespan. Kolb's work has influenced the field of action research, acting as a framework for life-long learning in a number of professions and giving rise to the idea of the learning organisation, a key concept in organisational management circles (Senge 1992).

It is becoming increasingly apparent that the future sustainability of the human species depends on adaptive, system-wide solutions to linked social, economic and ecological issues. It is becoming equally apparent that

Figure 1.3 Sustainability decision-making framework 1

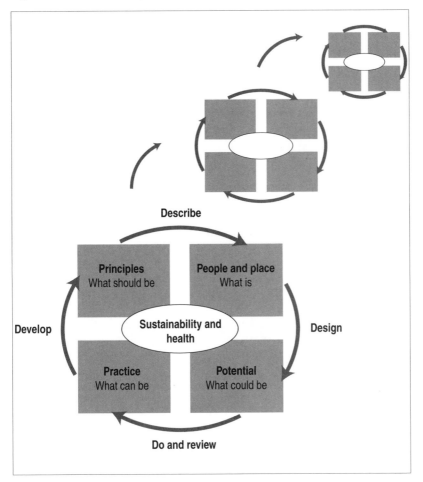

The principles by which we live, as private citizens or as expert practitioners, are based on some set of ethical values . . .

aids to understanding complex, inter-related ecological systems to improve decision-making will be needed to augment the prevailing analytical, single-factor thinking. Among such aids is the D4P4 decision-making framework designed to be used as a guide to local decision-making under conditions of system change toward sustainability (Brown 1997). The framework was first developed in partnership with local government authorities as a monitoring and evaluation model for local integrated state-of-the-environment reporting. Through the pursuit of grounded theory, which also follows the Kolb experiential learning cycle through ideas to practice to new ideas, the D4P4 framework became established as a useful tool in partnership with local government and their communities (Brown 1997). Since then the D4P4 framework, which links knowledge to action, has been used in a range of change management processes from land care communication and redesign of a curriculum in public health to regional state-of-the-environment reporting (Western Sydney Regional Organisation of Councils et al. 2000). By incorporating sustainable development principles into public health decision-making and so into public health education and practice, the change process goes through four stages of knowledge development and their related action. Kolb's experiential stages of develop, describe, design, and do (D4 in Figure 1.3.) enable the establishment of a knowledge base of principles, people and place, potential and practice, and subsequent review, thereby constructing a spiral learning process. This then gives us the 4 Ps in Figure 1.3.

Developing principles (what should be) to guide practice (what can be): applying new ideas

The principles by which we live, as private citizens or as expert practitioners, are based on some set of ethical values, whether the values are explicitly acknowledged or, more usually, taken for granted. The principles (what should be) drive our actions; for example, 'Since I value the sustainability of the human species, I should follow the precautionary principle. Because the risks from climate change are too great, this will mean reducing my energy use.' In the case of emergent concerns such as sustainability and health, longstanding values are not likely to change, but a fresh understanding of the situation may alter the principles that decide the type of action; for example, the shift in response to drought in Australia. Until a decade ago, it has been 'drought is a national disaster', with support to 'drought-stricken' families. The altered response is to 'drought as a normal event in the Australian climate', with support for 'responsibilities' of families to adopt different farming practices and/or leave the land, though some of the former response continues in parallel with the new approach. The ethical value of humane care for humans remains, but the accompanying principle for land care has dramatically changed, and so have the appropriate actions. The values underlying the key words 'health' and 'environment' are widely debated and indeed interpreted differently in different cultures and communities. The debate on the values underlying 'health' has been only partly resolved by the widely applied WHO definition: that health is the attainment of optimum bio-psycho-social wellbeing (World Health Organisation 1948).

This statement originally omitted 'spiritual wellbeing', leaving a gap criticised by many nation-states, formal religions and health professionals, to the extent that a recent World Health Assembly has recommended its inclusion (World Health Organisation 1999). The definition is also seen as lacking in that it does not consider environmental wellbeing as a necessary precondition for health. The value line exercise described in Activity 1.1 offers an example of the importance of identifying values and agreeing on some key principles before a mixed group of practitioners begins to work together.

Describing people and place (what is): reflecting and observing

Since public health practice now needs to respond to global environmental change, it is important that information on the status of sustainable development principles is included in most if not all public health teaching programs. Principles (what should be) will influence which aspects of health and environment (what is) are selected as content for training in evidence-based practice. Learning about sustainability and health is not primarily about information transfer, though it will require the best available information on people and place. The educational task lies in preparing for key roles as agents of change in the sustainable governance of our increasingly hazardous ecosystem. Environmental management then takes on a new significance as part of public health practice. Progress toward sustainability and health requires an accurate record of the status of inter-related changes in social, economic and environmental resources, and the cumulative effects of the interactions between them. The chapters that follow begin with an examination of the wide range of perspectives (environment-centred, people-centred, resource-centred) on the status of sustainability and health across the globe, and how these perspectives are being incorporated into the context of public health action. The situation varies from public health programs that fail to deal with sustainable development, to those where it is a central focus. Tools to help the public health practitioner understand the mass of background information and multiple options for action are needed in order to explore ways of moving forward.

Learning about sustainability and health is not primarily about information transfer . . .

Designing potential (what could be): abstract conceptualisation

In the emergent field of sustainability and health, practitioners are working with unpredictable outcomes and as yet largely unspecified practices.

At this stage of the early 21st century, the public health community is only just beginning to accept that sustainability is an important public health goal. Under these circumstances of uncertainty and change, the creative design of new ideas and strategic thinking, and new possibilities for practice, can well be of greater effectiveness than continuing to follow the precedents of established practice. This is not to suggest 'throwing the baby out with the bath water', but that there is a need to incorporate the new with the old, undoubted strengths of well-tried practice.

In this phase of the decision-making process, the ideas that will help realise the potential of human inventiveness and environmental resilience are also emerging. This knowledge is not already stored in libraries or professional practice records, but is being developed through the creative stimulus of changing environmental conditions, the interactions of globalisation, the technical capacity of the Internet and the warnings of impending crisis. The foundation for 'what could be' has been laid by deciding on shared principles and describing 'what is'. For this stage it will be most productive to begin a process that will lead decision-making groups to redefine sustainability and health. Open discussion will allow many viewpoints about the way forward to be considered. Public health practitioners will gain from working with the widest possible range of colleagues. During this phase, open dialogue in a creative, safe, non-confrontational environment as described by Bohm (1996) encourages entry of new ideas, and the synergy sparked by the interaction of different ideas provides the basis for learning. This returns the practitioner to the primary proposition underpinning Kolb's learning stages: learning is essentially individual and personal, and social learning proceeds from experiential individual learning. Chapters 4 and 6 explore the use of the rules of dialogue in practice, and Chapters 6, 7 and 8 address a range of ideas and possibilities for individual practitioners to expand their potential.

. . . the ideas that will help realise the potential of human inventiveness and environmental resilience are also emerging.

Doing and reviewing practice (what can be): concrete experience

Putting ideas into practice is the testing site of the whole decision-making process. Lack of such application is one of the most frequent complaints about the current management of the sustainability process, from the Kyoto principles on controlling greenhouse gases to the conclusions on lack of progress toward sustainability at the 2002 World Summit on Sustainable Development (Lonero 2002). Sustainability and health practitioners from public health cannot go it alone when it comes to practice; they need fellow practitioners from all the disciplines involved in this book. Chapters 5-8 cover the public health practitioner roles: acting for, delivering innovatively, and managing for sustainability and health.

Not only practice but also review of practice is essential for the effective practitioner. The scoping of what is intended to result from the practice and the context in which it is conducted need to be determined before the practice begins, otherwise the practitioner has no basis for making judgments on what works under what conditions; this is why the chapter on scoping is presented before the chapters on sustainability and health action. Traditional public health scoping practices include epidemiological profiles; for sustainability practice these need to be coupled with annual state-of-the-environment reports allowing for the observation of patterns that emerge. While all adult education in a changing society is education for change, the question remains of how change is expressed in the education and practice of public health professionals in an era of unsustainable change. The answer—or rather answers—to that question provide the foundation for the content, approaches and skills of a public health curriculum incorporating the principles of sustainable development. Such answers are emerging from a rapidly growing body of practical experience and theoretical debate on the pathways to achieving sustainability and health.

Putting ideas into practice is the testing site of the whole decision-making process.

Activity 1.3
Decision-making frameworks: how do we put knowledge into action?

Aim: to become familiar with the application of the D4P4 place-based decision-making framework as a public health diagnostic and planning tool.

Time: 2 hours.

Equipment: large sheet of paper, one transparency sheet and 7 felt pens for each group. In groups of 7-9, choose a sustainability issue that is important to where you are working; for example, genetically engineered crops, global warming, river flows, local pollution or waste issues.

Step 1. Place a large piece of butcher's paper on a table and on it draw a large version of the four boxes and connecting arrows of Figure 1.3.

Step 2. Fill in each of the boxes with the five major points answering the questions for your selected issue: Which principles are relevant here? *(Think of ESD, sustainability, Earth Charter etc.)*

What is the crucial and relevant information about people and place? *(Think of vulnerable populations, sensitive environments, sources of impact.)*

What initiatives would maximise the potential for sustainability? *(Think of local action, public health team-building, regulations change, policy development.)*

How would you go about putting the options into practice and evaluating them? *(Think of the resources, skills, strategies, and workforce needed.)*

Step 3. From the overview on the large sheet, prepare an action brief for a public health practitioner acting on the issue. What policies would they act under, who would be their clients, what change agency strategies would they choose, how would they put the strategies into action and what would be the criteria for success?

Step 4. Summarise the action brief for your group as the D4P4 cycle. Compare action briefs between groups.

1.5 Sustainability as public health practice: criteria for future-oriented practitioners

The move to incorporating sustainable development in socio-political structures worldwide has been slow, but is now accelerating under a new process of sustainability. Public health is one of the professions that needs urgently to reconsider its role in maintaining the health of human populations, in the light of current state of the world environment reports. Contemporary international events provide the teaching process with a clearly described and shared body of knowledge.

A recent report on public health education in the USA offers some rhetoric which could translate into producing practitioners who could comprehend the demands of these major changes (Institute of Medicine 2003). The report suggests that public health professionals 'must understand the theoretical underpinnings of the ecological model [of health] . . . to more effectively address the challenges of the 21st century' (Institute of Medicine 2003, pp. 6-7). The report built on earlier work emphasising the importance of the universal competencies together with the five core disciplinary areas (Fineberg et al. 1994).

Box 1.6 Universal competencies and core disciplinary areas in public health education

Universal competencies include:
- analytical skills
- communication skills
- policy development/program planning skills
- cultural skills
- basic public health science skills
- financial planning and management skills.

The disciplinary areas include:
- public health administration
- cultural competence
- epidemiology
- community-based participatory research
- biostatistics
- health policy and law
- behavioural sciences
- global health
- environmental public health
- ethics.

Source: Fineberg et al. 1994; Institute of Medicine 2003

While it represents a demanding repertoire of professional skills, the list in Box 1.6 offers the adaptability and openness to the new approaches needed for incorporating sustainability into an established profession. Sustainable development adds another perspective and body of content, much of it drawn from the field of environment governance, to the wide range of paradigms already existing in public health. Related fields include health risk assessment, social impact assessment, health promotion, health education, social justice, community development, epidemiology and the New Public Health and its vehicle of Healthy Cities, to name but a few (Hancock 2000, 2001; Baum 2002).

The content and skills of environmental management are equally well established, but not usually yet considered an integral part of public health. Environmental risk and impact assessments, environmental education and law, adaptive land management and Local Agenda 21 plans (from the 1992 UNCED *Agenda for Sustainable Development in the 21st Century*) are all grappling with the health implications of global and local environmental degradation (Hancock 2000). The overlapping sets of environmental and health activities described above lead inevitably to the conclusions that, of the two sets of information, each requires the other for effective decision-making; and that of the two sets of professional skills, each calls for close collaboration with the other. Each group of professional practitioners takes pride in its expertise and may well question the intrusion of others into its field; in neither group have sustainable development principles become fully established in professional education and practice. Yet between them, the arenas of environment and health already carry the expertise to implement all five of the principles of sustainability. In public health practice, equity within and between generations, precautionary action and monitoring play an integral part; while in environmental sciences, acting for the future, environmental integrity and monitoring form the basis of environmental management practice.

The content and skills of environmental management are equally well established, but not usually yet considered an integral part of public health.

Questions arise as to how best to address this new dimension of the established two-way relationship between environment and health. If public health practice now requires skills in environmental management and environmental management is increasingly addressing public health issues, does this mean:

- public health practice incorporates environmental management
- environmental management incorporates public health practice
- environmental health expands and takes responsibility for both; or
- a fresh form of all-encompassing professional practice is required?

The trend of the answers from sources in either environment or health is that all four options are waiting to be taken up. As in the *Hitchhiker's Guide to the Galaxy* (Adams 1979) we know the answer ('42'), but what is the question?

The degree of transformation needed to instigate well-documented strategies to move from global degradation to global sustainability requires changes not only in many professions but also in community practices and community services; so as far as the public health curriculum is concerned, sustainable development principles need to be included as:

- a recognised section of all specialised public health fields;
- a basis for collaboration with environmental professions;
- a part of core business for environmental health practitioners; and
- a form of professional expertise requiring research and development.

As well as forging a new combination from the parallel expertise of public health practice and environmental management, and supporting a strengthened environmental health profession, a sustainability and health curriculum faces a third and even more difficult task.

Public health and environmental health, both as professions and as research fields in general, remain narrowly scientifically based, while the solutions to problems in either field lie in understanding the social and environmental systems in which they operate (Lowe 2001). In both fields there is emerging exploration of transdisciplinary, systemic and future-oriented approaches to research and practice; that this remains tentative and far from the mainstream is evident in the criteria for research funding, duty statements for job applications, and most formal texts and resource files.

Many of the initiatives responding to health and environment issues and calling for new approaches are being described as 'sustainability science'. Lowe (2001) proposes developing **inside** science as an integrative method that is broadly multidisciplinary and systemic rather than the traditional unidisciplinary approach—a method that could be called sustainability science Mark 1. Others such as the US Academy of Science and a sustainability science research group at Harvard University go further and suggest that there is a need to go **outside** the research sciences and link to other sources of knowledge such as the community or strategic planners in positions of leadership. This new more inclusive direction could be labelled sustainability science Mark 2.

The future for public health practice involves working with other professions, communities and governments to incorporate sustainability science Marks 1 and 2 into everyday practice:

What will be required are significant advances in basic knowledge, in the social and technological capacities to utilise it, and in the political will to turn this knowledge and know-how into action. (United States National Research Council 1999)

The future for public health practice involves working with other professions, communities and governments to incorporate sustainability.

Public health was born out of the need for a transformation in civic responses to the movement of populations into cities in the 19th century (Ashton & Seymour 1988). The effect of a global population three times the size of that of the 19th century affecting the whole planet requires an equally major extension of current capacities to respond in all the professions, not only public health.

Developing principles and describing people and place

The education principles can be expressed as inquiry-based learning in sustainability and health . . .

The education principles can be expressed as inquiry-based learning in sustainability and health, applying the D4P4 decision-making for change framework outlined in Figure 1.3. Principles for guiding change are predetermined; applying sustainable development principles to public health is the aim of the enterprise. Place is also a given; sustainability and health issues arise from global environmental change. The condition of the planet and each locality is in a state of continual change, so that while the basic reference text is McMichael (2001), particular issues will need to be re-examined for each application of the curriculum or each locality where it will be applied.

Sets of principles that are discussed in this book include the principles of sustainable development and other anthropocentric frameworks, and the emerging more integrated meaning of sustainability and its relationship with the Earth Charter as an ecocentric framework (see Chapter 3).

Designing potential strategies and doing them in practice

The many potential directions for public health professional practice have been explored in a range of strategies, including the so-called New Public Health (now 15 years old), Local Agenda 21, Sustainable Communities, Common Ground and many others. Hancock (2001) provides reviews of current public health services addressing sustainability issues; Rees (2000) offers strategies for re-examining environmental resource use that include ecological and social needs for sustainable futures. Responding to the worldwide call for a wider scientific perspective on environment and health issues, Lowe (2001) offers an introduction to sustainability science, broadened by Brown et al. (2001) to include communities' local knowledge and government strategic directions (Chapter 4).

Reviewing possible strategic directions leads to decisions on which practical applications can best be tailored to conditions for sustainability and health. Such a review can produce:

- a curriculum (as in the present project);
- integrated strategic frameworks (Chapters 2-3);

- synthesis of all the evidence (Chapter 4);
- broad-based scoping capacity (Chapter 5);
- change-oriented public health practitioners (Chapter 6);
- an innovative public health program (Chapter 7); and
- a sustainability and health management strategy (Chapter 8).

Activity 1.4
Practitioner as change agent: continuum of change

Aim: for participants to identify their own position on change (a) in general; (b) for public health practice; (c) as part of a change team. It is assumed that all positions on the continuum will be found in any change process.

Time: 2 hours.

Equipment: Large sheets of paper, felt pens.

Participants form groups of five. Each group has a large sheet of paper with the change agents' options line (Figure 1.4).

Before discussion starts, each person puts a cross on the options for change line where they consider they stand generally on most things, and a tick where they stand on the changes towards sustainability and health recommended in this chapter. The group discusses the positions of the ticks and crosses, and the reasons for the pattern.

After 30 minutes discussion, the group writes the reasons they consider would place people in each position for changes towards sustainability and health on the paper line. Each person reviews where they consider themselves to be.

Leaving the options line paper on the table, the groups move to each table, where the responsible group explains their pattern.

Plenary discussion: Brainstorm the issues for change towards sustainability and health practice that need to be taken into account in any program for change. Note where they are covered in the text of *Sustainability and Health*.

Conclusion

At the turn of the century, many international events are addressing the adoption of sustainable development principles through the lens of

The move to sustainability worldwide has been slow, but is now accelerating.

structural change. It is now all but universally recognised that it is not only global economic resources and ecological balance that are at risk, but also the health of our species as a whole. International organisations such as the United Nations, the World Bank and globalised industrial corporations such as BHP and Shell have moved to initiate structural changes addressing the principles of sustainable development in their core operations. The move to sustainability worldwide has been slow, but is now accelerating. Public health is one of the professions that needs to reconsider as a matter of urgency its role in maintaining the health of human populations, in the light of the current state of the world environment. The following chapters expand on the issues and actions essential for public health practitioners to move into the era of sustainability and health.

Figure 1.4 Change agent continuum

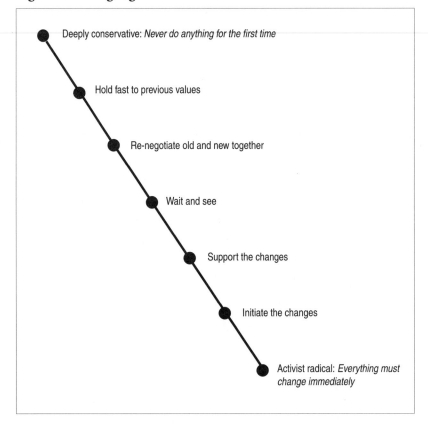

Deeply conservative: *Never do anything for the first time*

Hold fast to previous values

Re-negotiate old and new together

Wait and see

Support the changes

Initiate the changes

Activist radical: *Everything must change immediately*

References

Adams, D. 1979, *Hitchhiker's Guide to the Galaxy*, Pan Books, London

Ashton, J. and Seymour, H. 1988, *The New Public Health: the Liverpool experience*, Open University Press, Milton Keynes

AtKisson, A. 1999, *Believing Cassandra: An optimist looks at a pessimist's world*, Scribe Publications Pty Ltd, Melbourne

Baum, F. 2002, *The New Public Health*, 2nd edn, Oxford University Press, South Melbourne

Bohm, D. 1996, *On Dialogue*, Routledge, London

Brown, V. 1997, *Managing for Local Sustainability: Policy, problem-solving, practice and place*, National Office of Local Government, Canberra

—— 1998, 'The Titanic or the Arc?', *Measuring Progress: Is Australia getting better?*, ed. R. Eckersley, CSIRO, Melbourne

Brown, V., Grootjans, J., Ritchie, J., Townsend, M. and Verrinder, G. 2002, *Sustainability and Health Project Report 2002*, unpublished report to the Department of Health and Ageing, Canberra

Brown, V.A., Nicholson, R., Stephenson, P., Bennett, K.-J. and Smith, J. 2001, *Grass Roots and Common Ground: Guidelines for community-based environmental health action*, Regional Integrated Monitoring Centre, University of Western Sydney, Richmond

Brown, V.A., Ritchie, J. and Rotem, A. 1992, 'Health Promotion and Environmental Management: the partnership for the future', *International Journal of Health Promotion*, vol. 7, no. 3, pp. 219-30

Capra, F. 1983, *The Turning Point: Science, society, and the rising culture*, Fontana, London

—— 1996, *The Web of Life*, Anchor Books, New York

Department of Environment Sport and Territories 1992, *National Strategy for Ecologically Sustainable Development*, Australian Government Public Service, Canberra

Dovers, S. 1989, *Our Common Future: Australian implications and responses*, Centre for Resource and Environmental Studies, Australian National University, Canberra

Fineberg, H., Green, G., Ware, J. and Anderson, B. 1994, 'Changing public health training needs: Professional education and the paradigm of public health', *Annual Review of Public Health*, vol. 15, pp. 237-57

Flannery, T.F. 1994, *The Future Eaters: An ecological history of the Australasian lands and people*, Reed Books, Chatswood, New South Wales

Hancock, T. 1985, 'The Mandala of Health: A model of the human ecosystem', *Family and Community Health*, vol. 8, no. 3, pp. 1-10

—— 2000, 'IDRC and the management of sustainable urban development in Latin America: Lessons learnt and demands for knowledge', *Urban Ecosystems and Human Health*, vol.3, pp. 23-30

—— 2001, *Doing Less Harm: Assessing and reducing the environment and health impact of Canada's health care system*, Canadian Coalition for Green Health Care, Kleinberg

Institute of Medicine 2003, *Who Will Keep the Public Healthy? Educating Public Health Professionals for the 21st Century*, The National Academies Press, Washington

Kolb, D.A., Rubin, I.M. and McIntyre, J.M. 1974, *Organisational Psychology: An experiential approach*, Prentice Hall, New Jersey

Lonero, E.E. 2002, *Local Government and the Johannesburg Summit*, International Council for Local Environmental Initiatives (ICLEI), Toronto

Lowe, I. 2001, *Sustainability Science*, Australian Broadcasting Corporation, Brisbane

MacDonald, M. 1998, *Agendas for Sustainability: Environment and development into the twenty-first century*, Routledge, London

Mainieri, T., Barnett, E., Valdero, T., Unipan, J. and Oskamp, S. 1997, 'Green Buying: the influence of environmental concern on consumer behavior', *The Journal of Social Psychology*, vol. 137, no. 2, pp. 189-204

McMichael, A.J. 1993, *Planetary Overload: Global environmental change and the health of the human species*, Cambridge University Press, New York

—— 2001, *Human Frontiers, Environments and Disease: Past patterns, uncertain futures*, Cambridge University Press, New York

Meadows, D.H., Meadows D.L., Randers, J. and Behrens, W.W. 1972, *The Limits to Growth: A report for the Club of Rome's project on the predicament of mankind*, Potomac Associates, London

Pimentel, D., Tort, M. and D'Anna, L. 1998, 'Ecology of Increasing Disease', *BioScience*, vol. 48, no. 10, pp. 35-43

Prigogine, I. 1980, *From Being to Becoming*, Freeman, San Francisco

Rees, W.E. 2000, *The Dark Side of the Force (of Globalisation)*, Parklands Institute Conference, Edmonton

Senge, P.M. 1992, *The Fifth Discipline: The art and practice of the learning organisation*, Century Business, London

Soskolne, C.L. and Bertollini, R. 1999, *Global Ecological Integrity and 'Sustainable Development': Cornerstones of public health*, A Discussion Document, WHO European Centre for Environment and Health, Rome, http://www.euro.who.int/document/gch/ecorep5.pdf [22 January 2004]

Sustainability and Health Project Expert Advisors 2001, personal communication, audiotape of teleconference, December

United States National Research Council 1999, *Our Common Journey: A transition towards sustainability*, National Academy Press, Washington

Western Sydney Regional Organisation of Councils and University of Western Sydney, Brown, V.A., Love, D., Griffiths, R., Powell, J., Murphy, A. and Walsmley, A. 2000, *Western Sydney Regional State of the Environment Report 2000*, WSROC and Regional Integrated Monitoring Centre, University of Western Sydney, Sydney

Westra, L. 1998, *Living in Integrity: A global ethic to restore a fragmented Earth*, Rowman and Littlefield, Lanham, United Kingdom

World Commission on Environment and Development 1987, *Our Common Future: Report of the World Commission on Environment and Development*, Oxford University Press, Oxford

World Health Organisation 1948, *The WHO Constitution*, World Health Organisation Geneva

—— 1978, *Declaration of Alma-Ata*, World Health Organisation, Geneva

—— Health and Welfare Canada and the Canadian Public Health Association 1986, 'Ottawa Charter for Health Promotion', *Canadian Journal of Public Health*, vol. 77, no. 12, pp. 425-30

—— 1999, http://www.who.int/archives/who50/en/health4all.htm [13 February 2004]

World Summit on Sustainable Development 2002, *Health and Environment: Supporting Sustainable Livelihoods*, Towards Earth Summit 2002, Social Briefing No. 3 linkages, World Information Transfer, http://www.worldinfo.org [13 February 2004]

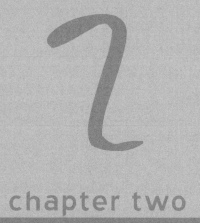

LISTENING

chapter two

Co-ordinating ideas on sustainability and health

John Grootjans, Mardie Townsend,
Colin Butler and Jane Heyworth

Summary

This chapter endeavours to equip public health practitioners and others with a critical understanding of a range of emerging conceptual frameworks with which they are likely to come into contact while working toward sustainability and health. The chapter will facilitate critical reflection on the many complementary and yet different theoretical perspectives related to sustainability and health. The improved understanding of different perspectives gained should lead to sustainability and health practitioners improving their ability to work in collaboration with stakeholders from wide-ranging backgrounds.

Chapter 2 Listening

Co-ordinating ideas on sustainability and health

John Grootjans, Mardie Townsend, Colin Butler and Jane Heyworth

Key words

Triple bottom line, deep ecology, cornucopian enchantment, biophilia, natural capitalism, voluntary simplicity, human ecology and health, indigenous perspectives, Keynesianism, eco-feminism, economic rationalism, ecological integrity, precautionary principle

Learning outcomes

On completion of this chapter public health practitioners and others will be able to:

- describe a range of theoretical perspectives on sustainability and health;
- describe the evolution of various theoretical perspectives in their historical contexts;
- compare, contrast and critically analyse a range of theoretical perspectives on sustainability and health;
- assess the implications of a range of theoretical perspectives on sustainability;
- discuss, critically reflect on and develop an argument to support his/her personal position on sustainability;
- explore seminal and critical literature related to a range of theoretical perspectives;
- apply a range of models designed for predicting future outcomes; and

- have come to a personal understanding of how he/she could work with people adopting each of these positions.

Outline

2.1 Sustainability and health
2.2 Sustainability and science
2.3 Sustainability and economics
2.4 Sustainability and environmentalism

Learning activities

2.1 Chinese whispers spiral
2.2 Where all the rivers flow: working collaboratively in complex ecological systems

Reading

Hawken, P., Lovins, A.B. and Lovins, L.H. 1999, *Natural Capitalism: The next industrial revolution*, Earthscan Publications Ltd, London

Mies, M. and Shiva, V. 1993, *Ecofeminism*, Spinifex Press, North Melbourne

Rees, W.E. 1998, 'How should a parasite value its host?', *Ecological Economics,* vol. 25, pp. 49-52

2.1 Sustainability and health

Chapter 1 set the sustainability and health practitioner on his/her learning pathway by giving a clear understanding of the issues that make ecological sustainability so important to the public health worker. Since the early Greeks we have known that our environment affects our health. The approach to the environment adopted by public health practitioners has focused on strong environmental controls to prevent disease. This approach has led to measured success and has come to underpin the attitudes and the actions of each professional working for people's health. For an excellent example of this approach one only needs to spend a few minutes in an operating room to see environmental control taken to an extreme; but this approach transferred to the environment outside the hospital contributes to the problem, not to the solutions.

Chapter 1 highlighted the issues emerging from this technical, control-oriented world-view. This chapter offers us an insight into a new way of looking at our environment as an ecological system with humanity as part of the system, with each element of the system in some way connected with every other element. The question for public health practitioners and others is, 'What is their role in a systemic ecological framework, and how is it different from the direct interventions advocated in an environmental control framework?' Chapters 2 and 3 take the public health practitioner through phase one of the D4P4 framework, 'describing people and place'.

Health workers often come from an action-oriented tradition where prompt and direct action is called for on a regular basis. Actions are dictated from experience and by firm protocols developed by authorities. The urgency in the health ecosystem is the need for caution and the consideration of options. The experience of a disturbed global environment is new, the options for action are many, and the need to carefully consider long-term, lifelong and multiple scale actions is great. Chapter 2 examines the many ways to describe the sustainability and health context: people and place. It describes a range of world-views (ie social constructions) and theoretical frameworks. Our aim is for public health practitioners and their colleagues to understand and value the perspectives of the people who have devoted their lives to understanding how we can make our future sustainable and humane, to find a perspective or combination of perspectives in which they are happy to work, and to be able to work with others who have different perspectives.

Since the early Greeks we have known that our environment affects our health.

A number of challenging and valuable approaches have emerged among sustainability advocates. Many of these approaches have developed considerable followings among scientists, world leaders and the community who bind themselves into loose affiliations, often using the labels even more loosely. Any such group is likely to be unfamiliar with the potential contribution or partnership potential of the other groups. There are many such groups and different names have been used to label similar groupings, leading to further confusion. For the purposes of understanding the field of sustainability and health, this chapter provides an introduction to a small number of the many interesting concepts being developed.

Working as sustainability advocates, it is important that public health practitioners and others avoid the risk of embracing only one of the emerging advocacy domains.

Working as sustainability advocates, it is important that public health practitioners and others avoid the risk of embracing only one of the emerging advocacy domains. In the past a new or creative idea has led to a school of thought and along with these emerging schools of thought, ivory towers have developed to administer the resources assigned to help propagate the thought, promoting rules for education and practice. Instead of encouraging a spiral of creativity, the result can be, and according to Illich invariably is, the reverse: the over-protection of certain ways of thought, limiting of new ideas and setting up silos of authority that inhibit the sets of ideas being linked (Illich 1969). The task of practitioners in sustainability and health is to understand as many as possible of the different viewpoints that exist, in order to incorporate as many as possible as supports for their own sustainability and health programs. Here we provide a stepping stone in this long and interesting task.

To facilitate understanding we would like the reader to follow a hypothetical case study through the different approaches being presented. Each new approach can be understood in relation to the case study. In some instances this is spelled out for the reader; in others the reader will need to discern the implications of the perspective or approach for the case study.

Imagine a health and sustainability practitioner working in a small community on the banks of a large river. The river, of course, is often the centre of attention to members of the community and will often come up in conversation. The river's flow is influenced by a range of people with differing perspectives: farmers, fishers, politicians, public servants, vacationers, water drinkers and so on. Each perspective is itself influenced by four elements from Hancock's (1985) 'mandala of health': personal behaviour, socio-economic environment, biophysical environment and human biology (see Figure 1.2). Using Hancock's Mandala of

Health allows us to understand that health outcomes are also the end result of complex, inter-related and random ecological events in the river system. River health will have a direct and significant impact on the wellbeing of people who live near and gain their livelihoods from it. Any action by government, farmers, or townspeople that affects the river will also affect the wellbeing of many people in the community.

Activity 2.1
Chinese whispers spiral

Aim: to demonstrate the need for listening skills.

Instructions: Arrange the participants in a line, sufficiently well spaced that each person is able only to communicate in whispers with one person on either side.

The first person thinks of a sentence relating to sustainability and health (preferably one that is not too simple), then whispers it to the person next to them, ensuring that no one else hears it. The next person whispers the sentence they thought they heard to the person next to them, and so on down the line. As each person completes their whisper, they move to the end of the line. The game continues until each person has given and received at least two whispers. At the end of the game, the last person announces to the group the sentence they received on their last turn and compares it with the original sentence, and a general discussion is held on how the message changed in the process of the game. (Each individual should be able to compare not only the beginning sentence and the one they first received, but also the change between their first and second turns.)

The game is most effective when the original message is relatively complex and when there is a large number of people participating.

2.2 Sustainability and science

As a respected member of the community the public health practitioner will often find him/herself talking about the river, because it is central to the lives of many of the people in the community. These people will come from many different world-views. As a professional in the health care system the practitioner will speak to many health professionals with a firm scientific education. The question is, how can the practitioner communicate in an ecological way that shows an understanding of the connection between the river and the health of the people?

The classical position has the public health practitioner as a health scientist talking about issues such as outbreaks of gastrointestinal disease caused by the quality of the water supply, a position well described in scientific journals. This scientific position has a history dating from Hippocrates and is entrenched in the world-views of health workers. Thinking ecologically allows the practitioner to consider economic and social factors as well as these important environmental considerations. As well, the practitioner must consider that events happening in his or her community are often the end result of global or national as well as local activities. As issues such as river toxicity emerge locally, the practitioner will need to immerse him/herself in literature about the complex web of interconnected issues associated with rivers. Fellow health professionals will, on the other hand, focus on medical/scientific explanations embedded in toxicology and bacteriology. While this is itself important information, it is unhelpful to see scientific information in isolation from the inter-relationships affecting the river and the health of people living with it.

Thinking ecologically allows the practitioner to consider economic and social factors as well as these important environmental considerations.

This section will help public health practitioners and others understand why rivers can become an important part of a health worker's life and how a health worker can come to understand the river ecologically.

The classical approach

Over the past 400 years a world-view underpinned by some basic principles has dominated science: it is based on reductionism, which looks at problems in small, solvable parcels; on objectivity, which attempts to reduce the impact of the researcher on what is being researched; and on empiricism, which suggests that research should be reduced to direct physical observations. What we have come to call truth is our evaluation of the sets of evidence available to us.

While there is no question that these principles have led to incredible technological development, many scientists have begun to question them (Bohm 1980; Capra 1996). The complexity of the new approach requires research methods that embed scientific problems in their complex contexts, accept that the observer has a direct impact on the findings, explore new metaphors to present findings other than numbers and recognise that truth is a social construct.

Our aim here is to search for fresh common ground in which all sets of workers in the field of sustainability and health can work constructively together. The ecoscience community holds adherents to each of the multiple world-views staking claims to the future. There are many examples of good science being rejected because of its commitment to one world-view or another. Lovelock's 'Gaia hypothesis' (1979) is a case in point where good science was marginalised as a type of mythology not relevant to the considerations of real science. Rachel Carson's *Silent Spring* (1963) underpinned the actions of the environmental movement for years, while scientists engaged in lengthy disputes over the scientific merit of the work.

Human health and ecology

The human health and ecology perspective acknowledges that human activity is changing ecosystems and that collectively these changes are endangering the health and future prospects of humans and other living creatures (Last 1998). It challenges the traditional approach to public health—one in which humans were viewed as a species separate from and superior to other species. In that approach, the interaction of humans with the environment was one in which humans were central and the environment was modified or managed to benefit human health.

The human health and ecology perspective acknowledges that human activity is changing ecosystems . . .

The ecological perspective on human health argues that humans are as dependent on the ecosystem as any other species (McMichael 2001).

> *Humans interact with each other as well as with other living creatures and these interactions can have important effects on the health of all partners in the complex closed ecosystem of our planet. We ignore this reality at our peril.* (Last 1998, p. 53)

The challenge is to manage the relationship between human activities and the physical, biological, social and economic environments in a way that protects and promotes health but at the same time does not threaten the integrity of the natural systems on which the physical and biological systems depend. This includes maintaining the availability of environmental resources, the functioning of natural systems that receive wastes produced by human society, and a stable climate. To achieve this 'sustainable transition' and thus avert the human health risks associated with overloading our biosphere, McMichael (2001, p. 364) suggests two essential strategies:

1. To consume nature's flows while conserving the stocks (that is, live off the 'interest' while conserving natural capital).

2. To increase society's stocks (human resources, civil institutions) and limit the flow of materials and energy.

The ecological perspective also requires that we think beyond the local and view health from a global perspective. A hundred years ago health problems tended to be local and effects tended to be acute rather than chronic. In the 1970s we became concerned about chronic effects of low-level exposure over a lifetime. Now we are realising that changes to our global environment are affecting our health and will affect the health of future generations to an even greater degree.

... so while improving the income and health status of the poor we must at the same time reduce consumption in developed countries.

When we consider health from a global perspective, McMichael argues that poverty is the greatest ecological challenge—so while improving the income and health status of the poor we must at the same time reduce consumption in developed countries. The human health and ecology perspective argues that we have exceeded Earth's 'carrying capacity'. The threat to human health arises from the increasing size of populations, increasing consumption and increasing use of environmentally damaging technologies (McMichael and Powles 1999). McMichael (2001) estimated that by the turn of the 21st century humans had already exceeded the planet's carrying capacity by about 30 per cent.

The challenge for public health practitioners and others is to change our way of thinking from a deterministic approach to health to a systems approach. Currently, when new environmental concerns are raised, policy-makers consider them harmless until research findings show otherwise. Many public health researchers accept the null hypothesis (the status quo) until it is disproved. The central theme of McMichael's book highlights the fallacy of this approach (2001, p. v):

> *Humankind's long evolutionary and historical experience shows how the social and natural environments affect patterns of disease and survival. Appreciating this ecological perspective on human population health—at a time when large-scale stresses are appearing in our world—is a prerequisite to achieving a sustainable future.*

An ecological approach requires that we take a precautionary approach. Hence we will be more reliant on models predicting future health effects rather than waiting for empirical evidence to emerge. Scientific methods will need to adjust and evolve to 'forecast the potential health consequences of anticipated but uncertain future changes in complex global environmental systems' (McMichael 2001, p. 330).

Yet what the precautionary approach means in practice is not clear. While the acute and medium-term health effects of an agent/technology/practice usually have been investigated prior to market placement, long-term health effects are often ignored until they emerge.

Likewise, Smith (2000) questions the dominance of environmental health issues by industrialised countries, suggesting that the increasing emphasis on the future impact of climate change on health may be diverting attention and resources from other current hazards such as air and water pollution. These hazards account for at least 15 per cent of the current global burden of disease, most of it in the least developed countries. Smith asks whether climate change would ever have such an impact on health, even in worst-case scenarios.

While the human health and ecology perspective acknowledges humans as just one part of an ecosystem, it is not clear that we have really moved beyond considering humans as central to this ecosystem. The articles written about the impact of climate change, for example, are predominantly about the impact on human health, although there is some regard for the health of future generations. However, this may simply be a reflection of political imperative by which human health has more influence over public policy.

Environmental scepticism

To confront the many non-government organisations and individuals undertaking informative environmental research around the world, a group of sceptics has emerged that has opened up a dialogue to present an alternative image to the so-called doomsday prophets. The sceptics attack the scientific basis of the findings being presented by these groups. Lomborg is the most recent author in the group of sceptics, with his book *The Skeptical Environmentalist* (Lomborg 2001).

Lomborg's criticism is with the litany of doom espoused by certain environmental activists. We have all heard the main points many times: natural resources are running out; the world's population is too big and growing at an alarming rate; rivers, lakes, oceans and the atmosphere are becoming dirtier all the time. Forests are being destroyed, fish stocks are collapsing, 40,000 species a year are becoming extinct and the planet is warming. The world is falling apart, in other words.

Lomborg attacks many of the concerns expressed by environmentalists. He suggests that these are just scare stories put about by ideologues and promulgated by the media. He makes these points:

While the human health and ecology perspective acknowledges humans as just one part of an ecosystem . . .

- air quality in the developed world has improved markedly over the past 100 years;
- human life expectancy has soared;
- the average inhabitant of the developing world consumes 38 per cent more calories now than 100 years ago;
- the percentage of people threatened with starvation has fallen from 35 per cent to 18 per cent;
- the hole in the ozone layer is more or less fixed;
- the global warming threat has been much exaggerated;
- the lifetime risk of drinking water containing pesticide residues at the EU limit is the equivalent of smoking 1.4 cigarettes.

In short, the world is not falling apart; rather, the doom-mongers have led us all down the garden path.

In other words, they say, Kyoto will buy us six years.

The sceptics point out that environmental intervention can also be costly. Implementing the Kyoto Protocol on carbon dioxide emissions is likely to cost $161-$346 billion dollars, and the average temperature of the Earth would probably be about the same in 2001 with Kyoto as in 1994 without it. In other words, they say, Kyoto will buy us six years. In contrast, several million deaths could be prevented each year by securing clean drinking water and sanitation for everyone at a one-off cost of $200 billion. To think that our politicians would abandon Kyoto and spend the saved money on wells and drains would be naive in the extreme, but in the view of the environmental sceptics the figures should cause every concerned individual to pause for thought. Lomborg's views continue to spark debate and to draw objections, with critics including respected scientists and environmentalists focusing particularly on perceptions that Lomborg manipulated the data to support his argument.

2.3 Sustainability and economics

Modern economic theory is usually traced to the 18th century, but economic arrangements between humans are as old as are human societies. Indeed, at least in simple forms, behaviours identifiable as 'economic' exist among many non-human species. The earliest economic arrangements among humans probably included mutual reciprocity and specialisation. In some societies these changed into more formal systems of barter and currency, used for trade and ceremonies. Simple forms of credit, interest and insurance can also be traced for millennia, including those in non-literate and non-agricultural populations.

Inequality and the exploitation of vulnerable individuals, genders, age groups and populations by those who are more powerful is also an ancient economic trait. The development of strongly hierarchical societies, including the holding of slaves, may be more common in economies with comparatively abundant resources rather than those that are purely subsistence. However, slavery and specialisation—once considered hallmarks of agriculturally based economies—existed in at least some non-agricultural economies.

The development of modern capitalism in the West, including the floating of the first public companies, was leavened by the age of exploration and fuelled by the speculative profits derived from discovery, plunder and trade. Initially, the most profitable commodities were spices and precious metals, but later came extensive trade in slaves and luxury crops such as sugar and cotton. The cost of these latter items was subsidised both by forced labour and the fertile land and abundant water resources appropriated by Europeans from indigenous populations.

Recently, inequality and exploitation of vulnerable individuals and groups has been exacerbated by globalisation. Globalisation is the 'process through which time and space are compressed as new technologies, information flows, trade, and power relations allow distant actions to have increased significance at the local level' (Almås & Lawrence 2003, p. 3). While globalisation is a commonly used term, the complexity of the mechanisms underpinning it contributes to a lack of understanding of its impacts on individuals and communities, their sustainability, health and wellbeing. Almås and Lawrence (2003, p. 8) argue that globalisation has quite concrete impacts at a local level in terms of 'employment and working conditions, industrial restructuring, local culture, and the environment'. The capacity of local communities to address and overcome the detrimental impacts of globalisation will depend on the promotion of 'interaction and linkages between policies, legislation, education, partnership and advocacy arrangements' (Hallebone et al. 2003, p. 237). Public health practitioners are in an ideal position to foster such interaction and linkages.

Today, economists do not speak with a single voice and by no means share a common world-view. There are many schools of thought, each of which defines the market system's relationship to the environment differently. Understanding the genesis and basic principles of the various economic

Recently, inequality and exploitation of vulnerable individuals and groups has been exacerbated by globalisation.

schools will help public health practitioners and others communicate with the different stakeholders, as they will all in some way be influenced by economic principles.

Economic liberalism

The school of thought called 'economic liberalism' matured in the 19th century, building on ideas initially proposed by the Physiocrats and Adam Smith, whose book *The Wealth of Nations* was published in 1776. These theories extolled the virtues of competition and deregulation, in reaction to the myriad government rules and tariffs that were commonly regarded as then stifling of economic development.

In recent decades a modern version of market deregulation has again become dominant.

In recent decades a modern version of market deregulation has again become dominant. In Latin America, market deregulation is often known as 'neoliberalism'. In several English-speaking countries the names were eponymous: 'Thatcherism' (UK), 'Reaganomics' (USA) and 'Rogernomics' (New Zealand). The most common term is 'economic rationalism'. Supporters of this school assert that the 'invisible hand' of the market—itself consisting of millions of individuals acting in their own self-interest—acts automatically (that is, without government intervention or regulation) to maximise economic efficiency and the production of goods and services. As a result, increases in conventional measures of economic progress such as gross national product (GNP) are claimed to be maximised.

Less explicitly, public welfare is also assumed to improve if the GNP increases. Supporters of market deregulation pay little attention to the distribution of goods and services, but when pressed often argue that any increase in inequality (if it occurs at all) is irrelevant, since a 'rising tide lifts all boats'. In other words, this school argues, as long as the real income (that is, income adjusted for inflation) of the poor is increasing, their relative position is irrelevant.

Simon Kuznets (1955), regarded as the father of the national account system that developed into the GNP, postulated that there is an inverse U relationship between income and inequality. Kuznets theorised that as income rises, inequality first increases but then falls so any increase in inequality (though undesirable) is a temporary phenomenon.

Unfortunately for supporters of the Kuznets theory, little evidence exists to support it as a general principle, even after five decades of study. Of interest to environmental policy practitioners, the concept of the

Kuznets curve was rejuvenated in the 1990s, following its appropriation by environmental economists to describe the putative increase, stabilisation and ultimate reduction in some pollutants as income increases.

In contrast to economic liberalist views that inequality is either ephemeral or irrelevant, critics of this approach argue that excessive inequality *does* matter and that beyond thresholds it leads to reductions in social capital (norms, networks, trust, cohesion) that threaten economic productivity. Holders of these views argue that economic productivity is enhanced by the rule of law, by the maintenance and upgrading of public infrastructure, and by institutions that act to serve and protect the public good.

They point out that excessive market deregulation damages public welfare. These commentators argue that unless restrained, market forces privilege the individuals and groups with the greatest pre-existing political and market power to create, modify and interpret society and its mores and laws in ways that magnify their advantages. This is an example of the law of increasing returns.

A tension thus exists: on the one hand, incentives *do* seem to stimulate and reward investment and innovation better (than do planned economies such as in the former USSR), but on the other hand public welfare— including public health—is reduced if inequality becomes excessive.

Social values are an important modifier of the impact of income and wealth inequality. For example, poverty can be reduced by redistributive measures, such as taxation, food supplements and subsidised health care. At the other extreme, market principles can be used to justify the displacement, starvation and even the killing of economically weak populations that lack market power (or entitlement), including to food.

Social values are an important modifier of the impact of income and wealth inequality.

The rise and fall of Keynesianism

The theories of John Maynard Keynes (1919), developed between the two world wars, became mainstream in developed countries in the early post World War II decades. Keynes wanted to modify the harsher aspects of laissez-faire capitalism, particularly its tendency to increase inequality, by harnessing political freedom and the economic dynamism of capitalism to maximise employment and provide a strong welfare state. Keynes also tried (far less successfully) to foster a fairer global economy through the fledgling Breton Woods institutions, especially the World Bank.

Keynesianism benefited from strong political and community support during the inter-war and post World War II period. In the United States the catastrophe of the Great Depression provided sufficient political support to erode the power of the free marketers, enabling significant redistributive policies, under President F.D. Roosevelt's policies of the 'New Deal'. After World War II, even Republican administrations in the United States were forced to support restrained forms of capitalism to be electable.

In Western Europe, too, the hardships of the Depression and World War II increased support for Keynes' policies and led to the introduction of strong welfare states, including the National Health Service in Britain. Keynesianism was influential in Australia and, arguably, the increased equality that it fostered contributed to decolonisation and efforts to promote development in the Third World. However, Keynesianism lost favour in the 1970s, in the face of increasing inflation, rising unemployment and sharp increases in the cost of oil. Supporters of more aggressive forms of capitalism used this crisis to call for the dismantlement of the welfare state and more deregulation, in order to foster renewed growth.

Market deregulation was promoted as a more effective way to attain social justice.

Simon Szreter (1997, pp. 693-728) argues that the political will to maintain Keynesian policies was eroded by the naïveté of electorates that were gradually forgetting the lessons that had led to the introduction of Keynesianism in the first place. He writes:

> . . . *citizens voted throughout the 1980s for governments promising the Fools' Gold of lower personal taxes in return for dramatic reductions in the provision of such public services. This was premised on the stigmatising argument that such public services were in some sense wasteful and parasitic (on the productive economy) and on the further presumption that there would be no important negative consequences flowing from the contraction of these public services and their 'elective targeting'.*

Market deregulation was promoted as a more effective way to attain social justice. It was claimed that this would occur through processes variously characterised as 'trickle-down' and 'increased capacity'. However, since 2000, the bursting of the dot.com bubble and the gradual unravelling of the corrupt web between companies, stock analysts, auditors and politicians has again called market deregulation into question. As well, the extent of the recent increase in inequality in deregulated economies is slowly being appreciated.

'The cornucopian enchantment'

As awareness and concern for the Third World grew in the decades after World War II, a consensus formed that rapid population growth in capital-poor countries harmed economic growth and in the worst case could trap populations in vicious cycles of poverty, disease, famine and conflict. Consequently there was strong support, including at the highest political levels in the rich and poor worlds, to aggressively promote family planning in the Third World. However, the success of the 'Green Revolution' led to an expansion of the global food supply through the 1970s and this, together with the value changes in the West that were eroding support for the welfare state, reduced support for measures that were designed to promote economic development and family planning in poor countries.

This changed perception reached its zenith in the writings of the American economist Julian Simon, who argued not only in favour of global laissez-faire economic policies but also global laissez-faire population policies. Simon (1981) argued that human beings are the 'ultimate resource' and that while every additional person created an environmental demand, they also could disproportionately increase the environmental supply because of the ingenuity of their minds and the capability of their hands. Thus, larger populations might *reduce* the harm wrongly attributed to over-population.

Environmentalists, ecologists and traditional demographers have consistently regarded this argument as simplistic to the point of absurdity. Nevertheless, faith in 'the cornucopian enchantment' has been influential in justifying reductions in foreign aid, including for family planning, and in obscuring the crucial role that the mismatch between environmental resources and population demand has played in the generation of many economic, political, health and food crises that have beset the Third World, especially since 1990.

. . . reduced support for measures that were designed to promote economic development and family planning in poor countries.

Ecological economics

Modern economics developed in a period when the impact of humanity on the natural world was modest. Harmful impacts, whether on distant, unseen or powerless populations or on faraway, unrecognised or future environments have long been recognised by economists and are known collectively as 'externalities'. However, until recently almost no effort has gone into their measurement. Effectively, the market price of goods and services has been and continues to be extensively subsidised by costs that are met by other people, other species and future populations. Ecological economists attempt to identify and measure these externalities; they also argue that the human economy is a subset of the natural economy and that damage to this wider economy will eventually damage the human economy.

The principles of ecological economists have so far had little overt influence on global economic policies; however, conventional economists are increasingly being forced to respond to key criticisms by ecological economists. So far their main response is that market forces will adequately protect critical environmental public goods; in other words, prices will rise as supply falls, enabling new equilibriums that not only reflect changed environmental realities but also human choice. Ecological economists argue that market mechanisms are inadequate not only because they ignore inertial effects but also because too few natural markets exist for crucial environmental public goods, including global climate systems and many ecosystem services.

Critics further argue that human decisions are not well informed but instead are manipulated by public relations techniques and biased media.

Critics further argue that human decisions are not well informed but instead are manipulated by public relations techniques and biased media. These critics identify a coalition between supporters of deregulated capitalism and non-ecological economics. They claim that market mechanisms and the continued disregard of externalities favour the accumulation of private goods for a wealthy and powerful minority at the expense of public goods, health and wellbeing of a comparatively poor and powerless majority, including future populations.

Natural capitalism

The concept of natural capitalism emerged during the late 1990s through the collaboration of Paul Hawken, and Amory and Hunter Lovins. Hawken, the author of *The Ecology of Commerce* (1993), recognised that if his hopes for the transformation of industry and government into systems that are 'inherently sustainable and restorative' (p. xiv) were to be realised, then industry and government would need to be provided with 'an overall biological and social framework within which the transformation . . . could be accomplished and practiced [*sic*]' (Hawken et al. 1999, p. ix). At the same time, according to Hawken et al. the view that a framework was needed to 'harness the talent of business to solve the world's deepest environmental and social problems' emerged in the minds of Amory and Hunter Lovins, who were working at the time with Ernst von Weizsäcker on the writing of *Factor Four: Doubling wealth, halving resource use* (von Weizsäcker et al., 1998). Natural capitalism, the business model developed by Hawken et al., is defined as 'capitalism as if living systems mattered' (1999, p. 9).

Four key strategies, elements or principles underpin natural capitalism.

A radical increase in productivity of resource use: natural capitalism requires that organisations adopt production systems and technologies that use resources more effectively. According to Hawken et al. (1999, p. 10), such a strategy will 'nearly halt the degradation of the biosphere, make it more profitable to employ people, and thus safeguard against the loss of vital living systems and social cohesion'.

A move towards biologically based production ('biomimicry'): by shifting to 'closed-loop' production systems, modelled on biological lines, Hawken et al. suggest that the whole notion of 'waste' can be eliminated. In such a system, every output can either be harmlessly returned to the ecosystem or be used as a valuable input for some other manufacturing process (Rocky Mountain Institute 2002). The benefits of this include a reduction in dependence on non-renewable resources, the elimination of waste and (often) of toxicity (Hawken et al. 1999; Rocky Mountain Institute 2002).

A shift from a 'production-consumption' model of business to a 'service-flow' model: natural capitalism calls for a shift away from the notion of wellbeing measured by the acquisition of goods to a notion of wellbeing based on the continuous receipt of quality, utility, and performance (Hawken et al. 1999, p. 10). Using this model, businesses would shift away from 'the sporadic sale of goods' to delivery of 'a continuous flow of services—leasing an illumination service, for example, rather than selling light bulbs' (Rocky Mountain Institute 2002). As well as focusing the economy on meeting customers' needs more effectively, producers will gain through more efficient use of resources, reduced waste, and reduced revenue fluctuations.

Investing in natural capital: natural capital 'refers to the resources and services provided by nature' (Lovins 2000b.) According to the Rocky Mountain Institute (2002), natural capital includes 'air and water purification, climatic stabilisation, waste detoxification, and so on—that make possible all economic activity, and indeed all life'. Within traditional industrial capitalism, the 'value' of the environment in capital terms has

Natural capitalism requires that organisations adopt production systems and technologies that use resources more effectively.

tended to be ignored. Natural capitalism challenges this approach, suggesting that 'any good capitalist reinvests in productive capital' (Rocky Mountain Institute 2002). Hawken et al. (1999, p. 11) call for business to reinvest 'in sustaining, restoring, and expanding stocks of natural capital', both those that are directly necessary to their operations and those that indirectly contribute to the maintenance of the ecosystem and the customer base.

The links between sustainability and health are inherent in the notion of natural capitalism. This is highlighted by Lovins (2000a):

> *Commerce requires living systems for its welfare—it is emblematic of the times that this even needs to be said. Because of our industrial prowess, we emphasise what people can do but tend to ignore what nature does. Commercial institutions, proud of their achievements, do not see that healthy living systems—clean air and water, healthy soil, stable climates— are integral to a functioning economy. As our living systems deteriorate, traditional forecasting and business economics become the equivalent of house rules on a sinking cruise ship.*
>
> *Natural Capitalism is based on respecting and learning from the natural order of things rather than replacing nature with human cleverness.*

The links between sustainability and health are inherent in the notion of natural capitalism.

Triple Bottom Line

The term 'triple bottom line' was coined by Elkington (1997) in *Cannibals with Forks: The triple bottom line of 21st century business* to describe the three elements (or 'prongs') of sustainability: economic prosperity, environmental quality and social justice. According to Elkington (1997, p. 74), the economic bottom line includes the *financial capital* of an organisation, its *physical capital* (such as plant and machinery) and *human capital* (the skills, experience and knowledge of the individuals in the organisation). Sustainability in relation to the economic bottom line revolves around cost competitiveness and projections about this into the future, demand (both current and future) for the organisation's products and/or services, profit margins and their sustainability, existing levels of human capital and how to maintain that into the future.

The environmental bottom line measures two main types of natural capital: 'critical natural capital', defined as natural capital that is essential to the maintenance of life and ecosystem integrity, and 'renewable, replaceable, or substitutable natural capital', which includes:

> *natural capital which can be renewed (eg. through breeding . . .), repaired (eg. environmental remediation . . .), or substituted or replaced (eg. growing*

use of man-made substitutes, such as solar panels in place of limited fossil fuels). (Elkington 1997, p. 79)

Elkington believes that for sustainability to be achieved, it is critical to achieve progress against the social bottom line—perhaps the most difficult of the triple bottom line components. This focuses on *social capital*, with Elkington adopting Fukuyama's understanding of social capital (Elkington, 1997, p. 85):

a capability that arises from the prevalence of trust in a society or in certain parts of it . . . the ability of people to work together for common purposes in groups and organisations.

In Elkington's view, for sustainability to be achieved trust will need to exist not only inside organisations but between organisations and their external stakeholders. Elkington (1997) notes that in the social bottom line, *human capital* also needs to be considered; in particular public health, skills and education, which are key measures of human capital, also relate to social capital.

In *Cannibals with Forks*, Elkington (1997) highlights the fact that full cost pricing (that is, including in the price of a product or service all the costs associated with its production and delivery)—an essential part of measuring progress toward sustainability—will require the development of ways of pricing values for which no market exists (for example, social capital, justice and equity).

Traditionally, companies have emphasised economic outcomes as the top priority, with social and environmental outcomes lagging behind in importance; however, adoption of a triple bottom line approach requires:

a new way of thinking, a way of making policy and a way of doing business which respects the integrity and interdependence of economic, social and environmental values, objectives and processes. (Wiseman 2002, p. 7)

In 1997 the Global Reporting Initiative was established, indicating that Elkington was not alone at the time in his focus on triple bottom line. Its June 2000 report states:

The Global Reporting Initiative (GRI) is a long-term, multi-stakeholder, international undertaking whose mission is to develop and disseminate globally applicable sustainability reporting guidelines for voluntary use by organisations reporting on the economic, environmental, and social dimensions of their activities, products and services. (Global Reporting Initiative 2000, p. 1)

. . . sustainability to be achieved, it is critical to achieve progress against the social bottom line . . .

The guidelines define the three elements of sustainability (the equivalents of Elkington's three components of the bottom line) as:

- Economic elements which include financial information relating to 'wages and benefits, labour productivity, job creation, expenditures on outsourcing, expenditures on research and development, and investments in training and other forms of human capital'.

- Environmental elements which include the 'impacts of processes, products, and services on air, water, land, biodiversity, and human health'.

- Social elements which include 'workplace health and safety, employee retention, labour rights, human rights, and wages and working conditions at outsourced operations'.

Elkington includes a checklist of key questions to be asked of organisations as part of a sustainability audit (1997, pp. 374-81), but does not define specific tools for measurement of performance. By contrast, the Global Reporting Initiative (2000, p. 18) sets out a hierarchy of performance information needed to report on triple bottom line status, as well as a detailed description of all of the variables required to be reported on.

The implications for health arising from a triple bottom line approach are obvious in the elements of each component, especially when we take into consideration the strong evidence of the negative impacts of poverty, environmental degradation and declining social capital on health. There is now a move to a single bottom line—a co-operative approach to avoid the traditional competitive edge between the social, economic and environmental sectors of organisations, government and educational institutions.

The result of this is that businesses and governments are quick to follow financial trends.

Single bottom line

It has been argued that triple bottom line indicators have the potential for problems (Gilding et al. 2002). Gilding et al. (2002) suggest that the self-reinforcing feedback loop inherent in financial indicators is overwhelmingly powerful and fast when compared to social indicators that are slow and weak. The result of this is that businesses and governments are quick to follow financial trends. Gilding et al. (2002) go on to suggest that the application of triple bottom line accounting tends to encourage separation of economic, social and environmental performance. What is needed are indicators which integrate the three concepts presented in the triple bottom line; this has become known as the single bottom line. Indicators are needed which highlight the interconnectedness of social, environmental and economic indicators.

Anielski (1998, 2002) has done a considerable amount of work in developing the genuine progress indicator (GPI). The GPI is an attempt to show with a single indicator the interconnectedness of several indicators of ecological progress. The GPI produces a single indicator based on human, social, natural, produced and financial capitals (Anielski 2002, p. 9). The benefits of Anielski's work can be seen in the human development index (HDI), which is a variation of the GPI and is used by the United Nations Development Program (UNDP) to produce annual reports on global progress which are available at http://www.undp.org/dpa/publications/hdro/98.htm.

The dialogue in the field of economics is extremely difficult because the positions taken are embedded in the certain language of mathematics superimposed on the uncertain language of social sciences. Arguments supporting different positions can seem to promote people's wellbeing while the reality of the local impact can be disastrous. It is with this local impact that public health practitioners will be most closely associated; for example, as deteriorating incomes lead to changes in diet, reduced access to education and deterioration of local environments (including water quality), health workers will be called on to address the flow-on health effects.

2.4 Sustainability and environmentalism

Under no circumstances could it be claimed that the environmental movement has a single world-view; members of environmental groups in the community will generally express opinions synthesised from a number of environmental positions. Some may advocate that the community must learn to live with the river and its ecosystem rather than forcing the river to fit into the human system. Others will take the position that the river has an essential quality whose integrity must be preserved intact and unchanged; yet another group will take the view that human intelligence can find a way out of any problem, and that environmental protection is simply a matter of developing appropriate technologies. It is the perception of polar opposite positions that tends to keep stakeholders from coming together. So learning to understand positions on either side will help public health practitioners and others to mediate between factions refusing to listen to each other.

Under no circumstances could it be claimed that the environmental movement has a single world-view . . .

Most countries have a wide range of environmental action groups that interpret action as any point along the full spectrum from policy development and lobbying to forest protests and media events. Their positions range from deep ecology (preserving all life, with humans not necessarily the most important) through sustainability (concerned with the future of the human/environment relationship) to the protection of human interests and human wellbeing from environmental hazards. Some are nationally based organisations. For example, the Australian Conservation Foundation is a national organisation which has a non-confrontational orientation to policy and practical research, and a broad remit covering both urban and wildlife issues. Similarly, there are various nationally based 'Wilderness Society' groups around the world which focus more narrowly on the ecosystems within their areas, and which mobilise the attachment people feel to threatened areas. Greenpeace, by contrast, is a global organisation dedicated to 'bearing witness'—that is, conducting highly visible public campaigns, though in recent years it has also addressed internal national policy issues. Greenpeace's major focus is on oceans and marine issues. The World Wildlife Fund is also an international body which has sizeable funds donated from firms that are happy to be associated with the preservation of endangered species—the main focus of the group.

In addition to these international and national organisations there is a range of local action groups, each with a particular approach or focus.

In addition to these international and national organisations there is a range of local action groups, each with a particular approach or focus. They include groups which: emphasise individual action; focus on homes and neighbourhoods; have an interest in local planning; campaign for better public transport and cycling facilities; promote renewable energy; and respond to local issues. There are environmental issue-based groups such as those concerned with water and those concerned with the coastal fringe, and there are health issue-based groups such as anti-pollution lobbies. There are also groups often not included in a list of groups acting for sustainability, such as breastfeeding support groups (for example, the La Leche League) and recreation-based groups (for example, the Surfrider Foundation) which have taken action leading to major policy changes such as pesticide bans and coastal protection. Altogether, whatever the local area of concern there will undoubtedly be a sustainability action group to help engage with the issue.

Individual action

Voluntary simplicity can seem an inappropriate name for this group; their lives appear to the outsider as anything but simple. Their efforts are often misunderstood by the general community as these people stand out as different, riding bikes, wearing handmade clothes and refusing to connect to town grids for water, sewerage and power. It is important for practitioners to consider their views, as they have often spent time trying to figure out an ecological balance for local circumstances. Achieving this local balance is extremely useful, but is often not understood by local townspeople.

Grounding oneself in the principles espoused by these groups is invaluable for understanding the ecological integrity of one's community, and thus is essential information for a public health worker interested in sustainability.

Voluntary simplicity is the label used to describe a movement where people are choosing to reduce their environmental impact. This movement is based on individual action that aims to take personal responsibility for global ecosystem collapse.

Gandhi suggested to the people of India that they should 'live simply, so others may simply live'. This statement resonates with the supporters of voluntary simplicity, especially in a world of depleting resources. There have always been groups willing to seek to better their lives by 'dropping out', with any number of utopian and religious movements based on simplicity. In the 1960s and 70s this orientation was exemplified by the 'hippy' movement, based around people who dropped out of society to set up communes/clusters whose lifestyles were based on self-reliance and on spiritual enlightenment founded on a variety of spiritual traditions including indigenous and Eastern religions. Their political structures were based on community participation and collaboration. These groups experienced various levels of success, and their experiences and learning inform proponents of voluntary simplicity.

This movement's lifestyle is in many ways difficult to maintain and requires continuing effort. The locations where people carry on the simple lifestyles are as often as not suburban households. In the past it was thought that to reduce one's impact on the earth, an individual would have to move away from urban lifestyles and take up residence on small rural plots. While people continue to make a choice to relocate, it is possible to reduce one's ecological impact no matter where one lives.

Henry Thoreau (1856) suggested that 'man is richest whose pleasures are the cheapest'. The inherent wisdom of this principle is not necessarily widely acknowledged today. While many people are attempting to reduce

Gandhi suggested to the people of India that they should 'live simply, so others may simply live'.

their own consumption, it is clear that the wealthiest 800 million people on Earth consume 1000 more calories—as well as over 80 to 90 per cent more protein—than the 4 billion people who make up the world's median income groups, not to mention the world's poorest people.

Globalisation leads to products that travel around the world before they reach markets. Attempts to keep the cost of these products low increase risks to both sustainability and health, including:

- increasing plantation sizes to achieve large-scale production at the expense of subsistence farmers, who relinquish their plots to work picking produce for agribusiness companies that pay low wages;
- exporting of agricultural products at the same time as famine relief is required;
- monoculture agriculture that depletes soil nutrients, requiring fertilisation to maintain yields, a process where costs further reduce the opportunities for small-scale farming and which also leads to a greater use of pesticides; and
- irrigation that wastes water and leads to aquifer pollution and depletion.

Globalisation leads to products that travel around the world before they reach markets.

The ecological cost is considered to be enormous. Fossil fuels are being soaked up to bring low-cost fruits to Australia from Argentina. In response to this the 'fair trade movement' advocates actions individuals can undertake to reduce the impact of such events:

- purchase of local food products that do not require extensive transport;
- eating seasonal foods rather than demanding year round supplies;
- demanding accredited green farm produce with no toxins and no ecological impact;
- demanding fair trade certification on all products; and
- producing for oneself.

As with any movement as large and relatively unorganised as the voluntary simplicity movement, corporate interests have begun to take an interest in this emerging market. Two concerns have arisen out of this interest in attracting 'green aware' buyers:

1. Companies are 'greenwashing'—claiming credentials which are not real. For example, one company claimed it was giving its Indonesian factory workers a 10 per cent pay rise. The reality was that the 10 per cent offered did not nearly compensate the workers for the prior fall in the value of the rupiah of more than 200 per cent.

2. Other companies have begun to produce products that do not meet

standards. One example is shower heads, for which claims of water reductions of up to 50 per cent are made but which (in some cases) on investigation fail to have any impact on water usage.

A central feature of decisions made by green consumers is their social conscience and concern for the depletion of resources, and for human suffering. In general, the green consumer attempts to analyse critically products being presented, but lack of accurate information may leave consumers at risk of being duped.

Technological action

Lovins (2000b) describes many technological innovations that enable people to reduce their ecological impacts, and von Weizsäcker et al. (1998) have hypothesised that a fourfold reduction in consumption of resources is possible without the introduction of new technology. Others suggest that a tenfold reduction in consumption is necessary to bring about sustainability (von Weizsäcker 1997). Technologies include solar cells, wind generators, energy-saving housing design, dry toilets, a return of water tanks to supply household water and sustainable transport. Some individuals are now moving to sustainable technology in planning and renovating their urban homes. Advocates of voluntary simplicity will argue that technology is not the answer on its own and promote other avenues that involve lifestyle changes leading to simpler ways of living.

Some individuals are now moving to sustainable technology in planning and renovating their urban homes.

Biophilia hypothesis

Thousands of tired, nerve-shaken, over-civilised people are beginning to find out that going to the mountains is going home; that wilderness is a necessity; and that mountain parks and reservations are useful not only as fountains of timber and irrigating rivers, but as fountains of life. (Fox 1981, p. 23)

While much of the discussion of the links between environment, sustainability and human health has in the past focused on environmental hazards, there is a growing recognition of the positive health benefits of human contact with the natural environment. Though the words of John Muir (and other earlier philosophers) indicate that the human health and wellbeing benefits of nature have been recognised throughout history, much of the impetus for the recent and mounting recognition can be traced to the publication of the book *Biophilia* by Harvard biologist Edward O. Wilson (1984).

Wilson articulates the view that human beings' 'innate tendency to focus on life and lifelike processes' (1984, p. 1) is not a matter of chance or even choice, but a response to a biological need that is part of the evolutionary history of the species, and essential to human physical and mental wellbeing. According to the biophilia hypothesis there was an evolutionary advantage in having knowledge about nature, an attraction to nature and respect for nature that contributed to the survival of early humans. For thousands of years, biophilia advocates say, humans have relied on an affiliation with nature to meet their physical, intellectual, emotional and spiritual needs (Gullone 2000; Kellert 1993, 1997; Suzuki 1997).

... there was an evolutionary advantage in having knowledge about nature, an attraction to nature and respect for nature that contributed to the survival of early humans.

While some of these nature-based benefits seem obvious (for example, physical or material benefits), others may be less so. Intellectual development (including cognition and critical thinking skills, and the accumulation of empirical knowledge and understanding) is claimed to have emerged 'because advantages accrued to those who nurtured this inclination to observe and understand . . . nature's extraordinary richness and diversity' (Kellert 1997, p. 62). Likewise, Kellert suggests, nature in the form of non-human creatures and landscapes have been crucial in 'nurturing . . . human capacities for affection, bonding, and companionship' (p. 108)—important aspects of human health and wellbeing (even survival) in evolutionary/historical terms and in modern society.

Since Wilson's book was published and further elaboration of the theory provided by Kellert and Wilson (1993), the merits of the theory have been widely debated and its implications studied. Kahn (1997, p. 54), studying children in the United States and Brazil, found that 'children have an abiding affiliation with nature, even in economically impoverished urban communities where such affiliations may seem least likely'. However, Kahn suggests there is a need to explore how childhood affiliations with and understandings of nature might influence adult attitudes and practices (1997, p. 54):

> *People may take the natural environment they encounter during childhood as the norm against which to measure pollution later in their lives. The crux here is that with each ensuing generation, the amount of environmental degradation increases, but each generation takes that amount as the norm— as the nonpolluted state.*

Other writers have highlighted the therapeutic benefits arising from exposure to natural environments (for example, Cordell et al. 1998; Ulrich 1993) and to animals (in the wild, in zoos and even domestic pets) (for example, Bustad 1996; Friedmann & Thomas 1995; Frumkin 2001; Katcher 2002).

These findings have implications for modern human health and wellbeing as well as for sustainability. Gullone (2000, p. 315) says 'there is substantial evidence to suggest that, as a species, our modern lifestyle may have strayed too far from that to which we have adapted'. Both Gullone (2000) and Heerwagen and Orians (2002) have drawn attention to the fact that human beings appear to have retained their fear of hazards (predominantly 'natural') relevant to their evolutionary past, yet failed to develop a sense of fear of the predominantly technological modern threats to safety. Given the evidence, this may prove a double whammy for modern health and wellbeing: we may fail to avoid modern hazards (including those associated with environmental degradation) and at the same time distance ourselves (because of outdated fears) from the beneficial effects of contact with nature.

Frumkin (2001), reviewing the evidence for 'salutary' (or beneficial) rather than 'toxic' (or detrimental) outcomes of environmental exposure, suggests that a new approach may be needed from professions as diverse as public health, urban planning, and landscape and interior design. Frumkin refers to these changes as 'the greening of environmental health', and says 'as we learn more about the health benefits of particular environments, we need to act on these findings' (p. 239).

Supporters of the biophilia hypothesis have highlighted the fact that human wellbeing is not about 'conquering' nature, but about sustaining nature (even if only for selfish reasons).

These findings have implications for modern human health and wellbeing as well as for sustainability.

Spirituality and the environment

Many people in the river community will speak with a passion that goes well beyond what other people might call a rational perspective. Many things in people's lives hold a much greater value than could be expected of a rational relationship between object and person: a spiritual connection. How can we as public health workers understand a farmer's relationship with their land; an artist's relationship with their art; the environmentalist's relationship with the river when we know that our spiritual connection is ephemeral and yet drives our every action? When working with these people, we as practitioners must understand that we are dealing with something that is not governed by reason alone. We cannot make the mistake of thinking that spirituality is something that is found only in a church. Human beings have a long history of developing spiritual connections with the environment, and this connection presents itself in many different ways. As public health workers we must learn to understand its different constructions within our communities.

Humanity's relationships with nature are deeply spiritual, a principle now adopted by many elements of the ecological movement. Feminist ecology, deep ecology and social ecology all describe the spiritual element of humanity's relationship with the ecosystem. Raising humanity's relationship with nature to the level of spiritual experience contributes to the heightened level of urgency in reversing recent environmental trends.

Humanity's relationships with nature are deeply spiritual, a principle now adopted by many elements of the ecological movement.

Ecological movements often refer to various indigenous communities for examples of the way forward in understanding spirituality. In *The Sacred Balance,* Suzuki (1997) describes current knowledge about indigenous spirituality and offers a useful introduction to the topic. The common theme that emerges in many indigenous forms of spiritual practice is the defining of Earth as deity in the form of mother. Lovelock for example chose Gaia, the ancient Greek name for Earth, as goddess and mother of all that is nature as a metaphor for his hypothesis of Earth as interconnected whole. Bianchi (1997, p. 93) expresses the emerging connection of the ecological movement to the sacred:

> *But the environmental challenge today is so great that it calls for a revised human consciousness of what it means to be a creature of earth. This demands a new spiritual understanding and experience of bonding with nature. It is what the socio-biologist, E. O. Wilson terms biophilia an attitude of profound respect for and attachment to our natural surroundings.*

Many indigenous communities describe a similar iconology to the early Greeks. The Earth as deity is described as the giver of life, giving our planet a deeply spiritual significance. It has been argued that the degradation of nature can be linked to the emergence of a masculine deity and corresponding emergence of a patriarchal hegemony which holds that the Earth is object, a resource for the improvement of the human condition, God is to be feared and worshipped, Earth is to be consumed (Merchant 1990; Plumwood 1993). Many indigenous frameworks express Earth as goddess, not to be worshipped and consumed but to be mutually beneficial through a relationship based on respect and worshipped through practice underpinned by a commitment to balance and harmony. When we watch a mother and child we see a mutually beneficial relationship where the child takes sustenance and the mother receives in return fulfilment. It is this balance that is the essence of the mother–child relationship and which indigenous spirituality attempts to emulate.

Christians around the world have contributed to thinking about spirituality and the Earth both within the various churches and the environmental movement. Thomas Berry, for example, is influential within both groups. Another example is Coehlo's (1994) book *By the River Piedra I Sat Down and Wept* in which Christians are reintroduced to the goddess through the power of a personal narrative. Their theses assist us in understanding, not a new Christian spirituality, but the re-emergence of a deeper understanding of human spirituality.

Environmentalists who underpin their actions by spiritual beliefs are exemplified in a comment in McPhee's (1971, p. 39) profile of environmental activist David Brower, in which resort developer Charles Fraser refers to environmentalists as 'druids':

A conservationist too often is just a preservationist, and a preservationist is a druid. I think of land use in terms of people. Ancient druids used to sacrifice human beings under oak trees. Modern druids worship trees and sacrifice people to those trees.

One tendency is for people with divergent perspectives on sustainability issues to attack the messenger. The preservationist platform that may confront the development lobby may be based on an urgent need to apply the precautionary principle; however, developers may swing public opinion in favour of development by labelling the messengers as 'druids' or 'freaks'. The argument often ends there, as one side wins and one loses, instead of following the more sustainable path of looking for common ground. Berry (1968, pp. 45-6) provides the public health worker with a word of caution when they begin to work with the deep essential feelings of the people they come into contact with around the river:

One tendency is for people with divergent perspectives on sustainability issues to attack the messenger.

Diversity is no longer something we tolerate. It is something we esteem as a necessary condition for a livable universe, as a source of the earth's highest perfection . . . To demand an undifferentiated unity would bring human thought and history itself to an end. The splendor of our multicultural world would be destroyed.

Feminism and sustainability

By grounding him/herself in the ideas of feminism, the public health worker will develop a better understanding of the genesis of many ideas that have underpinned a great deal of environmental activity. Both women and men contribute to every society, far beyond the basic child-rearing and gender roles. However, most societies have tended to give a higher profile and greater recognition to the social roles played by men. In Western society this is demonstrated in a highly gender-separated workforce (nursing, teaching and support administration are predominantly female roles, while engineering, computing and executive administration are male industries). Thus male and female living environments can differ sharply and so can their environmental perspectives on decision making (Mies & Shiva 1993). Feminism is the term frequently used for representing the often omitted experience and perspectives of women in a given society.

Both women and men contribute to every society, far beyond the basic child-rearing and gender roles.

In 1974, French feminist Francois d'Eaubonne coined the term eco-feminism. Historically, eco-feminism has not been a single set of clearly defined principles, but a dialogue that has led to an invigorating discourse that has moved into academic literature in its own right (for example, Plumwood 1993).

Eco-feminism is aligned with ecological schools of thought that are grouped under the headings of 'deep ecology' and 'social ecology'. As well, it has both drawn from and contributed to discourses around spiritual ecology and development ecology. One such insight has led to documenting the ways in which the oppression of women and the exploitation of the environment are interconnected in technological and patriarchal societies such as those of the Western industrial era, in which the contribution of both women and natural systems to the society have been undervalued and/or ignored. It is now considered that research and dialogue in one field will contribute to dialogue in the other. D'Eaubonne (1999, p. 179) has suggested:

> We must first put forward the principle that the abolition of patriarchy and the establishment of a relationship with the environment that is finally balanced are not only fundamentally linked, but also can only occur in a post-revolutionary and self managing society.

Some authors have suggested that women have a privileged understanding of nature through the direct experience of birth and immediate responsibility for nurturing of the child. In most subsistence cultural groups women take a primary responsibility for agriculture, which brings them closer to nature (see Mies & Shiva 1993). However, Merchant (1980) suggests that the feminine relationship to nature and therefore feminist ecology is historically a deeply spiritual experience. This position is contested because, as Twine (2001) suggests, this discourse retains a separation between culture and nature. The argument that women are closer to nature is underpinned by the principle that humanity is separate from rather than situated in nature. It is argued that this dialogue contributes to the discourse of patriarchal domination of both nature and the feminine, rather than providing an alternative.

Other authors contribute to the overall discussion by undertaking an historical analysis of 'women' and 'nature'. Throughout history the Earth and nature have consistently been feminised, a classic example being the term 'mother nature'. Feminists see this connection as a process by which both nature and women are dominated. The use of exclusionary dialogue controlled and dominated by the patriarchal hegemony contributes to the process of domination. This examination of power relationships and domination of both women and nature, which was commenced by Foucault (1972), has led to the inclusion of class and race as an interlocking and liberating discourse with nature and women. The feminist is participating in a postmodern dialogue to examine how women, nature, race and class are constructed throughout history to facilitate a new, liberating construction of all interconnected elements. As O'Reilly suggests:

In most subsistence cultural groups women take a primary responsibility for agriculture, which brings them closer to nature.

> Feminism is looking to become what one is, and doing what one wants to do as an individual, and not as a woman [one might add, 'or as a man']. (d'Eaubonne 1999, p. 182)

For d'Eaubonne a feminist revolution will bring about a collapse of the patriarchal hegemony over an economy based on over-consumption of resources. She states (1999, p. 184):

> The two principal factors in the rapid expansion of patriarchy, exhaustion of resources and global population growth, are the distant yet direct causes of the present-day ecological catastrophe.

The eco-feminist critique of the patriarchy revolves around a critique of dualism or a separation of woman and nature from the whole. This leads to efforts to bring about a non-reductionist discourse by women. Paradoxically, in the eco-feminist movement it is the ability of women to take themselves out of the picture and write as 'other' that enables them to engage in such an enlightening

The eco-feminist critique of the patriarchy revolves around a critique of dualism or a separation of woman and nature from the whole.

dialogue about humanity's and, more to the point, man's relationship with nature. By writing as other, the eco-feminist provides a mirror image of all that is unsustainable and of why the world will remain unsustainable until a new approach to nature emerges. It is difficult to see how such a comprehensive image of an unsustainable patriarchal society with an innovative approach to future directions could have been achieved from within.

Indigenous people and environment

Throughout countries such as Canada, the United States of America, Australia and New Zealand, in many small country towns, there are indigenous people. The long history of oppression of indigenous peoples by colonists has made the unlocking of knowledge held in that community almost impossible. And yet, public health practitioners and others will be in constant contact with this community; these people will more than likely take up half of the hospital beds, live in the worst housing and be in constant contact with the police. Experience tells us there will be only superficial communication between the health workers and the local indigenous community. Thinking ecologically, indigenous people are more than stakeholders in the river; they are key informants in understanding a balanced ecosystem: to work ecologically is to work to communicate with these people. This section provides an introduction to some indigenous thoughts on ecology.

Around the world, groups of indigenous peoples have maintained a balance with nature for millennia (Suzuki 1997). Flannery (1994) has suggested that indigenous groups have had a significant role in shaping the ecology of regions; for example, the 'fire stick farming' of Australia's indigenous peoples. In essence, once the ecosystem took shape in response to the arrival of the human species, a long and lasting harmony was established. While each indigenous group has developed a unique relationship with the ecosystem, there are features in common to all, which researchers such as anthropologists and ethnobotanists are attempting to discover. These researchers believe that within the culture, religion and lifeways of these groups it may be possible to discover a key to ecological sustainability.

One of the greatest dilemmas for humanity is the link between unsustainable consumption and individual wellbeing. In recent history there has been an increasing separation of consumers from the ecological impacts of their consumption. We no longer see the farm where our food is produced; we do not see the mine where our energy is produced; more recently we do not see the slave labour conditions in Indonesia and Mexico where our clothes are produced (Soskolne and Bertollini 1999). It is this blinkered lifestyle that enables the 800 million wealthy people of the world to act as parasites on the wellbeing of the 5 billion not so wealthy people, without compassion (Rees 1998).

Indigenous people consume; they consume to improve their wellbeing. This is no different from people from the more developed worlds. But their relationship with the environment has the effect of limiting the level of their consumption.

Once again in this simple act, governed by reciprocal kinship responsibilities, humanity is in balance with the ecology. In a similar vein, in 1967 the indigenous people of Arnhem Land in northern Australia were able to put a stop to the hunting of crocodiles, as the crocodile's brothers saw the dwindling numbers in the environment—an early example of species protection. In vain, environmental scientists such as Capra (1996) and Bateson (1979) have struggled to overcome the separation of humanity from nature, which was initiated by Aristotle 2500 years ago. While not all indigenous cultures have the same structures for achieving the reciprocal relationship described above, the different groups do have different systems that make it impossible to disentangle indigenous humanity from nature. This then becomes the first lesson for sustainability.

One of the greatest dilemmas for humanity is the link between unsustainable consumption and individual wellbeing.

Box 2.1 Indigenous knowledge

On one occasion, an experience helped me to understand the relationship of Australia's indigenous people to the ecosystem. While walking on the bank of the Katherine River with a friend, we strolled under a tree with a huge number of fruit bats hanging upside down, squawking and flapping their wings. My friend said: 'Ah, my nephew, you're so fat and I am so hungry; John, get a gun!' Well, I didn't have a gun, which was lucky for the bat, but can you imagine my horror at being asked to shoot my dinner in the middle of a National Park?

This passage goes some way to introducing the complexity of the relationship of Australia's indigenous people with their environment. At once we note an expression of kinship and an expression of the need for food for survival. The kinship locks people into a family relationship with all land, flora, fauna and people. Each person is related in some way to each other person. This complex set of familial relationships is expanded to include flora and fauna, then land. There is a mutual obligation that connects each entity; this obligation is controlled by a strict code of conduct that has become generically known by indigenous people around Australia as 'the law'. The 'law' governs what one eats and when one eats it; for example, certain groups of people do not eat certain foods. The 'law' also governs the way food is collected and prepared. The end result and, in fact, the purpose of this code of practice is to bring about a balance in nature, a balance achieved through reciprocal obligations between what is consumed and the consumer (Yunupingu 1994). For example, while collecting yams, a type of bush potato, I was scolded for being too greedy and not leaving enough yams in the ground for re-growth for next year.

Source: Yunupingu 1994

Activity 2.2
Where all the rivers flow:
working collaboratively in complex ecological systems

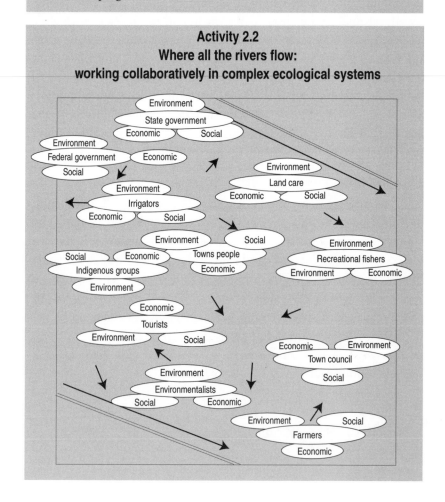

Explanation: This figure contains a lot of information and is meant to appear chaotic because that is a true representation of ecological systems. The wellbeing of the river and the people who live off the river is influenced by a large number of factors and stakeholders who affect the river in an almost infinite variety of ways. If public health practitioners and others are to succeed in complex ecosystems they need to learn strategies for working as part of complex systems rather than looking for order where there is none.

Learning outcomes: This scenario attempts to help the participant develop skills to work in complex ecological environments by:

1. developing skills in communicating with stakeholders who may have dissonant views; and
2. describing the connection between the relationships within the ecosystem and the wellbeing of people who live off the river.

Activity: Rivers around the world are now running dry as a result of many influences. What follows is an exercise in understanding the difficulties of environmental management through a look at river systems. This could be any river system around the world.

The diagram represented opposite is a model of a flowing river. The river is a composite of many molecules, a few of which are represented here. Each molecule has a different central atom, which is named. Each molecule shares the same three atoms, which we have called an economic atom, a social atom and an environmental atom, named after Hancock's 'Mandala of Health' (see Hancock 1985). These three atoms—which are common to each molecule—have varying impacts on the central atom, forcing each molecule to move in different directions leading to totally chaotic movement of molecules in the river flow. This represents a metaphor for river management systems. Using the Mandala of Health allows us to understand that health outcomes in the river system are also the end result of complex, interrelated and random ecological events. River health will have a direct and significant impact on the wellbeing of people who live near and gain their livelihoods from the river in so many ways. Any action by government, farmers, or townspeople that 'keeps the rivers flowing' is also an exercise that will affect the wellbeing of many people.

The participants will be divided into groups of four people who will form a special interest group, which represents one of the molecules presented in the diagram. Each member of the group will be allocated to one of the four atoms, environmental, economic, social and the central atom. This molecule group will need to meet prior to an all molecule (stakeholder) meeting, which will take place to discuss the river's flow. The three atoms in the outer ring will be expected to argue their case for the direction the central atom takes. You will meet and discuss the general direction your group will take, keeping in mind economic, social and environmental pressures while you make your decisions. One additional group will act as facilitators who will chair a meeting that has as its goal discussion of a government objective to keep the river flowing. The facilitator will begin with a five-minute talk on the importance of reducing the amount of water used for irrigation. This will open the meeting, which it is your job to chair.

Each group should develop a position on each of the following issues and be ready to argue their position at the large meeting.

Issues that will be on the agenda for the meeting will include:

Health: the influence of a healthy river system on the health of people.

Fertiliser use and eutrophication: algal blooms have become common features of several Australian rivers. These blooms lead to a build up of slime in portions of rivers which have ceased to flow. This bloom makes the water unpotable and unsafe for both human and animal consumption.

Fish stocks: numbers of native fish species in the rivers are low with certain species at the point of extinction. The fish are threatened by toxins in the water and introduced species.

Carp: carp are introduced species fish said to lead to riverbank deterioration.

Fishing: commercial and recreational fishing affect fish stocks.

Water skiers: some parts of the river are used for water skiing; this can have a negative effect on riverbanks and water quality.

Water wastage: in open irrigation channels up to 60 per cent of water drawn off for irrigation is lost through soakage and evaporation.

Indigenous sacred sites: to Aboriginal people rivers have been significant places providing people with plentiful food supply, religious sites and clan meeting places, and remain a significant part of Aboriginal people's lifeways.

Indigenous people: provide a pool of labour for the farmers during weed extraction (chipping) or cropping (picking) seasons. This places them at the forefront of occasional undisciplined use of pesticides and fertilisers, and it is this group of people that is the first to face the full toxic impact of bad farming practices. These toxins eventually enter the rivers and the atmosphere, working their way into every aspect of rural life.

Aesthetic sites: significant to tourism, rivers are beautiful places that provide locations for relaxation and enjoyment. Fencing for pastures and cropping limits access to special locations.

Water flows: it is sometimes said that the rivers flow backwards. This occurs when the amount of water drawn off leads to water flowing into them from downriver locations.

Town drinking water: many small communities rely on rivers for drinking water.

Sewage: in recent years water from sewage has been treated and then used in local irrigation programs. However, converting sewage is a slow process and many places dispose of sewage into rivers in early stages of treatment.

Land clearing: when trees are removed for creation of pasture the land becomes unstable, which leads to erosion and siltation of rivers.

Riverbank degradation: riverbank flora stabilise banks during floods. Clearing of riverbanks for parkland, housing or to provide access to water for cattle is having a significant impact on bank erosion and river siltation.

Stock fouling: stock will turn rivers that normally cease to flow during dry seasons into a series of turbid pools. This is made worse with the inclusion of nitrites from cattle waste.

Damming and weir control: rivers have been increasingly regulated to prevent floods and preserve water for irrigation. Flooding over the millions of years has created a unique floodplain ecology that is rapidly disappearing as water inundation is increasingly prevented.

The participants should complete the exercise by discussing:

- the difficulties of managing stakeholders with varying points of views and strategies for getting people to work together;
- the importance of the river as an ecological system to the health of people associated with the river.

Conclusion

Before taking any action, a thorough grounding in what has gone before is essential. This is a well understood but often neglected aspect of the process undertaken by the change agency that is promoting sustainability and health. While we accept that a comprehensive grounding in the story of sustainability science is impossible to achieve in the space provided, we have attempted to whet readers' interest and motivate them to go further. It is our hope that through this chapter and the further reading they have undertaken, public health practitioners and others will gain a broad understanding of the many perspectives on the links between sustainability and health. With that understanding as background, they will be in a position to develop a personal approach to sustainability and to develop strategies for working with people who adopt other approaches.

Before taking any action, a thorough grounding in what has gone before is essential.

The next chapter introduces some of the tools developed to make the job of advocates and actors for sustainability progress more smoothly. Any public health worker who wishes to take ecological action is bound to need one of these tools at some time during his or her activities, so understanding them during the preparation stage of the learning experience is important and makes up the content of Chapter 3. However, the record shows that these strategic frameworks are successful only to the extent that they incorporate the full range of possible contributing ideas and the people who hold them.

References

Almås, R. and Lawrence, G. 2003, 'Introduction: The global/local problematic' in *Globalisation, Localisation and Sustainable Livelihoods*, eds R. Almås and G. Lawrence, Ashgate Publishing Limited, Aldershot, pp. 3-24

Aneilski, M. 1998, *The 1998 US Genuine Progress Indicator Methodology Handbook*, Redefining Progress, San Francisco

—— 2002, *The Alberta GPI Blueprint: The Genuine Progress Indicator (GPI) Sustainable Wellbeing Accounting System*, Pembina Institute for Appropriate Development, Alberta, http://www.bgiedu.org/BGI-PDFs/Alberta%20GPI%20Blueprint.pdf%201.pdf [15 December 2003]

Bateson, W. 1979, *Problems of Genetics*, Yale University Press, New Haven

Berry, T. 1968, *Five Oriental Philosophies,* Magi Books, Albany

Bianchi, E.C. 1997, 'Trans-traditional Spirituality: Priets/Minister as Spiritual Seeker, Guide, Healer', *Corpus Reports*, September-October.

Bohm, D. 1980, *Wholeness and the Implicate Order,* Routledge, London, p. 93

Bustad, L.K. 1996, 'Recent Discoveries About Our Relationships with the Natural World' in *Compassion: Our last great hope—Selected Speeches of Leo K. Bustad, DVM, PhD*, Delta Society, Renton, WA

Capra, F. 1996, *The Web of Life*, Anchor Books, New York

Carson, R. 1963, *Silent Spring*, Hamish Hamilton, London

Coehlo, P. 1994, *By the River Piedra I Sat Down and Wept*, Harper Collins, UK

Cordell, K.H., Tarrant, M.A., McDonald, B.L. and Bergstrom, J.C. 1998, 'How the Public Views Wilderness: More Results from the USA Survey on Recreation and the Environment', *International Journal of Wilderness*, vol. 4, pp. 28-31

D'Eaubonne, F. 1999, 'What Could an Ecofeminist Society Be?', *Ethics and the Environment*, vol. 4, no. 2, pp. 179-84

Elkington, J. 1997, *Cannibals with Forks: The triple bottom line of 21st century business,* Capstone Publishing Limited, Oxford

Flannery, T.F. 1994, *The Future Eaters: An ecological history of the Australasian lands and people*, Reed Books, Chatswood

Foucault, M. 1970, *The Order of Things: An archeology of the Human Sciences*, Pantheon Books, New York

Fox, S. 1981, *John Muir and His Legacy,* Little & Brown, Boston, p. 23

Friedmann, E. and Thomas, S.A. 1995, 'Pet Ownership, Social Support, and One-year Survival After Acute Myocardial Infarction in the Cardiac Arrhythmia Suppression Trial (CAST)', *American Journal of Cardiology*, vol. 76, pp. 1213-17

Frumkin, H. 2001, 'Beyond Toxicity: Human health and the natural environment', *American Journal of Preventative Medicine*, vol. 20, pp. 234-40

Gilding, P., Hogarth, M. and Reed, D. 2002, *Single Bottom Line Sustainability: How a value centered approach to corporate sustainability can pay off for shareholders and society*, Ecos Corporation, www.ecoscorporation.com/think/sustainbusiness/single_bottom_line.pdf [15 December 2003]

Global Reporting Initiative 2000, *Sustainability Reporting Guidelines on Economic, Environmental, and Social Performance*, Global Reporting Initiative, Boston

Gullone, E. 2000, 'The Biophilia Hypothesis and Life in the 21st Century: Increasing mental health or increasing pathology?', *Journal of Happiness Studies*, vol. 1, pp. 293-321

Hallebone, E., Mahoney, M. and Townsend, M. 2003, 'Countering Localized Impacts of Globalisation: Some Rural Community Development Initiatives in Australia' in *Globalisation, Localisation and Sustainable Livelihoods*, eds R. Almås and G. Lawrence, Ashgate Publishing Limited, Aldershot, pp. 221-39

Hancock, T. 1985, 'The Mandala of Health: A model of the human ecosystem', *Family and Community Health*, vol. 8, no. 3, pp. 1-10

Hawken, P. 1993, *The Ecology of Commerce*, Weidenfeld and Nicolson, London

Hawken, P., Lovins, A.B. and Lovins, L.H. 1999, *Natural Capitalism: The next industrial revolution*, Earthscan Publications Ltd, London

Heerwagen, J.H. and Orians, G.H. 2002, 'The Ecological World of Children' in *Children and Nature: Psychological, sociocultural, and evolutionary investigations*, eds P.H. Kahn and S.R. Kellert, The MIT Press, Cambridge, Massachusetts, pp. 29-63

Illich, I. 1969, *Tools for Conviviality*, Fontana/Collins, London

Kahn, P.H. 1997, 'Developmental Psychology and the Biophilia Hypothesis: Children's affiliation with nature', *Developmental Review*, vol. 17, pp. 1-61

Katcher, A. 2002, 'Animals in Therapeutic Education: Guides into the Liminal State' in *Children and Nature: Psychological, sociocultural, and evolutionary investigations*, eds P.H. Kahn and S.R. Kellert, The MIT Press, Cambridge, Massachusetts, pp. 179-98

Kellert, S.R. 1993, 'The Biological Basis for Human Values of Nature' in *The Biophilia Hypothesis*, eds S.R. Kellert and E.O. Wilson, Shearwater Books/Island Press, Washington DC, pp. 42-69

—— 1997, *Kinship to Mastery: Biophilia in human evolution and development*, Island Press, Washington DC

Kellert, S.R. and Wilson, E.O. 1993, *The Biophilia Hypothesis*, Shearwater Books/Island Press, Washington DC

Keynes, J.M. 1919, *The Economic Consequences of the Peace*, Macmillan and Co., London

King, M.H. 1990, 'Health is a sustainable state', *The Lancet*, vol. 336, pp. 664-7

Kuznets, S. 1955, 'Economic development and income inequality', *American Economic Review*, vol. 45, pp. 1-28

Last, J. 1998, *Public Health and Human Ecology*, 2nd edn, McGraw-Hill, New York p. 53

Lomborg, B. 2001, *The Skeptical Environmentalist: Measuring the real state of the world*, Cambridge University Press, Cambridge

Lovins, A. 2000a, 'Natural Capitalism: Transcript of an Interview by Satish Kumar', *Resurgence Magazine Online*, Issue 198, January/February, http://resurgence.gn.apc.org/issues/lovins198.htm [2 April 2003]

—— 2000b, *Natural Capitalism*, Transcript of a presentation by Amory Lovins on the ABC Radio National documentary program 'Background Briefing', 8th October 2000, http://www.abc.net.au/rn/talks/bbing/stories/s196391.htm [2 April 2003]

Lovelock, J. 1979, *Gaia: A new look at life on earth*, Oxford, London

McMichael, A.J. 2001, *Human Frontiers, Environments and Disease: Past patterns, uncertain futures*, Cambridge University Press, Cambridge

McMichael, A.J and Powles, J.W. 1999, 'Human Numbers, Environment, Sustainability, and Health', *British Medical Journal*, vol. 319, no. 7215, pp. 977-80

McPhee, J. 1971, *Encounters with the Archdruid: Narratives about a conservationist and three of his natural enemies*, Farrar, Straus & Giroux, New York, p. 39

Merchant, C. 1980, *The Death of Nature: Women, ecology and the scientific revolution*, Harper, San Francisco

Mies, M. and Shiva, V. 1993, *Ecofeminism*, Spinifex Press, North Melbourne

Plumwood, V. 1993, *Feminism and the Mastery of Nature*, Routledge, London

Rees, W.E. 1998, 'How should a parasite value its host?', *Ecological Economics*, vol. 25, pp. 49-52

Rocky Mountain Institute 2002, 'What is Natural Capitalism?', *Research & Consulting*, http://www.rmi.org/sitepages/pid564.php [1 April 2003]

Simon, J.L. 1981, *The Ultimate Resource*, Martin Robertson, Oxford, UK

Smith, K.R. 2000, 'Environmental health—for the rich or for all?', *Bulletin of the World Health Organisation*, vol. 78, no. 9, pp. 1156-7

Soskolne, C.L. and Bertollini, R. 1999, *Global Ecological Integrity and 'Sustainable Development': Cornerstones of Public Health*, Rome, World Health Organisation, http://www.who.dk/document/gch/ecorep5.pdf [1 April 2003]

Suzuki, D. 1997, *The Sacred Balance: Rediscovering our balance in nature*, Allen & Unwin, St Leonards

Szreter, S. 1997, 'Economic Growth, Disruption, Deprivation, Disease and Death: On the importance of the politics of public health', *Population Development Review*, vol. 23, pp. 693-728

Thoreau, H. 1995 (1856), *Walden: Or, life in the woods*, Houghton Mifflin, Massachusetts

Twine, R.T. 2001, 'Ecofeminism in Process', www.ecofem.org/journal [24 February 2004]

Ulrich, R.S. 1993, 'Biophilia, Biophobia, and Natural Landscapes' in *The Biophilia Hypothesis*, eds S.R. Kellert and E.O. Wilson, Shearwater Books/Island Press, Washington DC, pp. 73-137

von Weizsäcker, E. 1997, *Factor Four: A key to sustainability*, Rio + 5 Special Focus Reports, http://www.ecouncil.ac.cr/rio/focus/summary/science.htm [1 April 2003]

von Weizsäcker, E., Lovins, A. and Lovins, L. 1998, *Factor Four: Doubling wealth halving resource use*, Earthscan, London

Wilson, E.O. 1984, *Biophilia*, Harvard University Press, Cambridge, Massachusetts

Wiseman, J. 2002, *Growing Victoria Together: Towards a triple bottom line work plan for government*, Department of Natural Resources/Catchment Management Authority Forum, Melbourne, 25 June 2002, p. 1

Yunupingu, M. 1994, 'Yothu Yindi: Finding the balance', *Voices From the Land, 1993 Boyer Lectures*, Australian Broadcasting Corporation, Sydney

GROUNDING   chapter three

Co-ordinating contexts for sustainability and health

John Grootjans and Mardie Townsend

Summary

Public health practitioners in many contexts are exploring their relationship with sustainability and health, personally and in the institutional framework, and facing the principles critical for a sustainable future. Newcomers to the dialogue on sustainability can become confused because the context varies considerably and the rules are still being formulated. This chapter grounds public health practitioners and others in these emerging contexts and helps her/him to reflect critically on the principles that are most relevant for particular contexts, programs and forms of practice. With this understanding, practitioners can more easily describe and analyse the potential for these principles to lead to stronger links between sustainability and health.

Chapter 3 Grounding

Co-ordinating contexts for sustainability and health

John Grootjans and Mardie Townsend

Key words

Declarations (human rights primary health care, environment and development), charters (Earth Charter, Ottawa Charter), treaties (local and global), conventions (indigenous rights, pollutants), protocols (Kyoto, Montreal), corporate codes of ethics and codes of practice

Learning outcomes

On completion of this chapter public health practitioners and others will be able to:

- describe a range of contexts in which practitioners can engage with sustainability and health;
- describe the evolution of various frameworks, international charters and resolutions in their historical contexts;
- articulate examples of how these can be used in a local context;
- compare, contrast and critically analyse a range of contexts in which sustainability and health can be an important consideration;
- assess the implications of how these contexts influence dialogue about sustainability;
- explore seminal and critical literature related to a range of contexts; and
- discuss the implications of the contexts described in planning for sustainability.

Outline

3.1   Frameworks and tools
3.2   Strategic frameworks
3.3   Health-based frameworks
3.4   Environmental frameworks
3.5   Holistic frameworks

Learning activity

3.1   Mind-mapping complex ideas

Reading

Earth Charter Initiative, *The Earth Charter*, The Earth Charter Initiative, http://www.earthcharter.org/earth charter/charter.htm.2003

United Nations 1948, *Universal Declaration of Human Rights*, United Nations http://www.un.org/ Overview/rights.html.2003

World Health Organisation 1978, *Declaration of Alma-Ata*, World Health Organisation, Geneva, http://www.who.int/hpr/background hp/almaata.htm

3.1 Frameworks and tools

This book has outlined issues related to sustainability, explaining why public health practitioners and others should consider engaging ecologically sustainable development in their everyday practice. One of the principles on which the book is based is that working for sustainability must be interdisciplinary. In Chapter 2 we introduced a variety of approaches that have emerged in the environmental movement and clarified some of the approaches that have emerged from different groups in the environmental movement. Each approach purports to be motivated by the goal of sustainability, and we presented some of the differences so practitioners can understand and value positions taken when in contact with advocates. Chapter 3 extends the work of Chapter 2 by presenting a number of national and international conventions that can be regarded as successful tools for those working for sustainability.

One of the principles on which the book is based is that working for sustainability must be interdisciplinary.

These conventions and frameworks contribute to the process of 'describing place', Phase 1 of the D4P4 model (see Chapter 1). In addressing the needs of public health practitioners and others working for sustainable development, considerable time is devoted to revealing the importance of what has gone before; this sharing is as broad as possible, not concentrating on any single strategy. This chapter focuses on providing a 'road map' of the relevant frameworks and highlights the resonances between the frameworks, rather than the complexity of the context.

Box 3.1 Our clients for this chapter

In Chapter 2 we facilitated the learning of public health practitioners and others by describing a hypothetical river town and how their role in achieving sustainability can be affected by many of the world-views about ecosystems. In this chapter we ask practitioners to imagine they are working with an urban indigenous community that, as the city's boundaries have expanded, has found itself on prime urban land. The people in this community are isolated by race, which affects almost every part of their daily lives: their schooling, health, housing and protection by the law. They are living in the 'Fourth World'; they suffer the morbidity and mortality of the Third World while in the midst of First World wealth and prosperity. Imagining working with this small but distinct community will help practitioners understand the importance of this chapter.

Over recent years there has been an increasing interest in issues of ecological sustainability. For example, in Australia since Agenda 21 (a blueprint for socially, economically and environmentally sustainable development, which emerged from the United Nations Conference on Environment and Development at Rio de Janiero in 1992) became part of the environmental health scene and local government authorities were given responsibility for implementing strategies to achieve its principles, policy statements have been produced at all levels of government to support its implementation. A national environmental council has taken leadership in policy development and in helping environmental health professionals achieve local and national goals of sustainable development. In the field of public health McMichael's books have endeavoured to put sustainability firmly on the public health agenda (McMichael 1993; 2001).

Over recent years there has been an increasing interest in issues of ecological sustainability.

Internationally many documents have emerged or been resurrected (including the Alma-Ata Declaration of 1978) that have direct relevance for the public health practitioner working for ecological sustainability. The practitioner should be aware that these documents often put forward propositions that are not only relevant to the health of populations, but that are also relevant to ecological sustainability in a global political context. In fact, many of the propositions in a document such as the Alma-Ata Declaration are timeless, although their idealism has meant that many of their targets have proved unattainable.

This chapter also introduces tools that can be useful for sustainability practitioners working in public health, and attempts to show how these tools are relevant to ecological sustainability and public health.

3.2 Strategic frameworks

Immediately following World War II the victorious nations came together to form the United Nations (UN), which was established in an effort to prevent a repeat of the conditions that led to war. Under the auspices of the UN several agencies were established with responsibility for overseeing economic, social and political conditions around the world.

The UN and its agencies have been active in developing and monitoring worldwide agreements on issues of concern. The United Nations Education Scientific and Culture Organisation (UNESCO) is the lead organisation in the development and implementation of agreements related to social justice.

One of its first agreements—and one that still has a major influence on global relations—is the *Universal Declaration of Human Rights.*

Equity is one of the lynchpins of agreements on both sustainability and health. In several countries indigenous people have found themselves in a minority with their human rights in conflict with the wishes of the majority. This often leaves communities needing to use systems in place to preserve equity and social justice, both locally and internationally, to settle disputes. Public health practitioners and others in a minority community need to understand the rights of the individual, and the mechanisms for preserving these rights becomes essential public health practice in working for sustainability.

The Universal Declaration of Human Rights

Both warring factions committed atrocities during World War II. Some of these were state sanctioned; others were perpetrated by individuals. The horror of the war years was that the world had lost its innocence: many of these acts were committed by educated people from the so-called civilised world. No longer could people hide behind the assumption that atrocities only happened locally, that they were perpetrated by uncivilised people and that they could be controlled by the triumph of good over evil. There was a clear sense amongst the world's leaders that a universal set of boundaries was essential.

To that end a benchmark on standards of human rights was established in 1948 as a guideline for nations to follow. The UN has proceeded to design and implement several conventions that clarify a person's basic rights. Once a nation becomes a signatory to these conventions, national courts can make decisions based on the principles set out in the conventions. In Australia, for example, while the Constitution sets out the rights of individuals, there is no specific human rights legislation; so UN conventions have proved useful for advocates of change. Australia's Constitution originally excluded Aboriginal people from constitutional rights. This was reversed by referendum in 1967. The original Constitution of the United States excluded slaves from the principle that 'all men are created equal' and it took a war—and many years of civil action—to change that situation.

There are examples of where legal precedent has been set using the guiding principles of UN conventions and where participation in the UN convention system has led to the enactment of local legislation—for

The horror of the war years was that the world had lost its innocence: many of these acts were committed by educated people from the so-called civilised world.

example, the *Racial Discrimination Act 1975* and the *Sex Discrimination Act 1984* in Australia.

Public health practitioners and others will come into contact with situations (sometimes perpetrated under the guise of being for the good of the majority) where an action reduces the rights of individuals. Understanding the Universal Declaration can have direct local relevance in pursuing ecological agendas for health. Inequalities in access to health, wealth, education and environmental protection are having major impacts on the health and wellbeing of populations; practitioners must take into consideration conventions to facilitate and support the actions of advocates for global equity. Using these tools effectively is one of the skills necessary for public health action.

What follows is a copy of the 30 Articles in the *Universal Declaration of Human Rights*.

Box 3.2 Universal Declaration of Human Rights

Article 1.

All human beings are born free and equal in dignity and rights. They are endowed with reason and conscience and should act towards one another in a spirit of brotherhood.

Article 2.

Everyone is entitled to all the rights and freedoms set forth in this Declaration, without distinction of any kind, such as race, colour, sex, language, religion, political or other opinion, national or social origin, property, birth or other status.

Furthermore, no distinction shall be made on the basis of the political jurisdictional or international status of the country or territory to which a person belongs, whether it be independent, trust, non-self-governing or under any other limitation of sovereignty.

Article 3.

Everyone has the right to life, liberty and security of person.

Article 4.

No one shall be held in slavery or servitude; slavery and the slave trade shall be prohibited in all their forms.

Article 5.

No one shall be subjected to torture or to cruel, inhuman or degrading treatment or punishment.

Article 6.

Everyone has the right to recognition everywhere as a person before the law.

Article 7.

All are equal before the law and are entitled without any discrimination to equal protection of the law. All are entitled to equal protection against any discrimination in violation of this Declaration and against any incitement to such discrimination.

Article 8.

Everyone has the right to an effective remedy by the competent national tribunals for acts violating the fundamental right granted him by the constitution or by law.

Article 9.

No one shall be subjected to arbitrary arrest, detention or exile.

Article 10.

Everyone is entitled in full equality to a fair and public hearing by an independent and impartial tribunal, in the determination of his rights and obligations and of any criminal charge against him.

Article 11.

(1) Everyone charged with a penal offence has the right to be presumed innocent until proved guilty according to law in a public trial at which he has had all the guarantees necessary for his defence.

(2) No one shall be held guilty of any penal offence on account of any act or omission, which did not constitute a penal offence, under national or international law, at the time when it was committed. Nor shall a heavier penalty be imposed than the one that was applicable at the time the penal offence was committed.

Article 12.

No one shall be subjected to arbitrary interference with his privacy, family, home or correspondence, nor to attacks upon his honour and reputation. Everyone has the right to the protection of the law against such interference or attacks.

Article 13.

(1) Everyone has the right to freedom of movement and residence within the borders of each state.

(2) Everyone has the right to leave any country, including his own, and to return to his country.

Article 14.

(1) Everyone has the right to seek and to enjoy in other countries asylum from persecution.

(2) This right may not be invoked in the case of prosecutions genuinely arising from non-political crimes or from acts contrary to the purposes and principles of the United Nations.

Article 15.

(1) Everyone has the right to a nationality.

(2) No one shall be arbitrarily deprived of his nationality nor denied the right to change his nationality.

Article 16.

(1) Men and women of full age, without any limitation due to race, nationality or religion, have the right to marry and to found a family. They are entitled to equal rights as to marriage, during marriage and at its dissolution.

(2) Marriage shall be entered into only with the free and full consent of the intending spouses.

(3) The family is the natural and fundamental group unit of society and is entitled to protection by society and the State.

Article 17.

(1) Everyone has the right to own property alone as well as in association with others.

(2) No one shall be arbitrarily deprived of his property.

Article 18.

Everyone has the right to freedom of thought, conscience and religion; this right includes freedom to change his religion or belief, and freedom, either alone or in community with others and in public or private, to manifest his religion or belief in teaching, practice, worship and observance.

Article 19.

Everyone has the right to freedom of opinion and expression; this right includes freedom to hold opinions without interference and to seek, receive and impart information and ideas through any media and regardless of frontiers.

Article 20.

(1) Everyone has the right to freedom of peaceful assembly and association.

(2) No one may be compelled to belong to an association.

Article 21.

(1) Everyone has the right to take part in the government of his country, directly or through freely chosen representatives.

(2) Everyone has the right of equal access to public service in his country.

(3) The will of the people shall be the basis of the authority of government; this will shall be expressed in periodic and genuine elections which shall be by universal and equal suffrage and shall be held by secret vote or by equivalent free voting procedures.

Article 22.

Everyone, as a member of society, has the right to social security and is entitled to realisation, through national effort and international co-operation and in accordance with the organisation and resources of each State, of the economic, social and cultural rights indispensable for his dignity and the free development of his personality.

Article 23.

(1) Everyone has the right to work, to free choice of employment, to just and favourable conditions of work and to protection against unemployment.

(2) Everyone, without any discrimination, has the right to equal pay for equal work.

(3) Everyone who works has the right to just and favourable remuneration ensuring for himself and his family an existence worthy of human dignity, and supplemented, if necessary, by other means of social protection.

(4) Everyone has the right to form and to join trade unions for the protection of his interests.

Article 24.

Everyone has the right to rest and leisure, including reasonable limitation of working hours and periodic holidays with pay.

Article 25.

(1) Everyone has the right to a standard of living adequate for the health and wellbeing of himself and of his family, including food, clothing, housing and medical care and necessary social services, and the right to security in the event of unemployment, sickness, disability, widowhood, old age or other lack of livelihood in circumstances beyond his control.

(2) Motherhood and childhood are entitled to special care and assistance. All children, whether born in or out of wedlock, shall enjoy the same social protection.

Article 26.

(1) Everyone has the right to education. Education shall be free, at least in the elementary and fundamental stages. Elementary education shall be compulsory. Technical and professional education shall be made generally available and higher education shall be equally accessible to all on the basis of merit.

(2) Education shall be directed to the full development of the human personality and to the strengthening of respect for human rights and fundamental freedoms. It shall promote understanding, tolerance and friendship among all nations, racial or religious groups, and shall further the activities of the United Nations for the maintenance of peace.

(3) Parents have a prior right to choose the kind of education that shall be given to their children.

Article 27.

(1) Everyone has the right freely to participate in the cultural life of the community, to enjoy the arts and to share scientific advancement and its benefits.

(2) Everyone has the right to the protection of the moral and material interests resulting from any scientific, literary or artistic production of which he is the author.

Article 28.

Everyone is entitled to a social and international order in which the rights and freedoms set forth in this Declaration can be fully realised.

Article 29.

(1) Everyone has duties to the community in which alone the free and full development of his personality is possible.

(2) In the exercise of his rights and freedoms, everyone shall be subject only to such limitations as are determined by law solely for the purpose of securing due recognition and respect for the rights and freedoms of others and of meeting the just requirements of morality, public order and the general welfare in a democratic society.

(3) These rights and freedoms may in no case be exercised contrary to the purposes and principles of the United Nations.

Article 30.

Nothing in this Declaration may be interpreted as implying for any State, group or person any right to engage in any activity or to perform any act aimed at the destruction of any of the rights and freedoms set forth herein.

Source: United Nations 1948

It is useful for practitioners to keep the principles set out in this declaration in mind. Practitioners should also keep in mind the obligations of nations which are signatories to other international conventions. These may prove useful in practitioners' activities to achieve public health. These conventions include:

- the International Convention on Civil and Political Rights;
- the International Convention on Economic, Social and Cultural Rights;
- the International Convention on the Elimination of All Forms of Racial Discrimination;
- the Convention Against Torture;
- the Convention on Elimination of All Forms of Discrimination Against Women; and
- the Convention on the Rights of the Child.

These conventions are available at http://www.un.org. As well, practitioners should become aware of various international treaties that have been written into national legislation. For example, in Australia legislation reflecting international conventions includes:

- the *Racial Discrimination Act 1975*;
- the *Sex Discrimination Act 1984*; and
- the *Crimes (Torture) Act 1998*.

Though the view has been expressed that any of these treaties are only as powerful as the UN General Assembly's and Security Council's willingness to implement punitive sanctions, enforcement mechanisms are in place for domestic legislation and international treaties. The instruments mentioned above have a range of enforcement mechanisms to support them; even the publicity surrounding breaches can be an effective tool for change. Sanctions have been successful against South Africa and the Serbian Republic. They were also used in Iraq in efforts to prevent the build up of weapons of mass destruction. There may also be circumstances in which a breach (or breaches) form part of the basis for military intervention.

Activity 3.1
Mind-mapping complex ideas

Aim: To find your own way of organising complex material so that it has meaning for you.

How do we do it?

Mind-mapping is a way of creatively arranging a collection of ideas and then organising them into a systematic order. As mind-mappers, we read a text such as the Human Bill of Rights or listen to a stimulating presentation. On a blank sheet of paper, we note down a key word anywhere on the sheet, as each interesting idea strikes us. We then add related words around each key word as our ideas evolve, drawing linking lines as we go. It is usual to have five to ten words radiating out around each key idea.

Why do we do it?

Education research has found that listeners and readers learn better when they organise their own material than when they take long notes. The exercise is innovative and creative; mind-expanding, not rote copying. Mind-mapping can strengthen our thinking skills.

Where and when do we do it?

Whenever we are faced with complex frameworks and interesting ideas, such as the Charters and principles in this chapter. Or in a good discussion where ideas are flying around.

However, scepticism relating to the effectiveness of international treaties and conventions seems to be supported by the failure of national governments to fulfil their obligations. For example, Australia has been found to be in breach of UN conventions on several occasions—making conventions seem toothless—but international pressure brought about by the breaches (for example, see Amnesty International's website) is an important consideration for those seeking an ecologically sustainable future.

3.3 Health-based frameworks

While international agreements alone are insufficient to protect human rights (including the right to health and wellbeing), two particular health-related statements have provided the basis for much international health promotion effort over the past 25 years. These statements also speak to people interested in acting ecologically. The authors believe these principles are signposts for moral, ecologically sustainable health action.

Around the world, the life expectancy of indigenous people is significantly shorter than that of the overall population in their societies.

Around the world, the life expectancy of indigenous people is significantly shorter than that of the overall population in their societies (Brown 2003). The reasons for this are complex. The benchmarks set by the documents that are introduced in this section are essential reading for public health practitioners and others working in urban indigenous communities. The principles set out in the *Declaration of Alma-Ata* (Box 3.2) if applied equitably in a population are a precursor to that population's health and wellbeing. Cuba and Kerala State in India are examples of places where governments have worked to achieve the principles of Alma-Ata. For practitioners working with minorities, knowing and understanding the principles of primary health care and their implications for local populations are essential elements of public health practice for sustainability.

The Declaration of Alma-Ata

The International Conference on Primary Health Care at Alma-Ata (Kazakhstan) in 1978 had among its participants ministers of health from more than 100 nations and representatives of 134 nations. Sponsored by WHO and UNICEF, the conference adopted the goal of 'Health for All by the Year 2000' (Werner et al. 1997).

According to McMurray (2003, p. 370), the conference declaration established three key principles:

1. That health is a fundamental human right, the achievement of which is not limited to efforts focused within the health sector.
2. That health inequities in and between countries are unacceptable, and social and economic development efforts are therefore required to reduce such inequities.
3. That appropriate planning and implementation of health care necessitates community participation, which is both a right and an obligation.

Box 3.3 Declaration of Alma-Ata

International Conference on Primary Health Care, Alma-Ata, USSR, 6-12 September 1978

The International Conference on Primary Health Care, meeting in Alma-Ata this twelfth day of September in the year Nineteen hundred and seventy-eight, expressing the need for urgent action by all governments, all health and development workers, and the world community to protect and promote the health of all the people of the world, hereby makes the following Declaration:

I. The Conference strongly reaffirms that health, which is a state of complete physical, mental and social wellbeing, and not merely the absence of disease or infirmity, is a fundamental human right and that the attainment of the highest possible level of health is a most important world-wide social goal whose realisation requires the action of many other social and economic sectors in addition to the health sector.

II. The existing gross inequality in the health status of the people particularly between developed and developing countries as well as within countries is politically, socially and economically unacceptable and is, therefore, of common concern to all countries.

III. Economic and social development, based on a New International Economic Order,[1] is of basic importance to the fullest attainment of health for all and to the reduction of the gap between the health status of the developing and developed countries. The promotion and protection of the health of the people is essential to sustained economic and social development and contributes to a better quality of life and to world peace.

---

[1] The 'New International Economic Order' is a document prepared in 1973 by developing nations, proposing changes in the international system that would allow less-developed countries the opportunity to build their way out of the never-ending cycle of poverty (Looney, 1999).

IV. The people have the right and duty to participate individually and collectively in the planning and implementation of their health care.

V. Governments have a responsibility for the health of their people which can be fulfilled only by the provision of adequate health and social measures. A main social target of governments, international organisations and the whole world community in the coming decades should be the attainment by all peoples of the world by the year 2000 of a level of health that will permit them to lead a socially and economically productive life. Primary health care is the key to attaining this target as part of development in the spirit of social justice.

VI. Primary health care is essential health care based on practical, scientifically sound and socially acceptable methods and technology made universally accessible to individuals and families in the community through their full participation and at a cost that the community and country can afford to maintain at every stage of their development in the spirit of self-reliance and self-determination. It forms an integral part both of the country's health system, of which it is the central function and main focus, and of the overall social and economic development of the community. It is the first level of contact of individuals, the family and community with the national health system bringing health care as close as possible to where people live and work, and constitutes the first element of a continuing health care process.

VII. Primary health care:

1. reflects and evolves from the economic conditions and sociocultural and political characteristics of the country and its communities and is based on the application of the relevant results of social, biomedical and health services research and public health experience;

2. addresses the main health problems in the community, providing promotive, preventive, curative and rehabilitative services accordingly;

3. includes at least: education concerning prevailing health problems and the methods of preventing and controlling them; promotion of food supply and proper nutrition; an adequate supply of safe water and basic sanitation; maternal and child health care, including family planning; immunisation against the major infectious diseases; prevention and control of locally endemic diseases; appropriate treatment of common diseases and injuries; and provision of essential drugs;

4. involves, in addition to the health sector, all related sectors and aspects of national and community development, in particular agriculture, animal husbandry, food, industry, education, housing, public works, communications and other sectors; and demands the coordinated efforts of all those sectors;

5. requires and promotes maximum community and individual self-reliance and participation in the planning, organisation, operation and control of primary health care, making fullest use of local, national and other available resources; and to this end develops through appropriate education the ability of communities to participate;

6. should be sustained by integrated, functional and mutually supportive referral systems, leading to the progressive improvement of comprehensive health care for all, and giving priority to those most in need;

7. relies, at local and referral levels, on health workers, including physicians, nurses, midwives, auxiliaries and community workers as applicable, as well as traditional practitioners as needed, suitably trained socially and technically to work as a health team and to respond to the expressed health needs of the community.

VIII. All governments should formulate national policies, strategies and plans of action to launch and sustain primary health care as part of a comprehensive national health system and in coordination with other sectors. To this end, it will be necessary to exercise political will, to mobilise the country's resources and to use available external resources rationally.

IX. All countries should cooperate in a spirit of partnership and service to ensure primary health care for all people since the attainment of health by people in any one country directly concerns and benefits every other country. In this context the joint WHO/UNICEF report on primary health care constitutes a solid basis for the further development and operation of primary health care throughout the world.

X. An acceptable level of health for all the people of the world by the year 2000 can be attained through a fuller and better use of the world's resources, a considerable part of which is now spent on armaments and military conflicts. A genuine policy of independence, peace, détente and disarmament could and should release additional resources that could well be devoted to peaceful aims and in particular to the acceleration of social and economic development of which primary health care, as an essential part, should be allotted its proper share.

The International Conference on Primary Health Care calls for urgent and effective national and international action to develop and implement primary health care throughout the world and particularly in developing countries in a spirit of technical cooperation and in keeping with a New International Economic Order. It urges governments, WHO and UNICEF, and other international organisations, as well as multilateral and bilateral agencies, non-governmental organisations, funding agencies, all health workers and the whole world community to support national and international commitment to primary health care and to channel increased technical and financial support to it, particularly in developing countries. The Conference calls on all the aforementioned to collaborate in introducing, developing and maintaining primary health care in accordance with the spirit and content of this Declaration.

Source: World Health Organisation 1978

The 'Health for All by the year 2000' strategy

In 1979, the resolution of the Alma-Ata conference was adopted by the World Health Organisation's Health Assembly through resolution WHA32.30, which endorsed the formulation and implementation of national, regional and global policies, strategies and action plans to achieve 'the attainment by all the citizens of the world by the year 2000 of a level of health that will permit them to lead a socially and economically productive life' (World Health Organisation, 1979). Key sections of the text of that resolution appear below (Box 3.4).

Box 3.4 Health for All by the year 2000
WHA32.30 Formulating strategies for health for all
by the year 2000

The Thirty-second World Health Assembly,

Recalling resolution WHA30.43 by which the Thirtieth World Health Assembly decided that the main social target of governments and of WHO in the coming decades should be the attainment by all the citizens of the world by the year 2000 of a level of health that will permit them to lead a socially and economically productive life;

Having considered the report of the International Conference on Primary Health Care;

Noting with appreciation the preliminary document of the Executive Board entitled 'Formulating strategies for health for all by the year 2000';

1. DECIDES that the development of the Organisation's programs and the allocation of its resources at global, regional and country levels should reflect the commitment of WHO to the overriding priority of the achievement of health for all by the year 2000;

2. ENDORSES the report of the International Conference on Primary Health Care including the Declaration of Alma-Ata, which:

    (1) states that primary health care, forming as it does an integral part both of countries' health systems, of which it is the central function and main focus, and of overall social and economic development, is the key to attaining an acceptable level of health for all;

    (2) calls upon all governments to formulate national policies, strategies and plans of action to launch and sustain primary health care as part of a comprehensive national health system and in coordination with other sectors;

    (3) calls for urgent and effective national and international action to develop and implement primary health care throughout the world, and particularly in developing countries, in a spirit of technical cooperation and in keeping with a New International Economic Order;

(4) recommends that WHO and the United Nations Children's Fund should continue to encourage and support national strategies and plans for primary health care as part of overall development, and should also formulate as soon as possible appropriate plans of action at the regional and global levels to promote and facilitate the mutual support of countries for accelerated development of primary health care;

3. CONSIDERS that, in accordance with the basic policy of adapting international activities to the real needs of countries, strategies and plans of action for attaining health for all by the year 2000 should be formulated first and foremost by the countries themselves, and that the regional and global strategies formulated on the basis of these national strategies, as well as on the basis of the strategies of regional groups formed by countries for practical reasons, should promote and facilitate accelerated development of primary health care in the Member States of WHO, as well as the attraction of substantial and continuing additional international resources for these purposes.

Source: World Health Organisation 1979

Twenty-five years on, health for all is still a distant dream. According to Werner et al. (1997), much of this failure can be attributed to the political context in which the Primary Health Care (PHC) programs launched to address the health inequities identified at the Alma-Ata conference were being implemented. Werner et al. (1997, p. 19) state:

> *It was foreseeable that in countries whose leadership was less than fully accountable to the people (that is to say, most countries), the liberating component of PHC soon resulted in resistance to its implementation.*

In their view part of the problem with the Alma-Ata Declaration lies in its language, which they claim was designed not to offend the governments that are its signatories. They suggest (p. 19) that the language of the declaration is open to interpretation and that this creates a situation where 'oppressive governments can translate it as they see fit' and that 'this undermines the essence and muffles the power of Alma-Ata's call for Health for All and the sweeping changes in power structures and economic systems that it requires'. Sadly, a review of worldwide health statistics supports their claim that 'the transformative potential of Alma-Ata remained largely on the drawing board'.

. . . the problem with the Alma-Ata Declaration lies in its language, which they claim was designed not to offend the governments that are its signatories.

Issues of social justice and inequalities, which were major principles in the Alma-Ata Declaration, re-emerged as major concerns in the Rio Summit almost 15 years later. Today the *Declaration of Alma-Ata* becomes a useful benchmark for public health practitioners and others against which to measure the performance of signatory nations and continues to be a useful resource for future planning.

The Ottawa Charter

Inherent in these strategies is recognition of the importance of contextual influences on health outcomes...

When the representatives of 38 nations met at the first International Conference on Health Promotion in Ottawa, Canada in 1986, it became clear that progress toward 'Health for All by the year 2000' had been limited. In response to this and in recognition of the shortcomings of the traditional health promotion approach focusing on lifestyle and behavioural approaches, the Ottawa Charter for Health Promotion was developed (Baum 2002; McMurray 2003). The charter (Box 3.5) recognised as prerequisites for health:

- peace;
- shelter;
- education;
- food;
- income;
- a stable ecosystem;
- sustainable resources;
- social justice; and
- equity.

(World Health Organisation et al. 1986, pp. 357-8)

Five major strategies for promoting health were identified in the charter:

- building healthy public policy;
- creating supportive environments;
- strengthening community action;
- developing personal skills; and
- re-orienting health services.

Inherent in these strategies is recognition of the importance of contextual influences on health outcomes, and on individual and community capacity to gain access to the resources to achieve and maintain health. The strategies also reflect the primary health care approach outlined in the Alma-Ata Declaration, and an 'ecological view of health' (McMurray 2003, p. 27).

Box 3.5 Ottawa Charter for Health Promotion

The first International Conference on Health Promotion, meeting in Ottawa this 21st day of November 1986, hereby presents this CHARTER for action to achieve Health for All by the year 2000 and beyond.

This conference was primarily a response to growing expectations for a new public health movement around the world. Discussions focused on the needs in industrialised countries, but took into account similar concerns in all other regions. It built on the progress made through the Declaration on Primary Health Care at Alma-Ata, the World Health Organisation's Targets for Health for All document, and the recent debate at the World Health Assembly on intersectoral action for health.

HEALTH PROMOTION

Health promotion is the process of enabling people to increase control over, and to improve, their health. To reach a state of complete physical, mental and social wellbeing, an individual or group must be able to identify and to realise aspirations, to satisfy needs, and to change or cope with the environment. Health is, therefore, seen as a resource for everyday life, not the objective of living. Health is a positive concept emphasising social and personal resources, as well as physical capacities. Therefore, health promotion is not just the responsibility of the health sector, but goes beyond healthy life-styles to wellbeing.

PREREQUISITES FOR HEALTH

The fundamental conditions and resources for health are peace, shelter, education, food, income, a stable eco-system, sustainable resources, social justice and equity. Improvement in health requires a secure foundation in these basic prerequisites.

ADVOCATE

Good health is a major resource for social, economic and personal development and an important dimension of quality of life. Political, economic, social, cultural, environmental, behavioural and biological factors can all favour health or be harmful to it. Health promotion action aims at making these conditions favourable through advocacy for health.

ENABLE

Health promotion focuses on achieving equity in health. Health promotion action aims at reducing differences in current health status and ensuring equal opportunities and resources to enable all people to achieve their fullest health potential. This includes a secure foundation in a supportive environment, access to information, life skills and opportunities for making healthy choices. People cannot achieve their fullest health potential unless they are able to take control of those things which determine their health. This must apply equally to women and men.

MEDIATE

The prerequisites and prospects for health cannot be ensured by the health sector alone. More importantly, health promotion demands coordinated action by all concerned: by governments, by health and other social and economic sectors, by non-governmental and voluntary organisations, by local authorities, by industry and by the media. People in all walks of life are involved as individuals, families and communities. Professional and social groups and health personnel have a major responsibility to mediate between differing interests in society for the pursuit of health.

Health promotion strategies and programs should be adapted to the local needs and possibilities of individual countries and regions to take into account differing social, cultural and economic systems.

HEALTH PROMOTION ACTION MEANS:

BUILD HEALTHY PUBLIC POLICY

Health promotion goes beyond health care. It puts health on the agenda of policy makers in all sectors and at all levels, directing them to be aware of the health consequences of their decisions and to accept their responsibilities for health.

Health promotion policy combines diverse but complementary approaches including legislation, fiscal measures, taxation and organisational change. It is coordinated action that leads to health, income and social policies that foster greater equity. Joint action contributes to ensuring safer and healthier goods and services, healthier public services, and cleaner, more enjoyable environments.

Health promotion policy requires the identification of obstacles to the adoption of healthy public policies in non-health sectors, and ways of removing them. The aim must be to make the healthier choice the easier choice for policy makers as well.

CREATE SUPPORTIVE ENVIRONMENTS

Our societies are complex and interrelated. Health cannot be separated from other goals. The inextricable links between people and their environment constitutes the basis for a socio-ecological approach to health. The overall guiding principle for the world, nations, regions and communities alike, is the need to encourage reciprocal maintenance—to take care of each other, our communities and our natural environment. The conservation of natural resources throughout the world should be emphasised as a global responsibility.

Changing patterns of life, work and leisure have a significant impact on health. Work and leisure should be a source of health for people. The way society organises work should help create a healthy society. Health promotion generates living and working conditions that are safe, stimulating, satisfying and enjoyable.

Systematic assessment of the health impact of a rapidly changing environment—particularly in areas of technology, work, energy production and urbanisation—is essential and must be followed by action to ensure positive benefit to the health of the public. The protection of the natural and built environments and the conservation of natural resources must be addressed in any health promotion strategy.

STRENGTHEN COMMUNITY ACTION

Health promotion works through concrete and effective community action in setting priorities, making decisions, planning strategies and implementing them to achieve better health. At the heart of this process is the empowerment of communities, their ownership and control of their own endeavours and destinies.

Community development draws on existing human and material resources in the community to enhance self-help and social support, and to develop flexible systems for strengthening public participation and direction of health matters. This requires full and continuous access to information, learning opportunities for health, as well as funding support.

DEVELOP PERSONAL SKILLS

Health promotion supports personal and social development through providing information, education for health and enhancing life skills.

By so doing, it increases the options available to people to exercise more control over their own health and over their environments, and to make choices conducive to health.

Enabling people to learn throughout life, to prepare themselves for all of its stages and to cope with chronic illness and injuries is essential. This has to be facilitated in school, home, work, and community settings. Action is required through educational, professional, commercial and voluntary bodies, and within the institutions themselves.

REORIENT HEALTH SERVICES

The responsibility for health promotion in health services is shared among individuals, community groups, health professionals, health service institutions and governments. They must work together towards a health care system which contributes to the pursuit of health.

The role of the health sector must move increasingly in a health promotion direction, beyond its responsibility for providing clinical and curative services. Health services need to embrace an expanded mandate which is sensitive and respects cultural needs. This mandate should support the needs of individuals and communities for a healthier life, and open channels between the health sector and broader social, political, economic and physical environmental components.

Reorienting health services also requires stronger attention to health research as well as changes in professional education and training. This must lead to a change of attitude and organisation of health services, which refocuses on the total needs of the individual as a whole person.

MOVING INTO THE FUTURE:

Health is created and lived by people within the settings of their everyday life; where they learn, work, play and love. Health is created by caring for oneself and others, by being able to take decisions and have control over one's life circumstances, and by ensuring that the society one lives in creates conditions that allow the attainment of health by all its members.

Caring, holism and ecology are essential issues in developing strategies for health promotion. Therefore those involved should take as a guiding principle that, in each phase of planning, implementation and evaluation of health promotion activities, women and men should become equal partners.

COMMITMENT TO HEALTH PROMOTION

The participants in this conference pledge:

- to move into the arena of healthy public policy, and to advocate a clear political commitment to health and equity in all sectors;
- to counteract the pressures towards harmful products, resource depletion, unhealthy living conditions and environments, and bad nutrition; and to focus attention on public health issues such as pollution, occupational hazards, housing and settlements;
- to respond to the health gap within and between societies, and to tackle the inequities in health produced by the rules and practices of these societies;
- to acknowledge people as the main health resource; to support and enable them to keep themselves, their families and friends healthy through financial and other means, and to accept the community as the essential voice in matters of its health, living conditions and wellbeing;
- to reorient health services and their resources towards the promotion of health; and to share power with other sectors, other disciplines and most importantly with people themselves;
- to recognise health and its maintenance as a major social investment and challenge; and to address the overall ecological issue of our ways of living.

The conference urges all concerned to join them in their commitment to strong public health alliance.

CALL FOR INTERNATIONAL ACTION

The Conference calls on the World Health Organisation and other international organisations to advocate the promotion of health in all appropriate forums and to support countries in setting up strategies and programs for health promotion.

The Conference is firmly convinced that if people in all walks of life, non governmental and voluntary organisations, governments, the World Health Organisation and all other bodies concerned join forces in introducing strategies for health promotion, in line with the moral and social values that form the basis of this CHARTER, Health For All by the Year 2000 will become a reality.

Source: World Health Organisation et al. 1986

These documents stand out in that the principles they advocate have direct relevance to today's global situation, and adherence to the principles they put forward will also be adhering to the principles of ecological sustainability. Health workers should become articulate in the principles set out in these documents and learn to use them as benchmarks against which public policy past, present and future can be measured.

3.4 Environmental frameworks

In the indigenous communities it is often local ecosystem degradation that is most stark.

So far we have examined the work of two United Nations organisations, UNESCO and WHO. Each has developed a number of international documents to support its work, often in response to a great deal of foundation work carried out by governments, individuals and non-government organisations and designed to represent the best interests of global populations.

After many years of lobbying by international environmental groups the UN has come to realise that early warning signs indicate that the world ecosystem is facing a crisis. In a response to these activities the UN has recognised that to sustain a healthy, wealthy and wise world population into the future will require world leadership—which can only be provided by the UN. The United Nations Environment Program (UNEP) advocates a sustainable future. Practitioners will need to work with these documents to bring about successful public health action. While WHO documents have a clear link to the health of populations, equality and environment are neglected aspects of public health action because politicians, government, funding bodies and thus public health practitioners seem to need immediate results, while action for equity or ecological sustainability needs perseverance over long periods with few short-term rewards. As well, action for equity or ecological sustainability requires sustained political activity that can bring the public health practitioner into conflict with the political leadership of the time.

In the indigenous communities it is often local ecosystem degradation that is most stark. Basic issues of water, sanitation and housing are often in chronic disrepair in contrast with the surrounding community. It is this often visible deterioration of ecosystems that confronts public health practitioners and colleagues. The principles set out in the documents in this chapter will have direct relevance to your work, as these communities seem to magnify the worst elements of ecosystem collapse with an obvious relationship to the health and wellbeing of community members. Understanding national and international negotiations on the environment is essential to public health practitioners and colleagues.

The Stockholm Convention on Persistent Organic Pollutants

For many years there has been lobbying to stop the use of persistent organic pollutants (POPs). Chemicals considered to be POPs include polychlorinated biphenyls (PCBs), DDT, dioxin, dieldrin, chlordane. While the full impact of these compounds on human health is not yet clear, some features of these chemicals have long indicated a need for precaution. These chemicals are persistent in the environment, resist breakdown and will remain in the environment for a long time. They are fat soluble and accumulate in the bodies of animals that come into contact with them; the higher up the food chain you are, the more POPs will accumulate in your tissue.

The precautionary principle should be well understood by sustainability and health practitioners . . .

Silent Spring by Rachel Carson (1963) first brought this issue to world attention in the 1960s, highlighting problems associated with the use of DDT. Lobbying since then led in 2001 to the Stockholm Convention, which attempts to remove 12 specific pollutants from the environment. However, it is important to recognise that this is a complex issue and that there continues to be debate about the risks and benefits of eliminating the use of these substances. Carson's (1963) work met with strong resistance from the agricultural, scientific and political sectors, and while the United States Environmental Protection Authority banned the use of DDT in 1972, even now DDT is still exported from America to other countries.

The story of POPs is interesting to public health practitioners and colleagues for several reasons. The first is illustrated by studying the campaign to see the end of production and use of POPs. The campaign involved years of lobbying by health, scientific and public interest organisations, including over 350 non-government organisations in 65 nations. It also required the co-operation of diverse international bodies such as the World Health Organisation, the International Labour Organisation, the Intergovernmental Forum on Chemical Safety and the United Nations Environment Program. The second is that most of the action on ending the reign of POPs is based on the precautionary principle, in that action preceded the completion of the collection of evidence. The precautionary principle should be well understood by sustainability and health practitioners; if, for example, public health practitioners need to rely on the accumulation of an enormous body of evidence (as in the case of cigarette smoking) before action is taken, in ecological terms remediation is more than likely to be impossible. It's essential that public health practitioners and colleagues realise this.

For the purposes of this book we have included Articles 1 and 3 of the convention, which explains to the practitioner the intent of the legally binding document (Box 3.6).

Box 3.6 Stockholm Convention on Persistent Organic Pollutants (and see Activity 4.2)

ARTICLE 1.

OBJECTIVE

Mindful of the precautionary approach as set forth in Principle 15 of the Rio Declaration on Environment and Development, the objective of this Convention is to protect human health and the environment from persistent organic pollutants.

ARTICLE 3.

Measures to reduce or eliminate releases from intentional production and use:

1. Each Party shall:
    (a) Prohibit and/or take the legal and administrative measures necessary to eliminate:
        (i) Its production and use of the chemicals listed in Annex A subject to the provisions of that Annex; and
        (ii) Its import and export of the chemicals listed in Annex A in accordance with the provisions of paragraph 2; and
    (b) Restrict its production and use of the chemicals listed in Annex B in accordance with the provisions of that Annex.
2. Each Party shall take measures to ensure:
    (a) That a chemical listed in Annex A or Annex B is imported only:
        (i) For the purpose of environmentally sound disposal as set forth in paragraph 1 (d) of Article 6; or
        (ii) For a use or purpose which is permitted for that Party under Annex A or Annex B;

(b) That a chemical listed in Annex A for which any production or use specific exemption is in effect or a chemical listed in Annex B for which any production or use specific exemption or acceptable purpose is in effect, taking into account any relevant provisions in existing international prior informed consent instruments, is exported only:

(i) For the purpose of environmentally sound disposal as set forth in paragraph 1 (d) of Article 6;

(ii) To a Party which is permitted to use that chemical under Annex A or Annex B; or

(iii) To a State not Party to this Convention which has provided an annual certification to the exporting Party. Such certification shall specify the intended use of the chemical and include a statement that, with respect to that chemical, the importing State is committed to:

(a) Protect human health and the environment by taking the necessary measures to minimise or prevent releases;

(b) Comply with the provisions of paragraph 1 of Article 6; and

(c) Comply, where appropriate, with the provisions of paragraph 2 of Part II of Annex B. The certification shall also include any appropriate supporting documentation, such as legislation, regulatory instruments, or administrative or policy guidelines. The exporting Party shall transmit the certification to the Secretariat within sixty days of receipt.

(d) That a chemical listed in Annex A, for which production and use specific exemptions are no longer in effect for any Party, is not exported from it except for the purpose of environmentally sound disposal as set forth in paragraph 1 (d) of Article 6;

(e) For the purposes of this paragraph, the term 'State not Party to this Convention' shall include, with respect to a particular chemical, a State or regional economic integration organisation that has not agreed to be bound by the Convention with respect to that chemical.

3. Each Party that has one or more regulatory and assessment schemes for new pesticides or new industrial chemicals shall take measures to regulate with the aim of preventing the production and use of new pesticides or new industrial chemicals which, taking into consideration the criteria in paragraph 1 of Annex D, exhibit the characteristics of persistent organic pollutants.

4. Each Party that has one or more regulatory and assessment schemes for pesticides or industrial chemicals shall, where appropriate, take into consideration within these schemes the criteria in paragraph 1 of Annex D when conducting assessments of pesticides or industrial chemicals currently in use.

5. Except as otherwise provided in this Convention, paragraphs 1 and 2 shall not apply to quantities of a chemical to be used for laboratory-scale research or as a reference standard.

6. Any Party that has a specific exemption in accordance with Annex A or a specific exemption or an acceptable purpose in accordance with Annex B shall take appropriate measures to ensure that any production or use under such exemption or purpose is carried out in a manner that prevents or minimises human exposure and release into the environment. For exempted uses or acceptable purposes that involve intentional release into the environment under conditions of normal use, such release shall be to the minimum extent necessary, taking into account any applicable standards and guidelines.

Source: United Nations Environment Program 2001

The Montreal Protocol on Substances that Deplete the Ozone Layer

To outline the chain of events that led to the setting up of this protocol, we have borrowed a statement from the United Nations Environment Program (UNEP) website (Box 3.7).

Box 3.7 Montreal Protocol on Substances that Deplete the Ozone Layer

In 1981 UNEP set up a working group to prepare a global framework convention for the protection of the Ozone Layer. Its aim was to secure a general treaty to tackle Ozone Depletion.

First, a general treaty resolved in principle to tackle a problem; then the parties got down to the more difficult task of agreeing on protocols that established specific controls. Even the first, relatively easy, step proved remarkably difficult. The Convention for the Protection of the Ozone Layer, finally agreed upon in Vienna in 1985, appears unexceptional. Nations agreed to take 'appropriate measures . . . to protect human health and the environment against adverse effects resulting or likely to result from human activities which modify or are likely to modify the Ozone Layer'; but the measures are unspecified. There is no mention of any substances that might harm the ozone, and chlorofluorocarbons only appear towards the end of the annex to the treaty, where they are mentioned as chemicals that should be monitored. The main thrust of the convention was to encourage research, co-operation among countries and exchange of information. Even so it took four years to prepare and agree. Twenty nations signed it in Vienna, but most did not rush to ratify it. The convention provided for future protocols and specified procedures for amendment dispute settlement.

With all its complications and seemingly endless disputes, the Vienna Convention set an important precedent. For the first time nations agreed in principle to tackle a global environmental problem before its effects were felt, or even scientifically proven.

As the experts began to explore for specific measures to be taken, the journal *Nature* published a paper in May 1985 by British scientists—led by Dr Joe Farman—about severe ozone depletion in the Antarctic. The paper's findings were confirmed by American satellite observations and offered the first proof of severe ozone depletion, making the need for definite measures more urgent. As a result, in September 1987 agreement was reached on specific measures to be taken and the Montreal Protocol on Substances that Deplete the Ozone Layer was signed.

Source: United Nations Environment Program 1987

Despite the difficulties outlined by UNEP in setting up the agreement, early signs suggest that signatories are complying with its guidelines. In addition, there is early indication that the hole in the ozone layer has at least stopped expanding.

The Rio Declaration on Environment and Development

In June 1992, the United Nations Conference on Environment and Development took place in Rio de Janeiro, Brazil. This conference built on the processes and understandings of the 1972 Stockholm Conference on the Human Environment, and on the work of the Brundtland Commission and its now famous publication *Our Common Future* (World Commission on Environment and Development 1987). Among the documents produced by the Rio conference were:

• the Rio Declaration on Environment and Development (Box 3.8); and
• Agenda 21 (a blueprint for socially, economically and environmentally sustainable development).

Both documents have significance for public health practitioners and colleagues. The Agenda 21 document is too long to include here, but should be read by anyone interested in the links between sustainability and health. It can be found at http://www.iisd.org/rio+5/agenda/agenda21.htm. The Rio Declaration is provided below.

Box 3.8 Rio Declaration on Environment and Development

The United Nations Conference on Environment and Development . . . with the goal of establishing a new and equitable global partnership through the creation of new levels of cooperation among States, key sectors of societies and people, working towards international agreements which respect the interests of all and protect the integrity of the global environmental and developmental system, recognising the integral and interdependent nature of the Earth, our home,

Proclaims that:

Principle 1
Human beings are at the centre of concerns for sustainable development. They are entitled to a healthy and productive life in harmony with nature.

Principle 2
States have, in accordance with the Charter of the United Nations and the principles of international law, the sovereign right to exploit their own resources pursuant to their own environmental and developmental policies, and the responsibility to ensure that activities within their jurisdiction or control do not cause damage to the environment of other States or of areas beyond the limits of national jurisdiction.

Principle 3

The right to development must be fulfilled so as to equitably meet developmental and environmental needs of present and future generations.

Principle 4

In order to achieve sustainable development, environmental protection shall constitute an integral part of the development process and cannot be considered in isolation from it.

Principle 5

All States and all people shall cooperate in the essential task of eradicating poverty as an indispensable requirement for sustainable development, in order to decrease the disparities in standards of living and better meet the needs of the majority of the people of the world.

Principle 6

The special situation and needs of developing countries, particularly the least developed and those most environmentally vulnerable, shall be given special priority. International actions in the field of environment and development should also address the interests and needs of all countries.

Principle 7

States shall cooperate in a spirit of global partnership to conserve, protect and restore the health and integrity of the Earth's ecosystem. In view of the different contributions to global environmental degradation, States have common but differentiated responsibilities. The developed countries acknowledge the responsibility that they bear in the international pursuit to sustainable development in view of the pressures their societies place on the global environment and of the technologies and financial resources they command.

Principle 8

To achieve sustainable development and a higher quality of life for all people, States should reduce and eliminate unsustainable patterns of production and consumption and promote appropriate demographic policies.

Principle 9

States should cooperate to strengthen endogenous capacity-building for sustainable development by improving scientific understanding through exchanges of scientific and technological knowledge, and by enhancing the development, adaptation, diffusion and transfer of technologies, including new and innovative technologies.

Principle 10

Environmental issues are best handled with participation of all concerned citizens, at the relevant level. At the national level, each individual shall have appropriate access to information concerning the environment that is held by public authorities, including information on hazardous materials and activities in their communities, and the opportunity to participate in decision-making processes. States shall facilitate and encourage public awareness and participation by making information widely available. Effective access to judicial and administrative proceedings, including redress and remedy, shall be provided.

Principle 11

States shall enact effective environmental legislation. Environmental standards, management objectives and priorities should reflect the environmental and development context to which they apply. Standards applied by some countries may be inappropriate and of unwarranted economic and social cost to other countries, in particular developing countries.

Principle 12

States should cooperate to promote a supportive and open international economic system that would lead to economic growth and sustainable development in all countries, to better address the problems of environmental degradation. Trade policy measures for environmental purposes should not constitute a means of arbitrary or unjustifiable discrimination or a disguised restriction on international trade.

Unilateral actions to deal with environmental challenges outside the jurisdiction of the importing country should be avoided. Environmental measures addressing transboundary or global environmental problems should, as far as possible, be based on an international consensus.

Principle 13
States shall develop national law regarding liability and compensation for the victims of pollution and other environmental damage. States shall also cooperate in an expeditious and more determined manner to develop further international law regarding liability and compensation for adverse effects of environmental damage caused by activities within their jurisdiction or control to areas beyond their jurisdiction.

Principle 14
States should effectively cooperate to discourage or prevent the relocation and transfer to other States of any activities and substances that cause severe environmental degradation or are found to be harmful to human health.

Principle 15
In order to protect the environment, the precautionary approach shall be widely applied by States according to their capabilities. Where there are threats of serious or irreversible damage, lack of full scientific certainty shall not be used as a reason for postponing cost-effective measures to prevent environmental degradation.

Principle 16
National authorities should endeavour to promote the internalisation of environmental costs and the use of economic instruments, taking into account the approach that the polluter should, in principle, bear the cost of pollution, with due regard to the public interest and without distorting international trade and investment.

Principle 17
Environmental impact assessment, as a national instrument, shall be undertaken for proposed activities that are likely to have a significant adverse impact on the environment and are subject to a decision of a competent national authority.

Principle 18
States shall immediately notify other States of any natural disasters or other emergencies that are likely to produce sudden harmful effects on the environment of those States. Every effort shall be made by the international community to help States so afflicted.

Principle 19

States shall provide prior and timely notification and relevant information to potentially affected States on activities that may have a significant adverse transboundary environmental effect and shall consult with those States at an early stage and in good faith.

Principle 20

Women have a vital role in environmental management and development. Their full participation is therefore essential to achieve sustainable development.

Principle 21

The creativity, ideals and courage of the youth of the world should be mobilised to forge a global partnership in order to achieve sustainable development and ensure a better future for all.

Principle 22

Indigenous people and their communities and other local communities have a vital role in environmental management and development because of their knowledge and traditional practices. States should recognise and duly support their identity, culture and interests and enable their effective participation in the achievement of sustainable development.

Principle 23

The environment and natural resources of people under oppression, domination and occupation shall be protected.

Principle 24

Warfare is inherently destructive of sustainable development. States shall therefore respect international law providing protection for the environment in times of armed conflict and cooperate in its further development, as necessary.

Principle 25

Peace, development and environmental protection are interdependent and indivisible.

Principle 26

States shall resolve all their environmental disputes peacefully and by appropriate means in accordance with the Charter of the United Nations.

Principle 27
States and people shall cooperate in good faith and in a spirit of partnership in the fulfilment of the principles embodied in this Declaration and in the further development of international law in the field of sustainable development.
Source: United Nations 1992a

The Kyoto Protocol on Greenhouse Gases

The relative success of the conventions on POPs and ozone depleting chemicals seems to have ended with attempts to limit greenhouse gases in the Kyoto Protocol. The Kyoto Protocol has been recognised as a very small first step for the world to take in reducing greenhouse gases. A factor four reduction in energy output is well recognised as necessary and achievable in current industrial capacity without any reduction in the quality of life (von Weizsäcker et al. 1998), yet the Kyoto Protocol attempts to get governments to commit to a much more conservative target. The freeze in progress toward sustainable development that this protocol has pre-empted is important for practitioners to consider in understanding change. The document states (Article 2):

> The ultimate objective of this convention and any related legal instruments that the Conference of the Parties may adopt is to achieve, in accordance with the relevant provisions of the Convention, stabilisation of Greenhouse gas concentrations in the atmosphere at a level that would prevent dangerous anthropogenic interference with the climate system. Such a level should be achieved within a time-frame sufficient to allow ecosystems to adapt naturally to climate change, to ensure that food production is not threatened and to enable economic development to proceed in a sustainable manner. (United Nations 1992b)

This objective is a very soft approach for governments, but it is now recognised that the emerging 'small government' agenda adopted by Australia and the United States among others (see Chapter 2) demands a reduction in government interference in markets. It is clear that even this minor greenhouse gas objective will need strong support from markets, which is not yet universally forthcoming. To that effect the progress of UNEP to putting the convention into practice is moving forward at a snail's pace. The following box (Box 3.9) sets out the Principles of the Kyoto Protocol. The detailed text of the Kyoto Protocol can be found at http://unfccc.int/resource/conv/conv_006.html.

Box 3.9 Kyoto Protocol on Greenhouse Gases

Article 2: Principles

In their actions to achieve the objective of the Convention and to implement its provisions, the Parties shall be guided, *Inter alia*, by the following:

1. The Parties should protect the climate system for the benefit of present and future generations of humankind, on the basis of equity and in accordance with their common but differentiated responsibilities and respective capabilities. Accordingly, the developed country Parties should take the lead in combating climate change and the adverse effects thereof.

2. The specific needs and special circumstances of developing country Parties, especially those that are particularly vulnerable to the adverse effects of climate change, and of those Parties, especially developing country Parties, that would have to bear a disproportionate or abnormal burden under the Convention, should be given full consideration.

3. The Parties should take precautionary measures to anticipate, prevent or minimise the causes of climate change and mitigate its adverse effects. Where there are threats of serious or irreversible damage, lack of full scientific certainty should not be used as a reason for postponing such measures, taking into account that policies and measures to deal with climate change should be cost-effective so as to ensure global benefits at the lowest possible cost. To achieve this, such policies and measures should take into account different socio-economic contexts, be comprehensive, cover all relevant sources, sinks and reservoirs of greenhouse gases and adaptation, and comprise all economic sectors. Efforts to address climate change may be carried out cooperatively by interested Parties.

4. The Parties have a right to, and should, promote sustainable development. Policies and measures to protect the climate system against human-induced change should be appropriate for the specific conditions of each Party and should be integrated with national development programs, taking into account that economic development is essential for adopting measures to address climate change.

5. The Parties should cooperate to promote a supportive and open international economic system that would lead to sustainable economic growth and development in all Parties, particularly developing country Parties, thus enabling them better to address the problems of climate change. Measures taken to combat climate change, including unilateral ones, should not constitute a means of arbitrary or unjustifiable discrimination or a disguised restriction on international trade.

Source: United Nations 1992b

Talloires Declaration

The Talloires Declaration (Box 3.10) is interesting because it directly relates to the role universities play in setting an example to the community and in the teaching of sustainability to practitioners. This document provides ample opportunity for public health practitioners and colleagues to explore issues of sustainability as these relate to their lives.

The declaration was a direct result of a conference of university chancellors from around the world who met to discuss the role universities can and should take in facilitating sustainability. The original group of signatories has grown over time, with other universities committing to the principles espoused by the original group. Practitioners can use the Declaration as a benchmark against which to measure their own campus and, more importantly, to find ways of becoming actively involved.

Box 3.10 Talloires Declaration

We, therefore, agree to take the following actions:

1) Increase awareness of environmentally sustainable development
    Use every opportunity to raise public, government, industry, foundation, and university awareness by openly addressing the urgent need to move toward an environmentally sustainable future.
2) Create an institutional culture of sustainability
    Encourage all universities to engage in education, research, policy formation, and information exchange on population, environment, and development to move toward global sustainability.

3) Educate for environmentally responsible citizenship
Establish programs to produce expertise in environmental management, sustainable economic development, population, and related fields to ensure that all university graduates are environmentally literate and have the awareness and understanding to be ecologically responsible citizens.

4) Foster environmental literacy for all
Create programs to develop the capability of university faculty to teach environmental literacy to all undergraduate, graduate, and professional practitioners.

5) Practice institutional ecology
Set an example of environmental responsibility by establishing institutional ecology policies and practices of resource conservation, recycling, waste reduction, and environmentally sound operations.

6) Involve all stakeholders
Encourage involvement of government, foundations, and industry in supporting interdisciplinary research, education, policy formation, and information exchange in environmentally sustainable development. Expand work with community and nongovernmental organisations to assist in finding solutions to environmental problems.

7) Collaborate for interdisciplinary approaches
Convene university faculty and administrators with environmental practitioners to develop interdisciplinary approaches to curricula, research initiatives, operations, and outreach activities that support an environmentally sustainable future.

8) Enhance capacity of primary and secondary schools
Establish partnerships with primary and secondary schools to help develop the capacity for interdisciplinary teaching about population, environment, and sustainable development.

9) Broaden service and outreach nationally and internationally
Work with national and international organisations to promote a worldwide university effort toward a sustainable future.

10) Maintain the movement
Establish a Secretariat and a steering committee to continue this momentum, and to inform and support each other's efforts in carrying out this declaration.

Source: University Leaders for a Sustainable Future 1999

Go to http://www.ulsf.org/programs_talloires.html for comprehensive information on Talloires activities.

Now that public health practitioners and colleagues have been grounded in the complex world of sustainability and have shared some of the tools available, we move to consider practitioners becoming directly involved in action for sustainability.

3.5 Holistic frameworks

The Earth Charter

The Earth Summit held in Rio de Janiero led to the creation of several important documents. One direct outcome was a commitment to develop the Earth Charter (Box 3.11), which would facilitate individuals, organisations and governments committing to a sustainable future.

Almost a decade after the Earth Summit recommended that a charter be prepared, the Earth Charter was finally completed. This document is relatively new but is progressively being adopted by more groups, so public health practitioners and others will need to become articulate in discussing the meanings and implications to the health of populations. It is important to recognise not only the content of the charter but also the process by which the charter was developed: a 'process of worldwide consultation and dialogue' (United Nations Educational, Scientific and Cultural Organisation 2001). When we consider the development of the frameworks examined above, the process of development of the Earth Charter seems to indicate an evolutionary process in the development of international frameworks for action on health and sustainability.

> **Box 3.11 Earth Charter Principles**
>
> I. RESPECT AND CARE FOR THE COMMUNITY OF LIFE
> 1. Respect Earth and life in all its diversity.
>   a. Recognise that all beings are interdependent and every form of life has value regardless of its worth to human beings.
>   b. Affirm faith in the inherent dignity of all human beings and in the intellectual, artistic, ethical, and spiritual potential of humanity.
> 2. Care for the community of life with understanding, compassion, and love.

   a. Accept that with the right to own, manage, and use natural resources comes the duty to prevent environmental harm and to protect the rights of people.

   b. Affirm that with increased freedom, knowledge, and power comes increased responsibility to promote the common good.

3. Build democratic societies that are just, participatory, sustainable, and peaceful.

   a. Ensure that communities at all levels guarantee human rights and fundamental freedoms and provide everyone an opportunity to realise his or her full potential.

   b. Promote social and economic justice, enabling all to achieve a secure and meaningful livelihood that is ecologically responsible.

4. Secure Earth's bounty and beauty for present and future generations.

   a. Recognise that the freedom of action of each generation is qualified by the needs of future generations.

   b. Transmit to future generations values, traditions, and institutions that support the long-term flourishing of Earth's human and ecological communities.

In order to fulfill these four broad commitments, it is necessary to:

II. ECOLOGICAL INTEGRITY

1. Protect and restore the integrity of Earth's ecological systems, with special concern for biological diversity and the natural processes that sustain life.

   a. Adopt at all levels sustainable development plans and regulations that make environmental conservation and rehabilitation integral to all development initiatives.

   b. Establish and safeguard viable nature and biosphere reserves, including wild lands and marine areas, to protect Earth's life support systems, maintain biodiversity, and preserve our natural heritage.

   c. Promote the recovery of endangered species and ecosystems.

   d. Control and eradicate non-native or genetically modified organisms harmful to native species and the environment, and prevent introduction of such harmful organisms.

   e. Manage the use of renewable resources such as water, soil, forest products, and marine life in ways that do not exceed rates of regeneration and that protect the health of ecosystems.

f. Manage the extraction and use of non-renewable resources such as minerals and fossil fuels in ways that minimise depletion and cause no serious environmental damage.

2. Prevent harm as the best method of environmental protection and, when knowledge is limited, apply a precautionary approach.

a. Take action to avoid the possibility of serious or irreversible environmental harm even when scientific knowledge is incomplete or inconclusive.

b. Place the burden of proof on those who argue that a proposed activity will not cause significant harm, and make the responsible parties liable for environmental harm.

c. Ensure that decision making addresses the cumulative, long-term, indirect, long distance, and global consequences of human activities.

d. Prevent pollution of any part of the environment and allow no build-up of radioactive, toxic, or other hazardous substances.

e. Avoid military activities damaging to the environment.

3. Adopt patterns of production, consumption, and reproduction that safeguard Earth's regenerative capacities, human rights, and community wellbeing.

a. Reduce, reuse, and recycle the materials used in production and consumption systems, and ensure that residual waste can be assimilated by ecological systems.

b. Act with restraint and efficiency when using energy, and rely increasingly on renewable energy sources such as solar and wind.

c. Promote the development, adoption, and equitable transfer of environmentally sound technologies.

d. Internalise the full environmental and social costs of goods and services in the selling price, and enable consumers to identify products that meet the highest social and environmental standards.

e. Ensure universal access to health care that fosters reproductive health and responsible reproduction.

f. Adopt lifestyles that emphasise the quality of life and material sufficiency in a finite world.

4. Advance the study of ecological sustainability and promote the open exchange and wide application of the knowledge acquired.

a. Support international scientific and technical cooperation on sustainability, with special attention to the needs of developing nations.

b. Recognise and preserve the traditional knowledge and spiritual wisdom in all cultures that contribute to environmental protection and human wellbeing.

c. Ensure that information of vital importance to human health and environmental protection, including genetic information, remains available in the public domain.

III. SOCIAL AND ECONOMIC JUSTICE

1. Eradicate poverty as an ethical, social, and environmental imperative.

    a. Guarantee the right to potable water, clean air, food security, uncontaminated soil, shelter, and safe sanitation, allocating the national and international resources required.

    b. Empower every human being with the education and resources to secure a sustainable livelihood, and provide social security and safety nets for those who are unable to support themselves.

    c. Recognise the ignored, protect the vulnerable, serve those who suffer, and enable them to develop their capacities and to pursue their aspirations.

2. Ensure that economic activities and institutions at all levels promote human development in an equitable and sustainable manner.

    a. Promote the equitable distribution of wealth within nations and among nations.

    b. Enhance the intellectual, financial, technical, and social resources of developing nations, and relieve them of onerous international debt.

    c. Ensure that all trade supports sustainable resource use, environmental protection, and progressive labor standards.

    d. Require multinational corporations and international financial organisations to act transparently in the public good, and hold them accountable for the consequences of their activities.

3. Affirm gender equality and equity as prerequisites to sustainable development and ensure universal access to education, health care, and economic opportunity.

    a. Secure the human rights of women and girls and end all violence against them.

    b. Promote the active participation of women in all aspects of economic, political, civil, social, and cultural life as full and equal partners, decision makers, leaders, and beneficiaries.

    c. Strengthen families and ensure the safety and loving nurture of all family members.

4. Uphold the right of all, without discrimination, to a natural and social environment supportive of human dignity, bodily health, and spiritual wellbeing, with special attention to the rights of indigenous peoples and minorities.

    a. Eliminate discrimination in all its forms, such as that based on race, color, sex, sexual orientation, religion, language, and national, ethnic or social origin.

    b. Affirm the right of indigenous peoples to their spirituality, knowledge, lands and resources and to their related practice of sustainable livelihoods.

    c. Honor and support the young people of our communities, enabling them to fulfill their essential role in creating sustainable societies.

    d. Protect and restore outstanding places of cultural and spiritual significance.

IV. DEMOCRACY, NONVIOLENCE, AND PEACE

1. Strengthen democratic institutions at all levels, and provide transparency and accountability in governance, inclusive participation in decision making, and access to justice.

    a. Uphold the right of everyone to receive clear and timely information on environmental matters and all development plans and activities which are likely to affect them or in which they have an interest.

    b. Support local, regional and global civil society, and promote the meaningful participation of all interested individuals and organisations in decision making.

    c. Protect the rights to freedom of opinion, expression, peaceful assembly, association, and dissent.

    d. Institute effective and efficient access to administrative and independent judicial procedures, including remedies and redress for environmental harm and the threat of such harm.

    e. Eliminate corruption in all public and private institutions.

f. Strengthen local communities, enabling them to care for their environments, and assign environmental responsibilities to the levels of government where they can be carried out most effectively.

2. Integrate into formal education and life-long learning the knowledge, values, and skills needed for a sustainable way of life.

    a. Provide all, especially children and youth, with educational opportunities that empower them to contribute actively to sustainable development.

    b. Promote the contribution of the arts and humanities as well as the sciences in sustainability education.

    c. Enhance the role of the mass media in raising awareness of ecological and social challenges.

    d. Recognise the importance of moral and spiritual education for sustainable living.

3. Treat all living beings with respect and consideration.

    a. Prevent cruelty to animals kept in human societies and protect them from suffering.

    b. Protect wild animals from methods of hunting, trapping, and fishing that cause extreme, prolonged, or avoidable suffering.

    c. Avoid or eliminate to the full extent possible the taking or destruction of non-targeted species.

4. Promote a culture of tolerance, nonviolence, and peace.

    a. Encourage and support mutual understanding, solidarity, and cooperation among all peoples and within and among nations.

    b. Implement comprehensive strategies to prevent violent conflict and use collaborative problem solving to manage and resolve environmental conflicts and other disputes.

    c. Demilitarise national security systems to the level of a non-provocative defense posture, and convert military resources to peaceful purposes, including ecological restoration.

    d. Eliminate nuclear, biological, and toxic weapons and other weapons of mass destruction.

    e. Ensure that the use of orbital and outer space supports environmental protection and peace.

    f. Recognise that peace is the wholeness created by right relationships with oneself, other persons, other cultures, other life, Earth, and the larger whole of which all are a part.

Source: United Nations Educational, Scientific and Cultural Organisation 2001

The Earth Charter can be used to promote responsibility among individuals, businesses and governments to adopt a more sustainable way of living. It can provide clear performance indicators for progress toward a sustainable lifestyle. The Earth Charter has also become an instrument to facilitate a critical and constructive dialogue between stakeholders about issues relating to ecological sustainability.

The charter is being used in organisational mission statements and strategic plans and has become a useful benchmark for businesses that adopt the triple bottom line as a principle of good management.

Endorsement of the Earth Charter by individuals or organisations signifies a commitment to an ecologically sustainable future. Endorsement also means the individual or organisation is willing to take part in a global partnership for change to implement Earth Charter values.

Achieving sustainability will depend ultimately on changes in behaviour and lifestyles, changes that will need to be motivated by a shift in values which are rooted in the cultural and moral precepts on which behaviour is predicated (Morin 1999). The Earth Charter is a purely voluntary document; adoption of its principles requires a real commitment to a sustainable future from the individual or organisation.

Often the meaning of documents such as the Earth Charter become obscured by reinterpretation, and it is the practitioner's responsibility to have a personal position on the meaning and importance of the document so it is possible to engage constructively and critically in the dialogue that follows.

. . . we recognise that for such policies and practices to be effective they will need to take account of the different ways in which people make decisions.

Conclusion

Building on the understanding of different perspectives relating to sustainability and health gained through Chapter 2, this chapter provides an understanding of the overarching frameworks (including strategic, health and environmental frameworks) in which practitioners and policymakers operate. The presentation and discussion of the various frameworks draws attention to the resonances between them, establishing a context conducive to the development of policies and practices to achieve sustainability and health. However, we recognise that for such policies and practices to be effective they will need to take account of the different ways in which people make decisions. Chapter 4 examines the ways in which individuals, communities, specialists, organisational strategists and holistic thinkers develop their viewpoints and deal with the viewpoints of others.

Resources

Amnesty International
http:web.amnesty.org ai.nsf/countries/australia

Earth Charter
http://www.earthcharter.org/

History of Lobby Groups on Persistent Organic Pollutants
http://www.oztoxics.org

Kyoto Protocol on Greenhouse Gases
http://unfccc.int/resource/convkp.html

Montreal Protocol on Substances that Deplete the Ozone Layer
http://www.unep.org/ozone/vienna.shtml

Ottawa Charter for Health Promotion
http://www.who.int/hpr/archive/docs/ottawa.html

Rio Declaration on Environment and Development
http://www.iisd.org/rio+5/agenda/agenda21.htm

Stockholm Convention on Persistent Organic Pollutants
http://www.pops.int/documents/convtext/convtext_en.pdf

Talloires Declaration
http://www.ulsf.org/programs_talloires.html

United Nations
http://www.un.org/Overview

United Nations Declaration of Human Rights
http://www.un.org/Overview/rights.html

World Health Organisation Declaration of Alma Ata
http://www.who.int/hpr/backgroundhp/almaata.htm

References

Baum, F. 2002, *The New Public Health: An Australian perspective*, Oxford University Press, South Melbourne

Brown, A. 2003, *Summary of Presentation at Indigenous Peoples and Socioeconomic Rights Expert Workshop, March 20-21, 2003*, www.cpsu.org.uk/downloads/Health%20issues.pdf [8 February 2004]

Carson, R. 1963, *Silent Spring*, Hamish Hamilton, London

Looney, R. 1999, *New International Economic Order*, material prepared for R.J.B. Jones ed., *Routledge Encyclopedia of International Political Economy* Routledge, London, http://web.nps.navy.mil/~relooney/routledge_15b.htm [8 February 2004]

McMichael, A.J. 1993, *Planetary Overload: Global environmental change and the health of the human species*, Cambridge University Press, New York

—— 2001, *Human Frontiers, Environments, and Disease: Past patterns, uncertain futures*, Cambridge University Press, Cambridge

McMurray, A. 2003, *Community Health and Wellness: A socio-ecological approach*, Mosby, Sydney

Morin, E. 1999, *Seven Complex Lessons in Education for the Future*, UNESCO, Paris

United Nations 1948, *Universal Declaration of Human Rights*, United Nations, http://www.un.org/Overview/rights.html.2003 [15 February 2004]

—— 1992a, *Report to the United Nations Conference on Environment and Development*, United Nations, Rio de Janiero http://habitat.igc.org/agenda21/rio-dec.html [15 February 2004]

—— 1992b, *United Nations Framework Convention on Climate Change (Kyoto Protocol)*, http://unfccc.int/resource/convkp.html [15 February 2004]

United Nations Educational, Scientific and Cultural Organisation 2001, *The Earth Charter Initiative*, http://www.unesco.org/education/esd/english/international/earthch.shtml [15 February 2004]

United Nations Environment Program 1987, *The Montreal Protocol on Substances that Deplete the Ozone Layer*, http://www.unep.org/ozone/pdfs/Montreal-Protocol2000.pdf [15 February 2004]

—— 2001, *The Stockholm Convention on Persistent Organic Pollutants*, http://www.pops.int/documents/convtext/convtext_en.pdf [15 February 2004]

University Leaders for a Sustainable Future 1999, *Talloires Declaration*, http://www.ulsf.org/programs_talloires.html [15 February 2004]

von Weizsäcker, E., Lovins, A.B. and Lovins, L.H. 1998, *Factor Four: Doubling wealth, halving resource use*, Earthscan, London

Werner, D., Sanders, D., Weston, J., Babb, S. and Rodriguez, B. 1997, *Questioning the Solution: The politics of primary health care and child survival*, HealthWrights, Palo Alto, California

World Commission on Environment and Development 1987, *Our Common Future: Report of the World Commission on Environment and Development*, Oxford University Press, Oxford

World Health Organisation 1978, *Declaration of Alma-Ata*, World Health Organisation, Geneva http://www.who.int/hpr/backgroundhp/almaata.htm [15 February 2004]

—— 1979, *Health for All by the Year 2000*, http://who.int/ism/mis/WHO-policy/hfadocs.en.htm [8 February 2004]

World Health Organisation, Health and Welfare Canada and the Canadian Public Health Association 1986, 'Ottawa Charter for Health Promotion', *Canadian Journal of Public Health*, vol. 77, no. 12, pp. 425-30

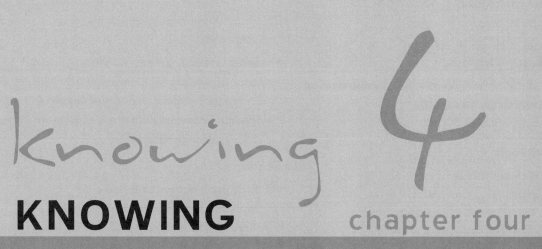

KNOWING

chapter four

Linking the knowledge cultures of sustainability and health

Valerie A. Brown

Summary

We have come to accept that, while the transition to sustainability requires changes in social values and alterations in population behaviour, continuing calls for integration, collaboration, and co-ordination in sustainability decision-making indicate that sustainability requires something more. Changes are needed in the differing and often competing ways we are constructing reality. In this chapter we discuss how we are currently compartmentalising knowledge and how that impedes public health practice in understanding sustainability and health. We explore the extent to which the five sectors whose collaboration is most often listed as essential to sustainability decision-making—individuals, community, specialists, organisational strategists and holistic thinkers—each work in their own knowledge regimes. We find that each sector forges its own internally accepted versions of reality and sets its own almost impermeable boundaries. To achieve the integrated decision-making being called for we offer practitioners in the field of sustainability and health a range of ways to unite these knowledge regimes.

Chapter 4 Knowing

Linking the knowledge cultures of sustainability and health

Valerie A. Brown

Key words

Knowledge cultures, synthesis, sustainability, accessibility, transdisciplinarity, ignorance, power, negotiation, knowledge brokers

Learning outcomes

On conclusion of this chapter the public health practitioner should be able to understand the ways evidence-based practice for sustainability and health involves five constructions of knowledge, and:

- working as an individual practitioner, will develop personal skills in the synthesis of his or her own community, specialist, strategic and holistic knowledge of an issue and develop professional skills in facilitating a synthesis for others;
- working with local knowledge, will have become familiar with ways of supporting the co-ordinated contribution of communities to resolving sustainability and health issues;
- working with specialist knowledge, will have the ability to select and apply frameworks from multidisciplinary and transdisciplinary studies that link contributions from environment and health-related disciplines, and other specialist areas according to the context;
- working with strategic knowledge, will have the capacity to design and take part in political and administrative actions that offer potential solutions to health and environment issues; and

- working with holistic knowledge, will have developed skills in working with community, experts and organisations to develop the potential for a shared focus for complex sustainability issues.

Outline

4.1 Evidence-based public health
4.2 Multiple knowledges
4.3 Strategies for synthesis
4.4 Tools for synthesis

Learning activities

4.1 Assessing the evidence: how do we tell the truth?
4.2 Linking the knowledges: case study of decision-making on persistent organic pollutants
4.3 Using the rules of dialogue: group negotiation exercise
4.4 Who do we involve in linking the knowledges?

Reading

McMichael, A. 2001, *Human Frontiers, Environments and Disease: Past patterns, uncertain futures,* Cambridge University Press, Cambridge, Chapter 1

Soskolne, C.L. and Bertollini, R. 1998, *Global Ecological Integrity and 'Sustainable Development': Cornerstones of public health,* WHO European Centre for Environment and Health, Rome, http://www.euro.who.int/document/gch/ecorep5.pdf

4.1 Evidence-based public health

Public health practice has long accepted the goal of being evidence based: that is, public health practitioners are committed to seeking a sound scientific basis for the decisions they have to make. However, while a scientific basis is certainly a necessary condition for evidence-based practice, we must ask whether it is enough for addressing the complex issues of sustainability and health. In addressing the complexity and uncertainty of sustainability issues they are rightly classified as 'wicked problems' by researchers such as Rittel (1972). Other forms of evidence such as those from affected communities and government agencies become of major importance. Issues of sustainability, like all issues of public health, invoke the precautionary principle, which requires acting or refraining from acting by evaluating the extent of the potential risk. The decision is made on the degree of risk regardless of whether the scientific evidence has been fully determined (Harding 1998). Such a decision involves evidence from sources other than science. It extends to information collected from individuals most at risk, from communities on their capacity to respond, from the sum of the appropriate specialist perspectives, from government policies and their degree of enforcement and from a concerted focus of all of these.

Public health practice has long accepted the goal of being evidence based . . .

Contributors to sustainability decision-making (identified as being key individuals, communities, specialist advisors and governments) currently draw on different sources of evidence in different ways (United States National Research Council 1999). The issue then becomes how to bring together the essential pieces of evidence that each can offer. Local knowledge of local conditions makes unique contributions to the design and implementation of precautionary programs. Scientific findings offer solutions that are practical and can be generalised, the overall goal of all specialised knowledge. An understanding of what is politically and administratively feasible is constructed in organisations such as governments, creating a knowledge base that can be best described as strategic knowledge. Less often identified but just as crucial as the local, scientific and government contributions are the insights of individuals as change agents, and a shared holistic understanding bringing a central focus to the complexity. For some decades now there has been consistent agreement that all these sources of evidence are the key to the transition to sustainability goals (Commission on Sustainable Development 1998; United Nations Conference on Environment and Development

1992; United States National Research Council 1999; World Commission on Environment and Development 1987; World Summit on Sustainable Development 2002).

What is largely ignored is that drawing on each of these different forms of evidence builds up a different construction of reality within each decision-making sector. We know that our knowledge—our interpretation of the ways in which the world works—is socially constructed (Berger & Luckmann 1971). What we each can know for ourselves with any certainty is built through a continuing dialogue between our direct experience and the social rules for knowledge and ignorance in which we are culturally immersed. The classic statement 'Inuit people have 24 words for snow' is but the tip of an iceberg. Local community, specialised, and organisational knowledges are constructed in different social systems with different languages and different interpretations of the same reality.

The groups do not necessarily share values or skills; and neither do they share the same knowledge base. Each of the groups who are contributing to integrated decision-making, individuals, a community, specialists and government, has their own language, set of priorities, sources of evidence and ways of testing it, all adding up to distinctive ways of constructing knowledge (Figure 4.1). Knowledge—'justified true belief about the way the world works'—(Honderich 1995 *Oxford Companion to Philosophy*) is constructed through testing new information and then incorporating it into one's previous mental framework. Reconciling the differences in the knowledge bases is at least as important as differences in values or skills for collaboration, co-operation and co-ordination, and other processes seeking some form of integration.

Holistic knowledge

Two knowledge constructions—individual and holistic—may be considered as bookends to the three more familiar and publicly recognised local, specialised and organisational or strategic knowledges. All construction of knowledge begins with the individual. If it is to last across generations it must eventually be carried forward into social rules through the construction of holistic symbols of 'correct' ideas and 'proper' behaviour. However, in Western cultures the capacity to encapsulate the heart of the matter in a single idea or symbol is so rarely explicitly recognised as a construction of knowledge, that the capacity for holistic thought is often considered to

> *We know that our knowledge—our interpretation of the ways in which the world works—is socially constructed.*

exist only in the artistic community. On the contrary, the ability to identify a holistic focus as a basis for our knowledge is inherently present in any individual or community; and whenever it is achieved, holistic knowledge is widely acclaimed. In many non-Western cultures, such as in Australian indigenous culture, holism is the dominant knowledge form. Aboriginal languages have no separate words for health or for environment; they are both expressed as the single word 'life'. The stories of the dreaming held by indigenous communities provide the means of constructing biophysical and social reality as one (Read 2000). Every member of the group carries the map of the terrain and the rules for social behaviour at the same time.

Holistic knowledge is an equally legitimate construction of knowledge to the other four (individual, local, specialised and organisational) that we are examining here, but since it can be so sharply rejected in rationalist Western thinking it requires rather more explanation. While it may be no more than equally essential than any of the more usually recognised knowledge constructions, that rejection ensures that it is most frequently the missing piece. In attempts to achieve collaborative decisions, sharing different holistic interpretations of the common concern can be the most effective step toward shared understanding. The mutual construction of what it is to belong to a nation or a profession is powerfully formed through the development of holistic icons and symbols: hence we have flags, logos, anthems and role models. Why else would companies seeking wide recognition spend a million dollars on an image such as a Coco-Cola bottle or McDonald's arches?

. . . a holistic focus as a basis for our knowledge is inherently present in any individual or community . . .

There is constant confusion in the application of the ideas of holism and the related ideas of synthesis, integration and co-ordination, not to mention the debates between proponents of hard (technical) and soft (people-based) systems (Midgley 2000) and participation and involvement (Arnstein 1969). These two pairs of concepts are concerned with technical and social perspectives and with forming collaborative relationships, respectively. We are using the term to refer to a construction of reality in the Smuts definition of holism (he invented the term): 'the tendency, as in nature, to form connected wholes' (Smuts 1936).

The language of synthesis can be confusing in a world that has concentrated on analysis. We differentiate them here as relationships between parts and wholes in the construction of knowledge, as follows:

- collaboration: working together cooperatively;

- co-ordination: linking working parts of a system;
- holism: finding the essence or core of the matter, considering the issue more than the sum of its parts;
- holarchy: an inter-related system of equivalent wholes;
- hierarchy: a graded set of diminishing parts;
- integration: putting parts together within the one system or explanatory framework;
- synthesis: putting parts together and generating something different or new; and
- synergy: new ideas, actions or energy generated through the process of synthesis.

Western science tends to define holism as the sum of all the other knowledges . . .

Western science tends to define holism as the sum of all the other knowledges, that is, claiming to know all the information on a topic, making it an impossible and even ridiculous task. Strategists often represent their task as holistic but are usually by definition co-ordinating the stages of implementing a single given value system, working to pre-set goals. Such an enterprise may well be integrative, but is rarely holistic. The concept of sustainability is so differently constructed and defined in each of the knowledge cultures that it is no surprise there is little concerted progress toward its achievement (Figure 4.2).

Individual knowledge

Our own individual knowledge is built from our personal, socially mediated learning experiences of local, specialised and strategic knowledge, as defined above. Consider, for example, the clothes you are wearing. They are your own choice within the limits of your own resources and the limits allowed by your community and your socio-political context. Imagine wearing the gear of the other gender, or the dress of another culture or time and place at this moment. What would be the response of your peers? Your organisation? What clothing (or absence of) would it take for your institution to censure you? What your clothing *is*, empirically, would be described quite differently by a cultural historian, a biochemist, an ethnobotanist, a sociologist, a psychologist, a designer and any three of your friends. The essence of what all that means, the holistic interpretation, might come from just one of those sources, or some combination in which they learn to listen to one another and to you. Box 4.1 contains an example of an individual's understanding of a sustainability theme being introduced into the public sphere.

The writer invokes each of the five different constructions of knowledge as he makes his case for being cautious of genetically modified crops.

Box 4.1 A letter to the editor: being scared of GM

Mr. A. Howe, Editor, *Sunday Herald Sun*, Melbourne

30 December 2002

Re: Scared of GM? An environmental scientist responds to 'GM scare hots up', *Sunday Herald Sun,* 29.12.2002, p. 30

Dear Mr Howe,

Being scared of GM may not be rational but it is reasonable. Here's why.

Humans are still very much taken by their apparent power over nature. The insights of science have heightened both the scope and extent of that power and genetic manipulation represents a quantum leap in both.

Now, science is not itself power. It is the careful attempt to theorise and build insight that stands the tests of repeated experimentation and open criticism over time and varied practice. The creation of theory is the domain of inspiration. Transforming theories into science, however, is the domain of rationality. It involves finding and running experiments that fit into what is already accepted as science and then subjecting the results to repeated criticism. In this effort, science is our most noble creation and so the SHS is to be congratulated for running its news article on poor science teaching in schools (29/12, p. 18).

For all that nobility, science is not and never can be, ultimate truth. It is the most reliable set of interpretations we have at any time and is, by the nature of science, always open to questions about its insights (laws and accumulated details) and methods. We definitely are not in a situation to say we have 'nothing to fear from GM foods'. We can listen when a proponent of GM foods says 'GM ingredients have been on our supermarket shelves for six years without a single scientifically reputable report of any adverse impact on human health'.

As a scientist myself I must have misgivings about how well such a proponent knows the field of writings on the topic and if he does know them, how he is interpreting those writings.

A more important concern with GM foods is one that goes way beyond the direct health implications to humans. It arises from the doubt we must always hold about scientific knowledge and the contexts within which it is applied. These are reasonable concerns but not rational ones; one cannot substantiate them with science because both come from outside science and its apparatus of proof.

> *They arise from our personal and social interpretations of the case.*
>
> *We are sufficiently powerful to suppress nature's attempts to reject us.*
>
> *As a still-living sufferer of an auto-immune disease (Crohn's) I am a living example of that power.*
>
> *We have become ourselves a global or nature-wide influence. This in itself may not be a problem; but we have now established world-spanning systems that make it difficult for nature as a whole to protect us.*
>
> *With only the shallow government assessment structures we currently have to judge what the market presents to us as GM foods, we are determining the future of something whose implications are very broad. And again, while this is not new—indigenous Australians transformed the continent with fire—we are currently wilfully disregarding the importance of these systems to our everyday lives and to the priorities that dictate what they should be. Of course, nature will prevail, but it may do so in ways that are unpredictable to us and we may not like them. Indeed much of nature may not like them either!*
>
> *Yours sincerely,*
>
> *A/Prof. Frank Fisher*
>
> *Director, Graduate School of Environmental Science*
>
> *Monash University*
>
> *Source*: Fisher 2002

Individual, community, specialists, organisational and holistic knowledge

Combining the different knowledges asks in turn for individuals with the capacity to unite these different interpretations of the issues within one cohesive framework.

For these four interpretations of sustainability to work together, a further construction of knowledge is needed. For individuals, community members, specialists and organisational players to work collaboratively toward a shared goal they require a shared holistic construction of that goal, an agreed interpretation of the essential core of each (undoubtedly complex and ambiguous) issue. Holistic knowledge was defined by the philosopher Berlin as 'relating everything to a single, central vision, one system more or less articulate and coherent, related by some central idea or principle' (Berlin & Hardy 1979, p. 3).

All this will still find individual practitioners socially conditioned into dividing what they know into the three boxes of community, specialised, and organisational knowledge. They can be expected to have little experience of holistic knowledge and will be struggling to re-integrate these kinds of knowledge in their thinking and their practice. Their personal knowledge will have been built from each individual's experience, skills, values, culture and learning, and perception styles. Becoming familiar with one's own ways of constructing the four public knowledges and reflecting on one's private knowledge is therefore a prerequisite for the sustainability practitioner. Kuhn (1970) demonstrated how each particular construction of knowledge, which he labelled a knowledge paradigm, develops its own body of content through its own methods of inquiry, tests for truth and frameworks for interpretation. In Figure 4.1 it can be seen that each of the constructions of public knowledge meets all these conditions.

Figure 4.1 Five paradigms of knowledge (after Kuhn 1970)
Modes of construction of knowledge in sustainability decision-making

Dimensions	Individual	Local	Specialised	Strategic	Holistic
Body of content	lived experience	shared experience	scientific disciplines	alliances	metaphors, images
Tools of inquiry	reflection	dialogue	observation	evaluation	imagination
Validation of evidence	self-referenced	memory	measurement	feasibility	recognition
Explanatory framework	identity	cultural expectations	cause and effect, systems design	democratic principles	core knowledge
Role model	*personal hero*	*good neighbour*	*inventor*	*good citizen*	*artist, poet, prophet*

> **Activity 4.1**
> **Assessing the evidence: how do we tell the truth?**
>
> *Aim: to identify the different constructions of knowledge.*
>
> **Materials:** letter to the editor in Box 4.1; the letters to the editor page of your local newspaper; Figure 4.1; groups of five people
>
> **Step 1.** Read the letter to the editor in Box 4.1. Discuss the forms of 'truth' that can be identified in the letter to the editor in Box 4.1. Can you identify the scientific, community, strategic and holistic positions? How are they constructed as truth? What are the forms of evidence on which each is based? What is the letter writer's position? Do you agree with it?
>
> **Step 2.** Follow the same process with the letter to the editor pages from different newspapers. Can you identify which sets of evidence you feel most comfortable with? Which in your opinion puts the best case? Or do you need them all?
>
> **Step 3.** As a group, what are your conclusions about the use of the various knowledges in presenting an argument for action on an issue?

Case study of knowledge of atmospheric lead

Lead levels in air can be taken as an example. Atmospheric lead is entirely a product of human industrial activity, so there is no room to doubt that health risks from lead are socially generated. The lifestyles and occupational options of those exposed to risk determine the extent of the resulting physiological damage and only those whose lived experience encompasses these can give a valid experiential account (individual and local knowledge). Biochemical tests determine the sources of lead and the dose; technical investigation will lead to the methods of reducing the emissions; economists will estimate the costs and benefits of different permissible limits; clinical specialists examine the extent of the physiological damage (multidisciplinary specialist knowledge). The feasibility of possible control measures requires a prior understanding and assessment of the political and administrative conditions needed to negotiate effective strategies between competing interests (strategic knowledge); the decision to remove lead from petrol in Australia was finally made 30 years after the original diagnosis of physiological harm from more than 20 micrograms of lead per litre of blood.

The final step rested on linking all the forms of evidence listed above in a cohesive, holistic explanatory framework accessible by all concerned (Berry et al. 1994). The decisions had to be made by a senior research committee of individuals whose personal knowledge had taken some time to adapt to the multiple knowledge perspective (Greene 2001). The five knowledges existing in isolation can and do lead to fragmentation and conflict as to who owns the 'truth'. Becoming linked to each other in a co-operative network at least allows the five sets of evidence to enrich one another, and at best provides the conditions for a new synthesis and a new synergy to allow new ways of addressing the issue to emerge.

The capacity to bring together these constructions of knowledge is still in its infancy. Reactions to the new form of public health challenge presented by the transition to sustainability are fragmented and polarised, with different solutions being advocated by often competing power structures. It is usual to find one issue (such as clean water) being dealt with simultaneously and separately in the environment and health sections of the same organisation with little contact and even hostility between the two (Brown et al. 2001). Further, the same division occurs routinely in education, policy, law and government, with little or no contact between the understanding of environment and of health that underlie their practice, and often with little contact with any other disciplines.

The capacity to bring together these constructions of knowledge is still in its infancy.

Divided knowledges in public health

None of this is in principle new to public health; the same division between specialist forms of knowledge occurs in the field between engineering and educational solutions to water pollution, for example. In sustainability issues the effect is magnified, partly because two well-developed professional fields are claiming the same territory (Brown et al. 2001), partly because sustainability issues are asking for a shift in the actual construction of knowledge from certainty to accepting ambiguity, and partly because sustainability necessarily involves the gamut of evidence from each of the five knowledges (Figure 4.2).

Experts and governments, industry and the public are trying separately and together—but often failing—to deal with the seriousness of this situation. The issues are most often approached as competing priorities between fresh water supplies, energy resources, employment levels, ecological integrity and the needs of the human population (World Bank 2002). Responses are channelled through the separate social, economic and ecological decision-making systems found in government, industry and community service organisations. Chapter 2 provides an overview of

Figure 4.2 Knowledge cultures within Western decision-making systems

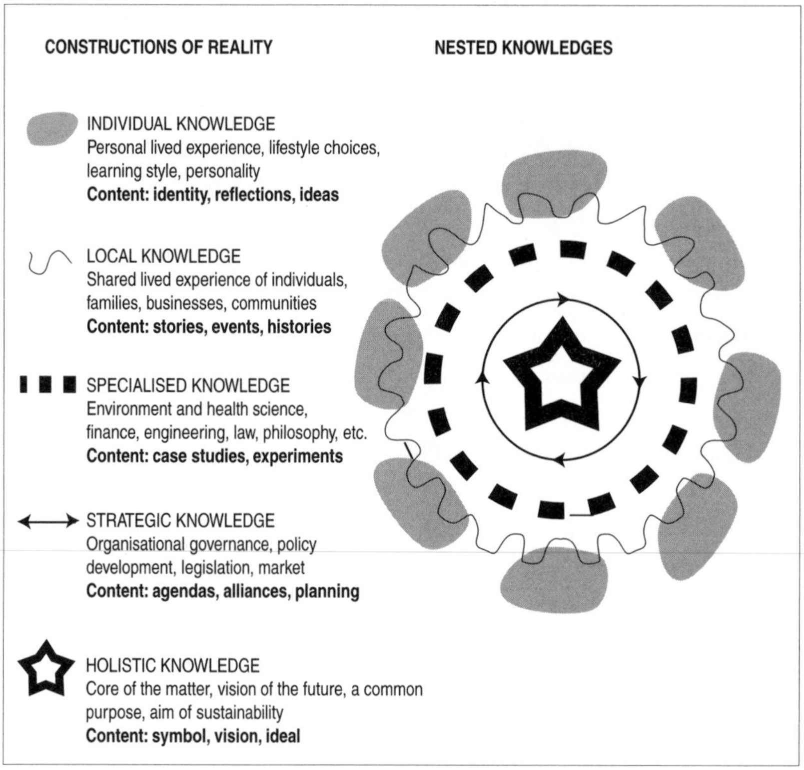

CONSTRUCTIONS OF REALITY

NESTED KNOWLEDGES

INDIVIDUAL KNOWLEDGE
Personal lived experience, lifestyle choices,
learning style, personality
Content: identity, reflections, ideas

LOCAL KNOWLEDGE
Shared lived experience of individuals,
families, businesses, communities
Content: stories, events, histories

SPECIALISED KNOWLEDGE
Environment and health science,
finance, engineering, law, philosophy, etc.
Content: case studies, experiments

STRATEGIC KNOWLEDGE
Organisational governance, policy
development, legislation, market
Content: agendas, alliances, planning

HOLISTIC KNOWLEDGE
Core of the matter, vision of the future, a common
purpose, aim of sustainability
Content: symbol, vision, ideal

strategies for sustainability and health generated from more than a dozen deeply held value positions along the human-environment continuum, each with merit but each pointing in a different direction.

It is no wonder review bodies consistently end their work with calls for collaborative, integrative, holistic, co-ordinating, co-operative, coherent, whole-of-government, whole-of-community decision-making, hoping to bring values, issues and actions into some form of commonly shared framework. But the fragmentation persists and the distinctions between the elements and forms of synthesis are rarely made clear. Collaborative and co-operative refer to interpersonal working relationships, as discussed in the chapters on 'acting' and 'learning'; co-ordination refers to the ways in which parts are related to one another in a logistics exercise, as in the co-ordination of a multidisciplinary taskforce.

The literature on sustainability repeatedly puts the case that it is overall structural change in organisational forms, in the construction of knowledge and in the human/environment relationship respectively, that is so badly needed. As discussed, this represents the full set of skills, knowledge and attitude that underlies all significant learning and change. The rest of this chapter examines how the sustainability transition can address these structural changes through the following changes in the construction of knowledge:

- developing skills in synthesis as well as existing skills of analysis;
- granting equal respect to individual, community, specialist, strategic and holistic knowledges; and
- seeking modes of collaboration and co-operation that allow for networking between knowledges.

The literature on sustainability repeatedly puts the case that it is overall structural change in organisational forms . . .

4.2 Multiple knowledges

About knowledge

Since the middle of the 20th century it has been widely accepted that our knowledge—that is, our understanding of how the world works—is not stored in libraries or issued as edicts from some expert source. Knowledge is socially constructed in the human head. Berger and Luckmann's (1971) *The Social Construction of Reality* called attention to the ways in which powerful ideas such as health, environment, time, sustainability and progress are constructed through social interaction. For example, during the peak influence of the biophysical sciences, health was regarded primarily as physical competence until its re-definition to 'optimum physical, mental and social wellbeing' in the constitution of the World Health Organisation, restated in the *Declaration of Alma-Ata* in 1978 on Primary Health Care. Meanwhile, health in Bali remains a matter of fitting seamlessly into traditional society and ill-health is treated as a social breakdown. In Aboriginal and Torres Strait languages health can only be translated as compatibility between life and land. Ill-health in an indigenous community calls for a diagnosis of how the land is failing to be protected and maintained (Mills 2000).

The Western cultural approach to knowledge places multiple hurdles in the way of redressing the fragmentation and polarisation of issues and solutions. Rules of analysis and hierarchical structure have become so firmly established that they remain the default option when facing pressures to change. Treating complex issues as open-ended and interconnected systems rather than as stratified and predetermined hierarchies requires a re-organisation of our patterns of decision-making. It also asks for reconsideration of our allocation of knowledge and ignorance and brings a much-needed respect for ambiguity and uncertainty to the black-and-white reasoning of right and wrong.

About ignorance

The Western cultural approach to knowledge places multiple hurdles in the way of redressing the fragmentation and polarisation of issues and solutions.

We spend much time in our education systems considering the construction of knowledge, but much less on the parallel construction of ignorance. Smithson (1989) identifies the ways in which the assignment of ignorance is a crucial step in the constructions of knowledge, a step by which we define what it is proper to know. In his taxonomy of ignorance he distinguishes between attributing ignorance to error or to irrelevance. Error may in turn be assigned to distortion or to incompleteness—familiar accusations from the specialised knowledge paradigm is that community knowledge is incomplete, since it refers only to the one case; that strategic knowledge is by definition a distortion because it seeks not to confirm but to alter reality; and that holistic knowledge is irrelevant since its methods of inquiry deal with complexity and ambiguity. On the other hand, communities can and do reject specialist knowledge as an incomplete portrayal of their lived experience, and strategic knowledge because it disturbs established ways of organising local reality.

A case in point is the frequent use of the three overlapping circle diagram of society, economy and environment to represent the essential elements of sustainability initiated by Hancock (1992), who has replaced it by the mandala in Figure 1.1. Isolating each of the three represents the way society is structured today, where separation has become part of the problem. By distinguishing them as separate systems they continue to fit with fragmented rather than collaborative frameworks for knowledge; in any organisation they will be competing with each other for resources, power and priority of action. The three circle approach assumes that the public's health can be summed up by the titles of the three research and resource sectors. The framework has worked well as an equity model in public health, where it promotes the assumption that affirmative action is needed to balance the currently unbalanced sectors.

We are seeking not one model as inherently better than another, since all have their strengths and weaknesses. Instead we look for frameworks that will allow for the contribution of multiple knowledges, movement forward into the uncertain or the ambiguous, and action-oriented links between progress and the knowledges. A change in thinking has transmuted the five strategies of sustainable development, drawn from *Our Common Future* (World Commission on Environment and Development 1987) and confirmed at the Rio Conference into the more synthesis-oriented 'sustainability'. Sustainable development offered to reunite the sustainability of ecosystems on one hand and economic development on the other. The two had been moving into opposition since the beginning of the industrial revolution. While the principles of sustainable development make up a comprehensive set, that set has seldom been implemented as a whole (Dovers 2001; MacDonald 1998). The original principles are also increasingly out-of-date: the economic and environmental gap between rich and poor is widening in every country so equity cannot be 'maintained' or even recovered (it is doubtful if it was ever realised). It needs to be the goal of affirmative action (World Resources Institute et al. 1996). Environmental equity between generations is now no longer possible given the estimated 300 to 500 years needed to halt (much less reverse) global warming (McMichael 2001). The best we can hope for is a new direction toward an as yet undetermined form of stability of human life-support systems.

We are seeking not one model as inherently better than another, since all have their strengths and weaknesses.

> ## Activity 4.2.
> ### Linking the knowledges: case study of decision-making on persistent organic pollutants (POPS)
> http://www.allenandunwin.com/sustainhealth

Since global ecological integrity has been breached and has now become identified as disintegrity (Pimental et al. 1998; Soskolne & Bertollini 1999), sustainable development goals need to be restated. Although begun with the best of intentions, the strategy of triple bottom line accounting (that is, valuing social and ecological costs as well as financial) has backfired, leading to stronger competition and fragmentation rather than collaboration. Even the concept of ecosystems services (valuing ecological systems for the services they provide), while valuable in bringing the question of natural resource use into the mainstream, avoids the point at issue. Social, economic and ecological factors are interdependent and cumulative in their effects, and complexity requires a far more sophisticated approach (Brown et al. 2001) (Figure 1.1).

The precautionary principle of acting beforehand to prevent risk and not acting at all where the risk from the action is too great appears to have stood the test of time. From this commonsense base a range of strategies and tools is emerging to address the integrity and the resilience of places, people and products. This interpretation has been symbolised by a move to using 'sustainability' rather than 'sustainable development' in policy documents, community programs and scientific literature (Australian Institute of Environmental Health 2003; IndoPacific Conference on Environment and Health 2002). In brief, this shift in concepts encapsulates the move from an analytical approach with distinct performance indicators to a more holistic framework with open-ended outcomes (a list of definitions and applications can be found in Box 1.4). An examination of the list identifies some of the key aspects of the new direction: first there are calls to bring together as a unit the activities of divided social, economic and environmental sectors; then follow equally consistent calls to combine community, specialised and organisational systems/sectors (industry and government) in holistic decision-making.

The precautionary principle of acting beforehand to prevent risk and not acting at all where the risk from the action is too great appears to have stood the test of time.

A change in the way we think about these issues is infiltrating every avenue of action for sustainability. Box 4.2 contains messages from each of the seven keynote speakers at the IndoPacific Conference on Environment and Health (2002); whether from the fields of systems thinking (Costanza), indigenous rights (O'Donoghue), social futures (Rapport), environmental epidemiology (McMichael), ecology (Waltner-Toews), public administration (Birch) or social ecology (Brown), their interpretation of sustainability is an integrative one (IndoPacific Conference on Environment and Health 2002). Each speaker found a different way to express the need to search for the essence of the issues—an essence that everyone could share whether presented as a systems diagram, an ethic, an administrative nexus, equity, policy, an overarching story, collaboration, trust or knowledge.

Box 4.2 Sustainability in action

Acting for sustainability means:

'Measuring, monitoring and valuing an essential relationship' (Robert Costanza)

'Recognising, respecting and learning from first people's care for country' (Loitja O'Donoghue)

'Integrating ministries, interlocking statistics and allowing inter-dependent sovereignties' (David Rapport)

'Addressing the different effects of global disintegrity on the poor and weak versus the rich and powerful' (Tony McMichael)

'Designing a great collective narrative' (David Waltner-Toews)

'Community-corporate trust' (David Birch)

'Reunion of the divided knowledge cultures' (Valerie A. Brown)

Source: All quotations are from keynote addresses at the IndoPacific Conference on Environment and Health 2002

The situation confirms Toulmin's (1977) interpretation of the construction of knowledge as a pendulum. Throughout history the dominant construction of knowledge has swung between cultures of analysis and cultures of synthesis. Eras of grand synthesis in the Western cultural tradition include Greek civilisation, the Renaissance and now, potentially, our present era in trying to achieve sustainability. After each major synthesis, a flood of analysis of the new ideas follows ever more refined pathways until eventually the collected information is so detailed that it (a) no longer makes collective sense and (b) no longer answers the major questions of the day. The pendulum has by then reached the end of its swing and seeks a new energy, a fresh synthesis that offers major answers to the dilemma. That synthesis generates new questions, and streams of analysis follow. In Kuhnian terms, analytical scientific discoveries have increasingly become a dominant paradigm or ruling framework since the last era of synthesis in the Renaissance (Kuhn 1970).

The synthesis discussed here is the search for methods of reconnection of the different constructions of reality by individuals, communities, specialists, governments and holists with respect to sustainability and health (Figures 4.1, 4.2). Only specialised knowledge has been recognised as a legitimate basis for decision-making for the 400 years of the industrial revolution (Toulmin 1977). Local community knowledge has long been dismissed as unreliable and trivial; the socio-political knowledge of organisational functioning as biased and self-serving; and holistic knowledge, identifying the essence of a matter, as probably impossible. On the other hand all these other constructions of knowledge have increasingly turned away from science, rejecting its contributions to their own form of knowledge as unrealistic, unrelated and offering a false promise of certainty. The gaps seem to grow wider, not narrower.

In the literature on professional knowledge there is little recognition of the importance of incorporating all five knowledges, and even less on the inherent relationship between the knowledges and their contributions to professional decision-making (Harding 1998). Yet logically it is essential for a profession's informed practice to include reflection on its own decision-making processes. Figure 4.2 summarises the relationships between the knowledges as nested knowledges, each building on the other. The symbols used to represent the boundaries reflect their origins. Individual knowledge is the almost invisible context or matrix for all other knowledge, since all knowledge is generated through human thought. However, individual knowledge is also the basis for all other constructions of knowledge. Individuals' privately generated knowledge becomes publicly shared through local social and place-based experiences that represent the local knowledge of each community. Communities' local knowledge taken together is of great variety, joined in the construction of a regional or national reality (hence the continuous wavy line). The source of the uniting thread may be place-, interest- or event-based. Since we are dealing with global ecological integrity and sustainability, the emphasis is on place-based community.

In the literature on professional knowledge there is little recognition of the importance of incorporating all five knowledges . . .

The collected experience of local knowledge, whether through individual interviews, observations of events or verbal history case studies, provides the source of data for each of the myriad perspectives of the research disciplines, represented in the diagram as distinct, unconnected packets of knowledge (the ring of boxes). In turn, the advice and the collected knowledge of those specialist disciplines inform the planning and organising capacity of administrations and governments. Scientists puzzle over why their advice is not taken by government (Costanza & Jorgensen 2002). One explanation is that organisational decision-making adds to that evidence from a very different source. The strategic reality of organisations is constructed through interpretation of the rules by which humans manage their worlds. Prime examples of how strategic knowledge has informed decision-making exist through the centuries in the Chinese *Art of Strategy*, the *Annals* of Confucius, Macchiavelli's *The Prince* and even the television series *Yes Minister*. Strategic knowledge has a given direction and a systemic relationship between the parts (the circle of arrows). The core of the knowledges, when they are explicitly connected at all, is some common purpose or shared perspective, represented as a guiding star. Throughout the present discussion the holistic core is assumed to be the goal of sustainability.

4.3 Strategies for synthesis

Collaborative action for sustainability requires not only goodwill between members but for all five constructions of knowledge to be linked together toward some concerted purpose. Individuals, communities, specialists and government agencies are all given to complaining somewhat bitterly of their exclusion from each other's decision-making, yet all have areas of operation in which they are legitimately the predominant decision-makers. Each, as we have discussed above, requires the others. We hear a great deal about the merit of bringing all five to the negotiating table and about empowering these partners equally, but little mention is made of the need to establish the conditions for the negotiations necessary for equal respect for their various distinctive constructions of knowledge. After all, negotiation, power and respect are intertwined.

To pursue these ideas further we need to go to the specialist literature. As Foucault (1970) identifies, until the end of the industrial revolution access to knowledge was power; in the globalised information era, access to the construction of knowledge is power; Foucault is as always equating knowledge with power: here he is comparing the quantity of knowledge held and the degree of access to it with the capacity to control its construction. The essential elements of that construction have been outlined in Figure 4.1 from a Kuhnian perspective. In the era of the industrial revolution, access to power meant gaining access to the use of technology and to professional skills, access strongly guarded by those controlling university entrance, program funding and peer review. In the information era, even the most specialised information and skills are open to everyone in cyberspace; access is limited only by the technological capacity of marginalised groups and nations. The result is that the knowledge of even the most advanced specialism is accessible, and access to its construction is now being challenged.

Two examples may be enough. The adage 'If I'm in a plane I want to be flown by a pilot who learned to fly in a proper training school' is being overtaken by on-line programs that can give more practice flying hours than any training school can afford. A national review of the surgical profession brought strong criticisms over the tight control by surgeons over entry to their qualification, limiting the workforce and resisting change (*The Australian* 2003). In the information era, the basis of those skills and the technologies is freely available outside previously heavily restricted formal sources. They

Collaborative action for sustainability requires not only goodwill between members but for all five constructions of knowledge to be linked together . . .

149

can be found on the Internet, in private institutions, in distance courses and through workplace education programs. There is still an influence of time and money on access to the information, but these are fast reducing. The key issue, as any website will reveal, is to evaluate the information contributed from research, professional, community and political perspectives. The issues arise from the incorporation of that information into knowledge.

In the information era, the basis of those skills and the technologies is freely available outside previously heavily restricted formal sources.

Bohm (1996) argues that all significant new knowledge comes through the generation of ambiguity and the recognition of paradox in the discussions between different interpretations of events. Not unreasonably, he suggests that knowledge exchanges between people who share the same construction of reality may expand their existing understanding, but are unlikely to generate new knowledge. This is reflected in the place-based decision-making (D4P4) framework in Chapter 1 (that is, the learning spiral of developing principles, describing people and place, designing potential and doing and evaluating practice). In Figure 1.2 it is assumed that the principles are already developed as sustainability principles. The description of people and place is based in all five of the knowledges. Generating design ideas of future potential requires shifts of thought linking the multiple knowledges. The Institute for Educational Studies has translated Bohm's ideas into a set of principles of dialogue (Box 4.3) which maximises the exploration of paradox in each of these dimensions (Gang 2000).

Box 4.3 Rules for dialogue in a multiple knowledge learning community

1. Remember that everyone (facilitators, general community, expert advisors and agency representatives) is an equal participant.
2. Take time to 'think and reflect' before responding to another's comments.
3. Make good use of all the tools for a learning community: sites for informal discussion, common themes, participants' passionate interests, technical help.
4. Use the dialogue creatively: introduce diagrams, pictures, sketches, photos, key points, summaries, and fresh ideas, without the need for a finished form. That can come later.
5. Treat the dialogue as a different medium of exchange, one that allows the exploration of issues and ideas in a non-adversarial manner.
6. Respect the rules of dialogue (for more detail see Bohm 1996, p.84).

Throughout the dialogue

1. Commit yourself to the process.
2. Listen and speak without judgment.
3. Identify your own and others' beliefs and assumptions.
4. Acknowledge the other speaker and their ideas.
5. Respect other speakers and value their opinions.
6. Balance inquiry and advocacy.
7. Relax your need for any particular outcome.
8. Listen to yourself and speak when moved.
9. Take it easy—go with the flow—enjoy.

Source: Gang 2000

Activity 4.3.
Using the rules of dialogue: group negotiation exercise
http://www.allenandunwin.com/sustainhealth

So far we have been discussing knowledge as 'in the head', but there comes a time when knowledge is translated into action: this is decision-making time, whether the decision is to act or not to act. The buffeting of real life events, the different value positions encased in the different knowledges, the perceived relevance of one knowledge over another are all matters that can restrict capacities for synthesis. The use of dialogue can generate the elements of a synthesis under conditions known to sponsor creativity, that is, security and trust. Trust is generated by confidence in the recognition that each contribution will be respected and valued. Security can be generated for the practice of synthesis, as it is for community or professional knowledge, by sharing a mutually generated framework that gives equal weight to all positions. There are many candidates for such a framework, from adaptive management and complex adaptive systems to the intuitive humanity of many spiritual systems. Here we are addressing the capacity for sustainability and health practitioners to use synthesis in their work. For that reason we have chosen the D4P4 decision-making framework, linking the construction of knowledge to experiential learning (Chapter 1) as a shared pathway to synthesis.

Different realities

Consider how sustainability strategies would be interpreted by the various stakeholders in the same river catchment by: a farmer struggling to make a living; a research hydrologist; the council's environmental health officer checking pollution; the estate agent supplying housing estates to people escaping from the city; and the regional development association, with the integrated catchment management committee, trying to guarantee a sustainable future. In one study of such a catchment eight farmers, environmental scientists and extension workers (who could be equated with local, specialist and strategic knowledge respectively) were taken in turn to three sections of a degraded water catchment and asked to describe what they saw. Discourse analysis of their replies found the three groups had identified different issues and their responses formed quite different verbal patterns (Ross et al. 1993).

There are many similar devices that can be used to identify the different realities in a way that allows all the players to hear each other.

There are many similar devices that can be used to identify the different realities in a way that allows all the players to hear each other. The Ross et al. study was based on the personal construct theory of George Kelly (Bannister & Francella 1993); but other effective processes include 'participatory rapid appraisal', pattern languages, and negotiation frameworks such as the Harvard Negotiating Process (Fisher & Ury 1987).

4.4 Tools for synthesis

Whole-of-community action

The community-based action web (Figure 4.3) is an integrative tool for whole-of-community-action developed through a year-long knowledge co-ordination process. This tool was the product of a workshop designed explicitly to bring all the knowledges together. The basis for the initiative was that the primary impact and management of any sustainability and health issue is at the community scale. The design and contents of that workshop drew on national policies and strategies already in place, including:

- principles of the National Environmental Health Strategy
  www.health.gov.au/pubhlth/publicat/document/envstrat.pdf;
- study of community perceptions of environmental health risk
  www.health.gov.au/pubhlth/publicat/document/metadata/envrisk.htm;
- study of environment and health professionals' perceptions of environmental health priorities (Cruickshank 2001);

Figure 4.3 Web of community-based action for sustainability and health

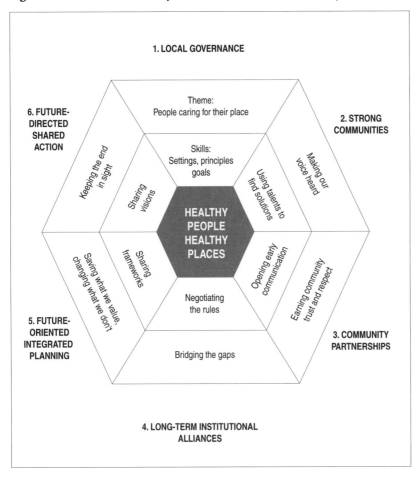

The basis for the initiative was that the primary impact and management of any sustainability and health issue is at the community scale.

Source: Nicholson et al. 2001

- guidelines for community-based environmental health action established through nationwide consultation expressly for the project: *Grass Roots and Common Ground www.uws.edu/research/rimc/cehaps*; and
- 30 public health practitioners at a writing workshop.

The web in Figure 4.3 and the resource book *Common Ground and Common Sense* from which it is drawn have a range of features designed to support synthesis and integration rather than analysis and compartmentalisation (Nicholson et al. 2001). The language used throughout the resource book was a shared use of language generated at the workshop and was edited by participants from all five of the knowledge bases. The elements of community-based action were also generated at the workshop using an open learning technique, which makes an open space for participants to spontaneously generate key issues and concerns and convene a group of colleagues to expand on them, using the rules of dialogue (Bainbridge 2002).

The approach to the generation of knowledge used in the action web process assumes that knowledge is emergent, not fixed (as in a formal workshop where prepared papers are read). It assumes that every participant has something of value to contribute to the generation of the new knowledge, rather than only a few leading specialists. The elements were expanded in terms of each of the knowledge cultures, with a strategic direction, a holistic focus and a method of inquiry for each. Finally, the web itself forms a whole from which no segment can be removed without impairing the action. The form of a web emphasises the point that the full set of strategic elements must be employed for any action to be effective. The relationship between each community and whole-of-community action is represented as a suite of negotiations in Figure 4.3 between the whole system of governance of a place (1.); between members of each community in that place (2.); between the set of local communities (3.); between the community and related organisations (4.); establishing a collaborative strategy for all the organisations together (5.); and committing to a long-term shared action on sustainability and health (6.).

Networking the knowledges

The process of making connections among the knowledges, generating synergies, is demonstrated in a regional change management strategy.

The process of making connections among the knowledges, generating synergies, is demonstrated in a regional change management strategy. The project originated in the planning department of a small coastal town in the Shoalhaven area of New South Wales (Brown et al. 1998). The goal was to develop a structure plan incorporating a community-preferred future that was both environmentally and socially sustainable. A change strategy was designed to redirect conflict within and between all five constructions of knowledge towards constructive collaboration and a shared purpose. At the beginning of an 18-month process, community groups supporting conservation and those supporting development were locked in traditional confrontation, arguing over incompatible specialised advice. Strategic frameworks differed between the political directions of councillors and the administrative directions of council. In addition, council staff seeking to manage change had to report to more than 25 state agencies, each with its own specialised strategic plan. Holistic direction was conspicuously lacking.

To address this situation an integrative, open learning process was designed to give full weight to each of the constructions of knowledge, incorporating groups from each on equal terms. Included in the process was a set of translation and negotiating processes and the D4P4 knowledge-into-action framework outlined in Chapter 1. A sub-district of Shoalhaven was able to achieve the following outcomes from the synthesis:

- developing shared principles: agree on a development plan that met the shared goals of farmers, conservationists and estate agents;
- describing people and place: argue constructively and successfully that a national highway scheduled to be constructed through the centre of their town should become a bypass;
- designing for potential: agree on a structural plan that determined the long-term future of the area, with 12 formal objections to the plan instead of the usual 200 to 300; and
- doing and reviewing practice: identify the indicators that would allow all parties (residents, outside experts, councillors and council staff) to monitor progress to their agreed future, and volunteer to collect the relevant data.

Activity 4.4
Who do we involve in linking the knowledges?
A stakeholder analysis

Aim: to determine who are the decision-makers in this place, and what you need to know from them (and they from you).

Time: could be three hours or three days, depending on the program.

Step 1. Take the issue you identified in Activity 4.3, in which you collected information and prepared a briefing paper. In this exercise you are setting up an action group to develop a forward program of work for the next 10 years. Identify who in your own community would be the members of the multi-skilled team representing all the interests. There are two challenges built in from the start:

- breaking down the normal loyalties in specialisations, professions, government agencies and community groups; and
- ensuring all the interests are properly represented.

Step 2. The challenge is to harness the interested parties in the project for collaborative, rather than conflicting, ends. Various interest groups provide information on and are capable of influencing the outcome of the project or process. If they are closely concerned with the issues for the project, then they must also be part of its resolution. While the number of such interests will be wide, their categories are predictable. There will be key players from policymakers, experts on facets of the physical and social environment, community agencies, influential individuals and the professions and trades that serve the area of emergency risk management. A stakeholder analysis as outlined below can be used to identify the main players of the significant interest groups.

The range of stakeholders can be readily identified within a number of societal dimensions. Consider the following list and any stakeholders you would add to the list.

Typical stakeholders in a sustainability issue

Dimension	Examples of stakeholders
Individuals	membership, age groups, socio-economic levels, ethnic groups, homeowners, underclasses
Community	workers, parents, residents, unemployed, church, industry management
Specialists	pollution control, urban planners, health surveyors, recreation officers, inhabitants
Strategy	prime minister, state premier, local councils, government and non-government agencies;
Services	emergency service providers, nurses, doctors, teachers, police, lawyers, welfare

Step 3. Check the list: have you included all the financial and political backers of the project or process; all the experts on technical matters; representatives of community and emergency service and regulatory authorities; consumers of services (both people 'at risk' and community leaders); local elected representatives; and representatives at officer level from local, state and/or federal governments?

Step 4. Use the D4P4 place-based decision-making framework to prepare an action plan that ensures there will be dialogue between the stakeholders at each stage.

Conclusion

Throughout this chapter we have put the case that each of the five constructions of knowledge involved in sustainability and health has its own form of valid and reliable evidence, its own conditions for synthesis and its own conditions for self-determination (Figure 4.2). In reviewing strategies and tools for their synthesis we have noted that each knowledge has its own internal mode of synthesis. Local knowledge can be collected as whole-of-community knowledge. Specialist knowledge uses multidisciplinary and transdisciplinary frameworks to link the separate disciplines. Organisational knowledge employs strategic thinking to harness political and administrative realities to potential solutions.

We have noted that the other two knowledges are inherently synthesising in co-ordination of evidence and compared them to bookends that link the other three. Holistic knowledge interprets any issue as an interconnected system greater than the sum of its parts, offering the synergy needed for the move to sustainability. Individual knowledge, innately constructed by each person from his or her lived experience of the interpretation of the other four, provides the vehicle for holistic interpretation. Multiple-knowledge synthesis for sustainability requires significant institutional and personal change, explored further in the following chapters.

The issue remaining is how to recreate this synthesis as a mainstream process for the global community facing long-term change in the transition to sustainability.

Like all extremes, the situation is generating its own antidote. Times of crisis and extreme pressure have regularly forced people to find ways in which the knowledges can become accessible to each other, their champions open to collaboration and their boundaries semi-permeable. London ridding itself of the yellow smogs of the 19th century and first half of the 20th century; New York pulling together as a city after the twin towers bombing; and the collaborative response of experts, governments and individuals around the globe and among nations to the epidemic of severe acute respiratory syndrome were each outcomes of combining strong local commitment to action, multidisciplinary specialised advice, and negotiation between different governance agencies, the driving force being the strong common purpose. Within each small community we find the same set of responses allowing rehabilitation after disasters such as fire or flood. The issue remaining is how to recreate this synthesis as a mainstream process for the global community facing long-term change in the transition to sustainability.

The two constructions of knowledge that offer the key to shared interpretations of reality, linking community, specialist and strategic knowledge, have been identified above as the individual and holistic constructions of knowledge. These offer links between the other three in a nested knowledge synthesis for the construction of reality (Figure 4.2) and as the inter-knowledge translation elements in a networked knowledge system (Figure 4.3).

Public health practitioners and colleagues will need personal access to integrative frameworks that allow them to link environment and health. They will need skills in exploring the core or essence of an issue. They will need to identify a community of fellow-practitioners in sustainability and health. In addition to these, they are left with three principal choices in knowledge management if they wish to contribute to a long-term partnership between sustainability and health:

Public health practitioners and colleagues will need personal access to integrative frameworks that allow them to link environment and health.

1. As specialists, maintaining their traditional population-based role of addressing the issues through epidemiology, case study examples and investigative skills;

2. As strategists, acting as multidisciplinary knowledge brokers linking the different specialist collections of knowledge in strategic ways that can be used by other professionals, the community and the politicians; or

3. As holists with a primary interest in developing an underlying coherent system in which all the knowledge sectors can work coherently within and between their own areas of interest.

For the specialist, generalist and holistic public health practitioner, you are joining an increasing company of practitioners from a range of fields who are working in between and around rather than within the disparate knowledge cultures. Depending on where you are working you will be called change agents as individuals, knowledge brokers within the disciplines, boundary spanners between organisations, and a polymath if you work between them all . . . and perhaps, as the skills in shared knowing develop, you may be called a synthesist.

References

The Australian 2003, 'Surgeons restrict entry', Sydney, 8 February, p. 3

Arnstein, S.R. 1969, 'A Ladder of Citizen Participation', *Journal of the American Institute of Planners*, vol. 35, no. 1, pp. 216-24

Australian Institute of Environmental Health 2003, *Journal Special Issues A and B: Sustainability in Environmental Health,* vol. 3, nos 1 and 2, Australian Institute of Environmental Health, Sydney

Bainbridge, B. 2002, *Open Space Institute Newsletter*, Open Space Institute, Adelaide, June

Bannister, D. and Francella, F. 1993, *Inquiring Man: The psychology of personal constructs,* 3rd edn, Routledge, London

Berger, P.L. and Luckmann, T. 1971, *The Social Construction of Reality: A treatise in the sociology of knowledge*, Penguin, Harmondsworth

Berlin, I. and Hardy, H. 1979, *Against the Current: Essays in the history of ideas*, Hogarth Press, London

Berry, M., Garrard, J. and Greene, D. 1994, *Reducing Lead Exposure in Australia. Volume 1: An assessment of impacts, final report. Volume 2: Technical appendices risk assessment and analysis of economic, social and environmental impacts*, National Health and Medical Research Council, Canberra

Bohm, D. 1996, *On Dialogue*, Routledge, London

Brown, V.A., Griffith, R. and Ohlin, J. 1998, 'A Great Place to Live with a Few Things to Fix: Sustainable health development in a small city in New South Wales' in *Tenth Anniversary Monograph, Developing Health*, ed. D. Broom, National Centre for Epidemiology and Population Health, Australian National University, Canberra

Brown, V.A., Nicholson, R., Stephenson, P., Bennett, K.-J. and Smith, J. 2001, *Grass Roots and Common Ground: Guidelines for community-based environmental health action*, Regional Integrated Monitoring Centre, University of Western Sydney, Canberra

Commission on Sustainable Development 1998, *Agenda 21: Work Program 1993-98. Meetings on Thematic Clusters*, United Nations, New York

Costanza, R. and Jorgensen, S. eds 2002, *Understanding and Solving Environmental Problems in the 21st Century: Toward a new, integrated hard problem science*, Elsevier, Oxford, United Kingdom

Cruickshank, M. 2001, 'Current Environmental Health Practice: Survey of people working in the field of environment, health and/or environmental health' in *Common Ground and Common Sense*, eds P. Nicholson, P. Stephenson, V.A. Brown and K. Mitchell, Department of Health and Ageing, Canberra, pp. 135-8

Dovers, S. 2001, *Institutions for Sustainability: Tela Paper*, Australian Conservation Foundation, Melbourne

Fisher, F. 2002, Letter to the Editor: Being Scared of GM, *Sunday Herald Sun*, 30 December, p. 8

Fisher, R. and Ury, W. 1987, *Getting to Yes: How to negotiate to agreement without giving in*, Arrow Books, London

Foucault, M. 1970, *The Order of Things: An archaeology of the human sciences*, Pantheon Books, New York

Gang, P. 2000, *Rules of Dialogue*, The Institute for Educational Studies Integrated Studies Program, Endicott College, Mass

Greene, D. 2001, *Where Have All the Policies Gone?: Analysis of policy implementation in Australia using lead as a case study*, Poola Foundation, New York

Hancock, T. 1992, 'Promoting Health Environmentally' in *Supportive Environments for Health*, eds K. Dean and T. Hancock, World Health Organisation Regional Office for Europe, Copenhagen, Figure 2 The mandala of health, p. 7; Figure 3 Interrelationships, p. 14

Harding, R. 1998, *Environmental Decision-Making: The roles of scientists, engineers and the public*, Federation Press, Leichhardt, New South Wales

Honderich, T. ed. 1995, *The Oxford Companion to Philosophy*, Oxford University Press, Oxford, p. 447

IndoPacific Conference on Environment and Health 2002, Sustainable Communities' Project, Edith Cowan University, Joondalup, Western Australia, November

Kuhn, T.S. 1970, *The Structure of Scientific Revolutions*, University of Chicago Press, Chicago

MacDonald, M. 1998, *Agendas for Sustainability: Environment and development into the twenty-first century*, Routledge, London

McMichael, A.J. 2001, *Human Frontiers, Environments, and Disease: Past patterns, uncertain futures*, Cambridge University Press, Cambridge

Midgley, G. 2000, *Systemic Intervention: Philosophy, methodology and practice*, Kluwer Academic/Plenum Publishers, London

Mills, P. 2000, *Strategic Plan for Far North Queensland Peninsula and Torres Strait Island Community Health Services*, FNQPTSI Community Health Services, Thursday Island

Nicholson, R., Stephenson, P., Brown, V.A. and Mitchell, K. eds 2001, *Common Ground and Common Sense: Community-based environmental health planning*, Commonwealth of Australia, Canberra

Pimental, D., Tort, M. and D'Anna, L. 1998, 'Ecology of Increasing Disease', *BioScience*, vol. 48, no. 10, pp. 35-43

Read, P. 2000, *Belonging: Australians, place and Aboriginal ownership*, Cambridge University Press, Cambridge

Rittel, H. 1972, *On the Planning Crisis: Systems analysis of the first and second generation, reprint no. 107*, The Institute of Urban and Regional Development, University of California, Berkeley, California

Ross, H., Abel N. and Manning, M. 1996, 'Farmers, Scientists and Extensions Workers: Understanding and communicating about environmental processes on farm land' in *Landcare Languages*, ed. V.A. Brown, Commonwealth of Australia, Canberra, pp. 271-81

Smithson, M. 1989, 'The Changing Nature of Ignorance, and Managing in an Age of Ignorance' in *New Perspectives on Uncertainty and Risk*, ed. J. Handmer, Centre for Resource and Environmental Studies, Australian National University, Canberra, pp. 5-66

Smuts, J.C. 1936, *Holism and Evolution*, Macmillan, London

Soskolne, C.L. and Bertollini, R. 1999, *Global Ecological Integrity and 'Sustainable Development': Cornerstones of public health*, WHO International Workshop, WHO European Centre for Environment and Health, Rome Division, Rome 3-4 December 1998, http://www.euro.who.int/document/gch/ecorep5.pdf [20 February 2004]

Toulmin, S.E. 1977, 'From Form to Function: The philosophy and history of science in the 1950s and now', *Daedelus*, summer

United Nations Conference on Environment and Development 1992, *Agenda 21: A blueprint for survival into the 21st century*, United Nations Environment Program, Rio de Janeiro

United States National Research Council 1999, *Our Common Journey: A transition towards sustainability*, National Academy Press, Washington

World Bank 2002, *Sustainability Report*, World Bank, New York

World Commission on Environment and Development 1987, *Our Common Future: Report of the World Commission on Environment and Development*, Oxford University Press, New York

World Resources Institute, United Nations Environment Program, United Nations Development Program and World Bank 1996, *World Resources 1996-97*, Oxford University Press, New York

World Summit on Sustainable Development 2002, *Health and Environment: Supporting sustainable livelihoods*, *Towards Earth Summit 2002*, Social Briefing No. 3 linkages, World Information Transfer, http://www.worldinfo.org. 2002 [15 March 2003]

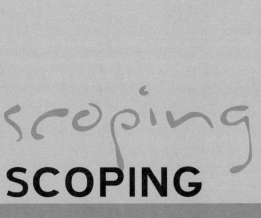

SCOPING

Designing and monitoring sustainability and health programs

Valerie A. Brown, John Grootjans,
Jan Ritchie and Helen Jordan

Summary

The scope of sustainability is wide, with its interconnected themes and concerted action towards systemic social change. Designing and monitoring programs in an uncertain, complex and dynamic system requires collaborating with others in deciding what is most important, and developing change-oriented visions, aims, strategies and outcomes. The scoping framework has to take account of all of these. This chapter emphasises the importance of involving key individuals, community members, specialist advisors, government agencies and integrative processes in program planning, negotiation of outcomes, data collection and evaluation, from the very beginning of a program.

Scoping takes place at every stage of the place-based decision-making (D4P4) process, through:

- articulating a shared local vision of people and place: local integrity is the basic unit of global sustainability;
- local community stakeholders collaborating with experts to design potential for local action;
- local health and environmental services and the community putting their designs into practice and monitoring the outcomes by collecting and collating data; and
- local community stakeholders using local data against global indicators to evaluate the principles for the way forward.

Chapter 5 Scoping

Designing and monitoring sustainability and health programs

Valerie A. Brown, John Grootjans, Jan Ritchie and Helen Jordan

Key words

Monitoring, scoping, assessing, evaluating, sustainability, local/global systems, information files, cross-referenced grids, networking systems, learning spiral

Learning outcomes

From the material in this chapter, public health practitioners and students will be able to:

- develop strategies which facilitate groups articulating their vision of a sustainable future;
- design a program on sustainability and health based on processes that expand the potential for systemic change;
- identify the sets of decision-makers (key individuals, the community, the professions and government agencies) that need to collaborate in any decision-making system;
- involve the full set of decision-makers in the design, delivery and review of the program through:
  - developing the principles driving the action;
  - describing the people and places involved;
  - designing change-oriented programs; and
  - developing and applying an effective set of indicators for monitoring change.

Outline

5.1 Monitoring strategies: what we believe we need to know

5.2 The decision-making spiral: what we know we need to know

5.3 The file, the grid and the cycle: what we know we don't know

5.4 Working with others: what we don't know we don't know

5.5 Scoping the program stages: what we now know we need to know

Learning activities

5.1 Synoptic workshop designs

5.2 Participatory rapid appraisal

5.3 Sharing ideas: brainstorming

5.4 Scoping and grounding: guided visioning exercise

Reading

Briggs, D. and Wills, J. 1999, 'Presenting Decision-Makers with Their Choices: Environment health indicators for NEHAPS' in *Environmental Health for All*, eds D.J. Briggs, R. Stern and T.L. Tinkler, Kluwer Academic Publishers, Dordrecht, pp. 187-201

Brown, V.A. 2001, 'Monitoring Changing Environments in Environmental Health' in *Environmental Health*, vol. 1, no. 1, pp. 21-34

International Institute for Sustainable Development: Bellagio principles on assessment of sustainable development, http://www.iisd.org/pdf/bellagio.pdf [20 February 2004]

5.1 Monitoring strategies: what we believe we need to know

The need to consider the full scope of any sustainability and health initiative, in its broadest context, from start to finish and even on to the next step is a key part of the 'business as very unusual' that is sustainability and health (Box 1.4). While it is quite usual to monitor a program throughout its life (process evaluation) and essential to evaluate the final outcome (summative evaluation), scoping includes both of these and more.

Working towards sustainability and health means to incorporate flexibility and innovation, to bring together multiple experts and community stakeholders, and to recognise relationships and the need for change. Scoping is the name of the mapping process, which begins by identifying all these dimensions, then following their dynamic changes throughout the life of a program and concluding by deciding what should happen next. What should happen next is but one more step on the endless spiral of working with change.

Strategies for scoping sustainability and health programs need to not only take account of, but also be actively responsive to, the complex and dynamic context in which they must function.

Strategies for scoping sustainability and health programs need to not only take account of, but also be actively responsive to, the complex and dynamic context in which they must function. This context includes the diversity of perspectives that will need to be involved in a constructive collaboration (Chapter 2), and the potential frameworks from which to choose the program guidelines (Chapter 3). It also means incorporating the different constructions of knowledge by the key decision-making sectors of individuals, community, specialists, government and holistic thinkers (Chapter 4).

As they seek to organise this complexity, practitioners are likely to be misled by two aspects of current practice. One of these is the tradition of a search for certainty in the collection of scientific evidence. The other is the emphasis on right thinking as being solely deductive thinking, that is, working within a predetermined rule. Each of these can be counter-productive in a future-oriented and dynamic problem-solving context. Each can make us believe we already know what we need to know, when the enterprise of moving towards sustainability requires creatively breaking new ground in knowledge construction, problem solving and professional skills.

A key principle of sustainability is the precautionary principle (Box 1.5): acting with caution to avoid potential harm and taking positive action to prevent harm, without waiting for scientific certainty. This principle establishes a decision-making arena in which there is limited ability for the data to provide us with certainty. For example, we know many things about the impact of persistent organic pesticides on human health, including the finding that there is a high probability above a certain dose of developing cancer of the liver. Because of mediating circumstances we cannot point to any one individual and say that if that person has a high exposure, then they will be the individual who will get liver cancer.

But we still need to act to protect the population as a whole.

But we still need to act to protect the population as a whole. There may be a cancer cluster that is of great concern to local farming families who use the pesticide, but is too small to give a significant level in an epidemiological investigation. The degree of local concern means that it is reasonable for the local government to take preventive action and control the use of the pesticide. Such lack of certainty to support their actions has on many occasions given people, organisations and governments excuses to escape the need to be reasonably cautious.

As Harremoës et al. (2002) point out, the environment is continually impacted on by events whose hazards to health and ecosystems are underscored by risk, uncertainty and ignorance. Monitoring of interventions designed to lower or prevent such impacts has to take account of this uncertainty. It must follow interactions between events, maintain constant feedback loops, and take account of possibilities and potential rather than seek certainty. With sustainability and health, the hoped-for outcome is to achieve sound, even wise decision-making for the long-term, not merely to be 'right' for the moment. In the words of a senior ecologist, 'we have oceans of data, rivers of information, some pools of knowledge, but only a very few drops of wisdom' (Nix 1993).

The strength of traditional monitoring methods, such as risk assessment and environmental and social impact assessments, is underpinned by the quantitative and deductive approaches of science, typified by measurement and a set formula of inquiry. However, science is broader than that, and the issues presented by sustainability and health require the practitioner to add qualitative and inductive modes of collecting evidence as well (Funtowicz & Ravetz 1990). This in turn calls on unfamiliar skills, skills that have not traditionally been included in either health or environmental monitoring.

Inductive as well as deductive problem-solving and use of qualitative as well as quantitative methods of collecting data need to be factored in to the scoping exercise.

Ezzy (2002) describes deductive methods of problem-solving as starting with a set of fixed expectations or an accepted explanation or theory, and asking questions arising from that theory. Results are tested against the expectations or predictions of the original accepted framework or theory, but are not used to test the theory itself. Ezzy goes on to describe the inductive process as starting with an open question that seeks answers from direct observation, and then uses the answers to build or test a theory which will be confirmed, added to or altered by collecting more data. The results are used to confirm an existing theory or construct a new explanation of events.

Figure 5.1 Deductive and inductive problem-solving

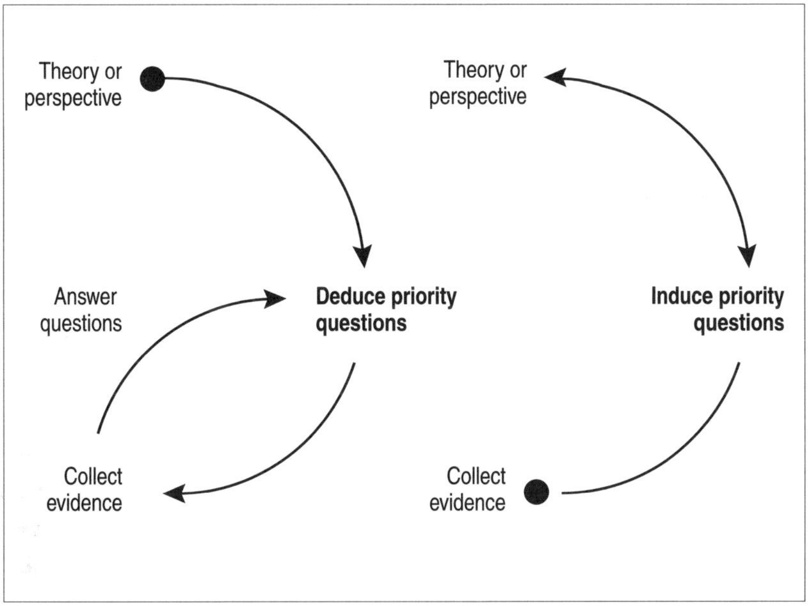

When we see these two approaches side by side in Figure 5.1 it is self-evident that together they make up a complete thinking process, a conclusion that has interesting parallels with action and participatory research methodologies and the D4P4 decision-making process outlined in Chapter 1. Kolb et al. (1974) suggest that learning is incomplete unless learners move through a complete cycle of observation, reflection, application and review. In developing indicators that can be used to monitor progress towards the goals of every stage of this problem-solving cycle, we unite the inductive and deductive, which for too long have been treated as if they were separate activities.

Kant (1995) in his book *Critique of Pure Reason* long ago made the point that deductive reasoning cannot establish that something exists—you have to assume something about reality before you start. What scoping presents in this chapter does not challenge this self-justifying cycle, but adds to it. Deductive thinking allows biophysical measurements and socio-cultural observations to be collected in the light of what we know now. Both provide 'the facts', that is, the evidence which can inform the inductive development of a new explanation or theory. The facts cannot speak for themselves—they are always interpreted within a prior framework.

Science usually advocates keeping the twin steps of deduction and induction separate. With the incorporation of relativity and chaos theory, uncertainty is now accepted as part of the scientific endeavour, and uncertainty requires both inductive and deductive processes since the theory or perspective can no longer be regarded as 'fixed', that is, known beforehand (Figure 5.1). The initial step in sustainability problem-solving is to recognise that there is already a real world out there, but any explanation of how that world works is being derived from within the chosen framework and existing expectations of the problem-solvers themselves.

Figure 5.2 A Rose is a rose is a rose

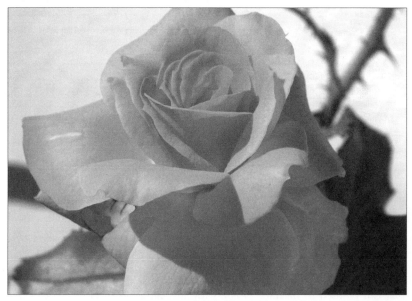

In Figure 5.2 we can see a flower which, Kant would argue, exists as *a priori knowledge*, that is, before the observer looks at it. So as far as Kant is concerned the observations can only be tested against a theory that exists in isolation from the actual observation: the object may be a thing of beauty, an unwanted weed, a token of love, a bearer of thorns and a member of the botanical family Rosaceae. Each person who sees the flower has their impressions coloured by social, political, historical, family and cultural perspectives that give the flower a unique interpretation in the minds of each observer. In agreeing with others about our interpretation, the object becomes socially as well as physically constructed. This unique individual interpretation, which we term a person's 'world view', informs human attitudes and behaviours towards that flower (Checkland 1993). Acknowledging our own personal and professional world-view is essential in approaching the changes needed to progress towards sustainability. What we believe we need to know is only the entry point to scoping sustainability action.

5.2 The decision-making spiral: what we know we need to know

In designing a sustainability and health program there will be more than one perspective involved in defining the problems, and each may well have their own preferred framework or theoretical position. Scoping is therefore not a one-track process, as in the simplified drawings in Figure 5.1. The activity of scoping will bring together several of the perspectives reviewed in Chapter 2 and at least one of the frameworks in Chapter 3.

Scoping is therefore not a one-track process . . .

At this point you, the reader, may wish to review Chapters 2 and 3 to decide which perspectives you are most comfortable working with, and which framework you would choose to adopt in your work. What ideas would you then need to include in a scoping process? Now go back to the same chapters and consider the ideas that might need to be incorporated if acting from an economic perspective, and one that is consistent with the framework of the Earth Charter. Do the questions change?

When you have determined the framework and the range of perspectives you wish to use, you have begun scoping the sustainability issue. The next step is to enlarge the orbit of what you already know (deductive reasoning, lateral thinking). The visioning exercise in Activity 5.4 is appropriate here.

In response mode, with a known problem and fixed resources, the parameters may appear to be fixed, as in cleaning up an oil spill for instance. For most issues of sustainability and health, however, that is not enough. We need to consider how to prevent another oil spill ever again (inductive reasoning). The origins of the interaction are wide and diffuse, linking local to global events and local council to national interests. There are multiple goals involving social and physical dimensions of change, as well as fixed measures. Resources for action depend on collaboration and are spread through the whole community, not contained within one profession or jurisdiction. Preventing future oil spills requires a broad review of the evidence leading to a potential change in the explanatory framework.

Preventing future oil spills requires a broad review of the evidence leading to a potential change in the explanatory framework.

How can we both identify the range of biophysical and socio-political data we will need, and find the best theory/framework/perspective to use in seeking resolution? There is no one-fits-all right answer. In this chapter we propose a synoptic problem-solving framework, one that can combine these diverse interests and arrive at an inclusive understanding rather than to continue the confrontational, one-right-answer mode that has been the dominant process. To be synoptic is to take full account of each key perspective on the same issue and then consider the collected understanding they convey, a whole that is greater than the sum of the parts. One parallel is the synoptic weather chart, in which the temperature, humidity, terrain, climate, history of weather events and statistical probabilities are combined to give a prediction of future conditions.

In deciding how to construct the synoptic problem-solving framework, the criteria are that it be adaptive, inclusive and future oriented. In Chapter 1 we suggested that the basic framework for a sustainability and health practitioner needs to be a learning framework. This involves accepting that there is continual change, and continual opportunity to build on the learning from that change. The same spiral applies to scoping an action program, but in this case there will be a range of interested parties. Thus in Figure 5.3 we return to the sustainability decision-making cycle, this time as a synoptic problem-solving basis for scoping a program. This time the learning is not that of the single practitioner, but the mutual learning of the five key knowledge cultures.

The need to involve all five of the decision-making sectors (individuals, community, specialists, government and holists) is argued in Chapter 4. Here we build on that argument to assume that, whatever the individual

Figure 5.3 Sustainability decision-making framework 2: decisions-into-practice (D4P4)

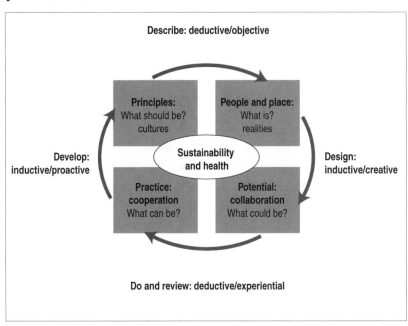

value systems of the participants (development, conservation, or spiritual), the five sectors, each of which represent a distinctive knowledge culture, must each be taken into account in scoping any action for sustainability and health. Figure 5.3 expands considerably from Figure 1.3 in Chapter 1, incorporating the appropriate form of evidence at each step.

The D4P4 decisions-into-practice cycle assumes that the program design begins with checking that the principles for action are already developed within each of the decision-making sectors through a review of interest groups concerned, exploring their value positions and goals in relation to both sustainability and health and the proposed program. Then comes collection of evidence on people and place, the basic information available on social and ecological conditions. So far, the process has been deduction after collecting existing information.

The next stage taps into the potential for change, and the process moves to an inductive mode. The creative phase requires appropriate visioning and foresighting techniques such as in the activities provided for this chapter, synoptic workshops, brainstorming, participatory rapid appraisal and structured visioning. Each of these activities is grounded in the idea that all participants from all decision-making sectors validly know what they know, and can justify the evidence on which they make their decisions. What is often missing at the beginning of a project is the creative leap that allows the decision-making sectors to combine what they know, and move forward together to discover fresh solutions.

Activity 5.1
Synoptic workshop designs
(either role play or real problem-solving)

Background: Understanding any complex problem requires careful scoping, in order to identify the key variables needed to interpret the complexity. Just as important are the relationships between the variables, and the framework within which the problem is to be understood. In contrast to all the methods reducing the number of variables to be considered to a minimum, and assuming the relationship between them is linear cause and effect in open-ended matters such as sustainability, the need is to scope the maximum relevant issues and treat the connections between them as opportunities for collaborative learning.

Aim: To bring together key decision-makers on a sustainability issue, within a framework and a process that will allow maximum contributions from each participant working together towards a deeper understanding of the whole, for the group as a whole and for their own particular interest.

Time: Three hours to three days (30 minutes to half-day debrief).

Resources: Round tables for five to ten people, marked *Individual, Community, Specialist, Strategic* and *Holistic*. On arrival have refreshments for general mingling, and ask each person to choose the table that most closely represents their interest in the issue.

Process A: Minimum: one hour. Identify a serious sustainability issue for the locality or region in which you are placed. Invite equal numbers of interested workshop participants from the categories of key individuals, community, specialist, strategic and holistic.

Note: People may not identify with the category in which they are placed and/or may feel they belong in more than one. Allow participants to arrange things as they wish. This may leave unequal numbers or a request for an extra in-between table.

Give each table the same case history of the issue, prepared using the synoptic scoping framework. Each table is asked to appoint a reporter and an observer, and a chair if they wish. Ask each table to come up with a synoptic ten-point action plan on the issue which includes each of the other groups (45 minutes). They present the plan to the whole group as an overhead slide in 3 minutes (15 minutes per group).

Discussion (30 minutes): Effectiveness of each group's action plan (group members), adequacy of proposed collaboration (other groups), distinguishing characteristics of the process of each group's analysis of the issues (participant observer).

Process B: one hour. Reform the tables with mixed groups, one person from each of the decision-making sectors. Each table takes one action plan and, using the synoptic planning framework, develops a set of goals, a situation analysis, potential innovative directions and a resource list and timetable (45 minutes). Finally, the group will decide when and how the process will be monitored and evaluated. Each group presents for 3 minutes (15 minutes).

Discussion (30 minutes): Whole group discussion on comprehensiveness of coverage; equality of participation; maximising resources; new learning; and practicality of each design. Ideally, construction of a composite design.

5.3 The file, the grid and the cycle: what we know we don't know

In trying to think creatively in searching for new directions, new ideas surface that may send the participants back to the previous stage in the synoptic framework, collecting further information from all parties both biophysical and social. If the visioning, forecasting, brainstorming or other method of exploration has been successful, there will be valuable new ideas and new avenues for action well worth exploring (see Activities 5.1 and 5.4). Finding out what we do know, not re-inventing the wheel and being alert to recognising what we don't know are essential elements of scoping.

Once we have re-examined what we need to know, with fresh minds about our scoping styles and asking new questions prompted by the decision-making spiral, we are in a position to find out what we do know. After we are confident about what we do know and what we need to know, it is time to decide what we don't know. Finding out what we don't already know is easier than ever before, in this information era with its World Wide Web, rapid travel and supposedly open societies. The synoptic scoping framework discussed above will only be as strong as the reliability and validity of the information available to back it up.

The three main options for collecting the information needed in scoping sustainability and health programs are the file, the grid and the cycle (Figure 5.4). Each format contributes to the knowledge needed in a very different way. With modern information technology, information files are larger and more accessible than ever before. But however comprehensive the Internet and however reliable the information, it is still an information file that has to be interpreted and evaluated before it can be applied to each project. It is not yet knowledge. In comparison, a similar increase in the capacity for cross-referencing data using modern computing technology has allowed an increase in interpretation of data and so in knowledge. The increases in understanding range from local population behaviour to the global sweeps of climate change.

The three main options for collecting the information needed in scoping sustainability and health programs are the file, the grid and the cycle

The cycle is increasingly the favoured mode for data presentation in designing and monitoring sustainability programs. The cycle is able to build on the file and the grid, and allows for the inclusion of a time sequence of events. It links easily to strategic knowledge (Figures 4.3 and 4.4). If the cycle is regarded as open rather than closed, it is able to allow for inductive reasoning and new interpretations of the data.

Thus each of the three information formats contributes different components of the scoping system, and each format has its own strengths and weaknesses (Figure 5.4). The file ensures the safe storage and retrieval of data and acts as a reliable repository, but it can also be a control mechanism since there is a tendency for the custodians of information to restrict access. Specialised language can form a barrier to access, and so can lack of respect for information from knowledge cultures other than one's own.

The grid allows a large number of possibilities to be canvassed, and offers unexpected insights into relationships. Unless there is an agreed value basis for ranking priorities, the interaction between the variables can be overwhelming and directionless. The detail of a grid makes it easier to identify any particular interest, position and appropriate action, but more difficult to recreate an idea of the whole.

The most commonly used way of turning files into knowledge is cross-referencing two sets of files to form a decision-making grid (column 2,

Figure 5.4). In the health field this means linking risk factors, disease states and interventions; in the environmental field it involves monitoring human activities in relation to their impacts on environmental processes. Since sustainability and health programs address the interface between the two, they will need to build on both sets at once. This requires at least a grid; for most sustainability decision-making it will require a systemic, cyclical approach.

From Figure 5.4 we can identify the appropriate use of each of the possible formats, their principal purpose, explanatory frameworks, type of content, uses, time scale and type of indicators. The cycle provides the opportunity to monitor the complex interactive health/environment system over time, allowing for illuminative evaluation (feedback throughout the program delivery) as well as summative (final outcome) evaluation. The cycle offers the opportunity to actively monitor progress, to integrate different knowledge cultures and to consider the future. There is, however, a considerable difference between the closed information cycle and the open-ended decision-making spiral, as we shall find from the examples that follow.

Figure 5.4 Information sources for environment and health reporting (adapted from Brown 2001)

Design elements	The file	The grid	The cycle
Principal purpose	data collection	risk management	action guide
Frameworks	biophysical state of humans and the environment (separately)	pressure-state-response indicators (transactions), epidemiological profiles	pressure-state-response-potential (transformation), driving force-pressure-state-exposure-effect-action
Content	qualitative and quantitative data	social, economic and environmental information sets	integrative indicators of system change
Uses	Reference	environmental management decisions	integrated decisions about the future
Time scale	present record	moving away from the past	moving toward future goals
Indicators	scientific data	level of risk	signs of progress

Files

The wealth of descriptive data collected in health and environmental sciences can readily be found in local and national information collections, and on comprehensive websites. The difficulty is no longer access, but that information is collected under different sets of assumptions and held in different archives. Heath statistics in 2003 take no account of long-term feedback effects on health from environmental change, even though health sources predict increased spread of vector-borne diseases, and epidemiologists have calculated that 40 per cent of the global human disease burden has environmental causes (Pimental et al. 1998). Nor do many environmental state-of-the-environment reports make more than passing reference to effects on human health (for example, the Australian National State-of-the-Environment Advisory Council 2001) although there are exceptions such as Canada (Environment Canada 2002).

Each sector therefore needs to know what information the other holds. For health you can expect to make use of epidemiological profiles (Abbott 1990), the biennial reports of the country's Institute of Health and Welfare or equivalent, and local health profiles and epidemiological reports. Most countries follow OECD advice and publish a *State of the National Environment* every few years. It is also becoming common for local government authorities to issue a similar annual report (Brown 2001).

When social and biophysical indicators are aggregated in this way, the single figure can carry a strong social message as well as a measurement function.

The characteristics of an information file are listed in column 1 of Figure 5.4. Information is collected in a reference frame, building on existing content according to the skills of the collectors and with certain uses in mind. All of these are taken for granted in each discipline or speciality, and the information continues to serve its traditional users well. Geographic information systems (GIS) and large-capacity personal computers make searching files a new possibility for even minor projects. Lists of useful websites are provided at the end of this chapter. Aggregate indicators are constructed through cross-referencing a number of different information sources, and the final result incorporated into a single aggregated file. When social and biophysical indicators are aggregated in this way, the single figure can carry a strong social message as well as a measurement function.

One of the best known and most widely used of the aggregate measures is the ecological footprint developed by Wackernagel and Rees (1996)—see websites of other integrated indices—which has been used to calculate national regional, local and personal natural resource use, that is, their footprint on the Earth (see Chapter 6 for the calculation). The Genuine Progress Indicator (Hamilton 2002) and the General Progress Indicator (Wackernagel 2002) each total social, economic and ecological trends in a single number. Unless the various contributions to the cross-referencing are understood in context, and so are accessible to decision-making, the final number becomes information and its collection format a file.

There is a large family of integrative decision-making indicators using holistic symbols to connect the indicators with strategic decisions and involve the local community. One of the classic sets is for Sustainable Seattle, which AtKisson (1999) developed into COMPASS. Dashboard uses the concept of the indicators on a car dashboard. It is free software, available on http://www.esl.jrc.it/envind/dashbrds.htm. There are sustainable communities indicators; indicators for ethical businesses (the Valdez Principles), for university campuses (the Talloires Convention) and for industry (the Balaton Framework). The most recent edition of each of these can best be found through net searches on their titles.

Sets of comparisons between environment, health and sustainability indicators were developed during a joint meeting on environmental monitoring between the United States and Canada. This outline gives the public health practitioner a good indication of the type of empirical data that can and should be collected to show the relationship between the environment and health of populations. Uses of environmental, health and sustainability indicators (separately and together) are:

- assessing the current risks and responses, documenting trends in the condition over time (goal indicators);
- anticipating hazardous conditions before adverse impact (early warning indicator);
- identifying causative agents to specify appropriate management action (diagnostic); and
- demonstrating interdependence between indicators (correlational indicator).

(US-Canada International Joint Commission 1996, cited in Cole et al. 1998)

There is a large family of integrative decision-making indicators using holistic symbols to connect the indicators with strategic decisions and involve the local community.

Grids

Cross-referenced decision-making grids are usually contained within a single discipline. For issues of sustainability and health, cross-referencing is needed between a wider number of sources, at the least the environmental, social and economic disciplines and the individual, local, strategic and holistic knowledge cultures. Taking an example from a project to set up monitoring systems for a polluted lake project, stakeholders from varying backgrounds will argue that the quality of the water is based on different parameters. Public health practitioners will measure the concentration of a bacterium, *Escherichia coli*, which can cause diarrhoea and which indicates the level of faecal organic matter in the water. But however sick the presence of *E. coli* may make humans, for the biologists organic matter may in fact increase the fertility of the water ecosystems. Environmentalists will measure biological oxygen demand—the amount of oxygen in the water available to supply the photosynthesising plants that supply food to the lake ecosystem. The decay of high levels of rotting plant matter removes the oxygen and the system fails; this represents death for the ecosystem, but can mean that the upper levels of the water are free of biological matter and more attractive to swimmers.

For issues of sustainability and health, cross-referencing is needed between a wider number of sources ...

For most of the life of public health as a professional practice, environmental risk monitoring has been assigned to the environmental health sector and the form of monitoring has been the grid; that is, documenting the elements of health risks as a matrix of contaminating agent and health status. A widely used example is the DPSEEA (driving force-pressure-state-exposure-effect-action) conceptual framework (Figure 5.5). Briggs and Wills (1999, p. 200) recommend that appropriate measures need to be defined for each of the DPSEEA factors and that the following considerations need to be made:

> *The relatively demanding criteria and design specifications . . . mean that most environmental health indicators are use-specific. Indicators developed in relation to one issue cannot normally be applied to others. Specific indicators usually need to be designed for specific environmental hazards and health outcomes. This means that it is rarely appropriate to try to develop a small and permanent set of environmental health indicators [that] can suit all requirements.*

The long-standing diagram representing sustainability issues is the three interlinked circles of society, economy and environment, as in Figure 5.6, developed by Trevor Hancock in 1992 (Hancock also designed the more complex Mandala of Health in Figure 1.1). The use of the circles has ensured recognition that all three sets of resources are required in planning for a sustainable future. The intersections between the circle identify the 'action areas' of sustainability: sustainable communities, supportive environments and sustainable development.

Figure 5.5 DPSEEA grid for environmental health monitoring

Issue	Water-borne infections					
	Driving force	**Pressure**	**State**	**Exposure**	**Effect**	**Action**
Factors/ processes	increasing livestock numbers	increasing leakage and runoff of livestock wastes	increased levels of microbiological contamination in streams and drinking water	increased exposure to microbiological contaminants while bathing and in drinking water	increased incidence of gastro-intestinal infections	improved water treatment: control of livestock wastes
Indicators	livestock numbers	number of reported pollution incidents due to livestock wastes	percentage of stream water quality samples failing guideline value for faecal coliforms	estimated personal exposure to faecal coliforms in bathing and drinking water	Incidence of gastro-intestinal infections in general population	number of prosecutions for contamination of waters by livestock wastes

Source: Briggs & Wills 1999, p. 199

Figure 5.6 Three-circle diagram of sustainability (after Hancock 1992)

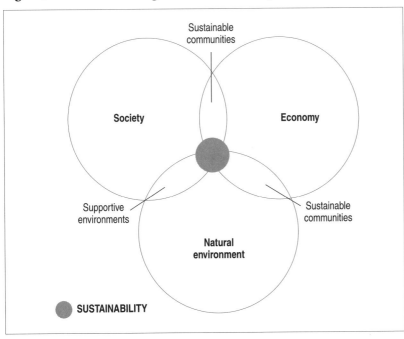

Over the years of applying this Venn diagram approach to sustainability issues, the limitations of what is essentially a grid have become apparent. The diagram gives no scope for connections between the three, leaving the information or actions separate, to be cross-referenced (National Research Council 1999). The three were originally identified for monitoring purposes as the so-called triple bottom line. If not followed by some form of synthesis, this tripartite view can serve to strengthen, not reduce, the competitive boundaries between them. More recently, there have been projects identifying the triple bottom line plus one (and including governance), and/or the single bottom line, the integrated goal of sustainability.

Cycles

The scoping and monitoring tools for environmental health (DPSEEA) and environmental management (PSR) each began as a grid and have more recently been developed into a cycle (column 2, Figure 5.4). In some ways each still functions as a grid, that is it cross-references the decision-making components rather than reviewing the relationships between them. As tools originally designed for monitoring, however, each still captures a snapshot rather than the dynamic interactions between the parts.

The closed circles of most impact and risk assessments and other monitoring schemes do not usually incorporate the social learning and transformational change dimensions that are the hallmarks of sustainability, though they have begun to include the connections between the sectors of health and of environment. Emphasis is given to collaboration, creativity and change in the decision-making for participatory practice (D4P4) spiral outlined above (Figure 5.3). The four steps in the D4P4 framework combine and extend the environment and health DPSEEA framework, if:

- the driving force for human activities (the pressure) is accepted as being driven by principles;
- the state of the environment includes people as well as place;
- the potential for change is included; and
- the cycle moves on to action and then to revisiting the principles.

A global iterative process over time has shifted the way we think about monitoring change in the environment. Files of data were turned into grids that provided us with information about relationships between factors. These grids were then developed into cycles in order to highlight the dynamic nature of sustainability. More recently sustainability science has demanded that cycles be further developed into spirals to highlight the need for innovation and ongoing change as we now accept there is no single answer, such as technology or economics; the best we can hope for is ongoing improvements in the situation.

Under the guidelines prepared for the World Health Organisation's Health and Environmental Analysis for Decision-making, Linkage Analysis and Monitoring Project (HEADLAMP), the DPSEEA framework has been further developed as a source of decision-making indicators, using a cycle (Figure 5.6). The various stages of the DPSEEA framework form a logical causal chain; that is, DPSEEA organises the concepts in a way that links them into an intuitive series of related steps that incorporate the elements of the environmental sector's pressure-state-response framework discussed below. The framework is flexible and becomes a cycle in that one may enter it at any stage, though it works best if one begins by considering driving forces first.

A global iterative process over time has shifted the way we think about monitoring change in the environment.

The pressure-state-response (PSR) framework, a tool for monitoring progress toward implementing sustainable development, was developed by the Organisation for Economic Co-operation and Development (1993a; 1993b) (Figure 5.7). The PSR model of environmental decision-making is now routine for all OECD countries (the OECD sends a monitoring team to each member country in turn to evaluate progress). Australia (every four years), almost all states (annually) and all local government authorities in New South Wales (annually) use this framework. As a closed circle, cause and effect model it is effective for selecting and applying indicators for sustainable development principles.

The original PSR framework allows for evaluating the interaction between environmental risks and social activities, but not social risks. While it is cyclical in recognising the continuing interaction between the three factors of human activity, environmental condition and human response, it links the three in a cause and effect mode without addressing the form of the interactions. Decisions about moving toward sustainability require that the monitoring process assess the current state of the environment, identify the pressures and match them to effective responses. Further, for sustainability and health practice, the framework needs a feedback loop acknowledging that pressure on the environment is pressure on human health as well. It is also important to acknowledge the need for the whole system to change in order to move toward a more sustainable state (Figure 5.7). National and

Figure 5.7 Framework for developing environmental health indicators

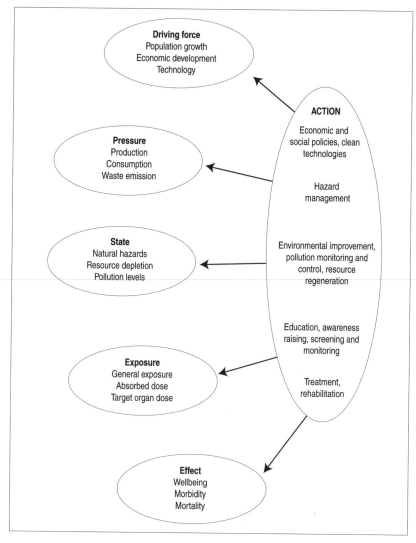

Source: Modified from Briggs & Wills 1999

local state of the environment reports have begun to add 'implications' to the cycle for this purpose.

Recent work has added an open-ended 'potential' category to the closed PSR cycle, and replaced the simple cause and effect link between the categories by the scoping actions required (Brown 2001; Brown et al. 2000). The new spiral has a close similarity to the synoptic decision-making spiral.

Figure 5.8 Extended pressure-state-response framework

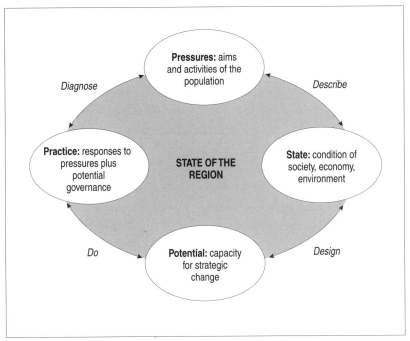

Source: Brown 2001; Organisation for Economic Cooperation and Development 1993a, 1993b; Brown et al. 2000

Activity 5.2
Participatory Rapid Appraisal (PRA)
http://www.allenandunwin.com/sustainhealth

5.4 Working with others: what we don't know we don't know

Qualitative research methodologies, such as focus group expressions of concern about environmental impact, can be used alongside quantitative methodologies in the form of cancer research studies to inductively inform the development of new theory about sustainability options. Qualitative research methodologies, such as regional action groups, can be used alongside quantitative methodologies to deductively test the reliability of theory. Scoping for sustainability advocates a partnership of methods. We can't know what we don't know unless we have a wider framework, which alerts us to our areas of ignorance. Working with key individuals, the relevant community, a range of specialists, organisations in government and industry and some holistic thinkers is the framework recommended here.

Such a mix of approaches carries its own problems as well as its strengths. In Chapter 4 we saw that each of the knowledge cultures of community, specialists, strategists and holists has its own knowledge systems, mode of setting priorities and ways of protecting its borders. If all five groups of stakeholders are to contribute to a program, active steps will be needed to encourage their inclusion as respected equal partners. Data collection methods differ between the knowledge bases: individuals draw on their experience, the community tells stories, experts use case studies, strategists work to their agenda and holists create an icon or goal that acts as a synthesis for all the others. The first requirement of a competent scoping monitoring system for informed decision-making is to value the contributions of all five forms of knowledge, thereby constructing a networked knowledge system that builds on the file and the grid (Figure 5.4) and is involved in an open learning system (Figure 1.3).

Scoping for sustainability advocates a partnership of methods.

Following the cycle in Figure 5.3, scoping begins with selecting the priority sustainability and health issue; this can be at any scale from cleaning up a polluted lake, reducing city waste, or a national greenhouse gas abatement program to reduce global warming. In filling the first box, developing principles, we find that there are established principles for public health regarding the absolute value of human life, professional relationships and client rights. In environmental matters there are equally established principles on the value of life and on the integrity of ecological systems from the food chains to global systems. In sustainability and health both sets of values operate, sometimes with a conflict of interest—as we recognised in the value line, the first activity in Chapter 1. The interdependency of human health and the health of the biophysical environment brings an overarching set of values into play, demonstrated in the principles of the Earth Charter in Chapter 3 and the New Public Health, explored in acting and innovating below.

Having decided which principles operate in your project, the second step is to move on to scoping a description of people and place related to those principles. For example, if the issue is a polluted lake and the key principle is long-term local responsibility for local sustainability, the description of people should include factors that enhance or reduce their capacity to act for themselves and the approaches of local industry to the clean-up. The description of place will include the cumulative impacts of local sources of pollution. Once you have the relevant description of people and place—of what is happening on site now—then the third step, designing the program with a built-in potential for change, comes into play.

A planning framework does not itself provide a method for developing indicators; it shows where they will be needed. How to design, define or quantify an indicator is best left to the people affected to decide, based on past research and experience and current knowledge and practice. A framework does set the parameters within which the goals can be set, and indicators can be developed and subsequently interpreted. The logic of the monitoring process has changed from a cause and effect approach to a continuous scoping cycle of a systemic interaction between multifaceted parts, addressing an as yet unknown future.

A planning framework does not itself provide a method for developing indicators; it shows where they will be needed.

In the case of a polluted lake, opportunities for effective and long-term change could include lobbying all polluter sources, innovative methods of local community education on pollution sources and their risk levels, and reviews of the need for new government regulation and monitoring. Indicators will need to be developed for progress on each of these. The final step in this round is the implementation and review of the program in the light of the principles and the potential you have identified. Indicators for outcomes at each stage of the cycle/spiral should by now have been included in the program design. Indicators of success from consumer and government perspectives will be different, and both should be included; for example, pollution may have been lowered this year, but have community understanding and government action increased enough to reduce the pollution next year?

Circumstances can change and unexpected events occur at any time in the social learning process involved in working toward sustainability goals, so we need to check decisions against the original principles at the end of each cycle, to decide what to do next. It may be that a new or different principle can be included for the next round; for example, the community core principle can change from citizen responsibility for the clean-up to citizen responsibility to influence government policy, or to take citizen action on polluting industries. Or the same principle may apply, but the implementation strategy fail and have to be redesigned. Thus the cycle turns again, and is in fact a spiral.

Circumstances can change and unexpected events occur at any time in the social learning process involved in working toward sustainability goals

. . .

After first scoping the principles, issues, potential and practice for your public health team you will have an idea about the project from your own perspective. During this first round of scoping it will be useful to complete the stakeholder identification exercise in Chapter 4 (Activity 4.4). From this list you identify the key team members (including at least one from each of the knowledges) you will recruit to work with you. It is important to have the organising group work together on this collaborative scoping exercise, which then sets the framework for the project; in this way everyone is familiar with each other's goals, approach and resources from the beginning. It is also important to use the rules of dialogue throughout this and subsequent meetings so people from the different decision-making sectors can hear and be heard.

If the project is a major one, has potential for conflicts of interests or will be long term, it is of value to consider a more extensive team development process for the program management team. The team will have been selected through the stakeholder process. In scoping the program with your fellow practitioners it is also desirable to clarify the organising group's 'rules of engagement' (Aslin & Brown 2004); this includes commitment to the rules of dialogue, agreement about meeting procedures and potential group problem-solving processes. If members of the group have previously been involved in conflict or are likely to be (which is quite possible in the field of sustainability and health), it is worth including some negotiation exercises in the scoping phase so the group is familiar with a negotiation technique if tensions arise.

This stage of the project is of particular importance, because for long-term change it is necessary for the stakeholders to develop ownership of the problem and any solutions that may come from the group's work. Attention should be paid by practitioners acting as facilitators to building trust between stakeholders who in the past have been viewed as competing rather than collaborating. The concept of trust becomes very important in a scoping exercise where patience and perseverance are essential in actively allowing all positions to be heard, no matter how 'far out' they seem. Activity 5.2 offers a collaborative exercise that may help reduce tensions before they emerge.

The impact of lead on human health has been known as an objective reality since the ancient Romans first used it extensively in their daily lives, and yet at the turn of the century lead was added to paint and petrol as a cost-effective means of improving performance. Objective science, especially in the last 100 years, has built up what should have been an undeniable body of evidence to support the removal of lead from petrol and paint, however there were 50-year delays in having lead removed from these products (Brown et al. 2001). This simple analogy makes it imperative for researchers to better understand lead objectively in order to unravel the physiological reaction of the body to lead poisoning; at the same time this analogy leads us to see that it is imperative to undertake research which helps us to understand the relationship between lead and the community. Scoping provides us with the proposition that by integrating methodologies these time delays in building evidence and achieving results in case examples such as lead may be reduced. All of this requires working closely with decision-making sectors other than your own.

The concept of trust becomes very important in a scoping exercise where patience and perseverance are essential in actively allowing all positions to be heard . . .

5.5 Scoping the program stages: what we now know we need to know

This chapter has discussed many of the issues that should be considered when developing indicators to monitor the outcomes of the decision-making stages in response to local or global risks to the environment and to health combined. It has avoided setting fixed rules for public health practitioners on methods they should use. What we are presenting here are the issues you should consider and the strategies you can use to scope the entire issue, necessary steps before you reach the stage of identifying locally appropriate indicators.

Scoping the potential for change is the first step in the delivery of a sustainability and health program that aims to engage the whole of a community in reconstructing some aspect of its management of local and global ecosystems. The program will by definition be about changing the biophysical environment in addition to introducing social change. Since sustainability goals are open-ended and as yet uncertain, the operation of scoping is much like the first step in a research process. Scoping is therefore:

- the first task in all sustainability decision-making and program design;
- the essential grounding of the action in people and place;
- the basis for exploring the potential for systemic change; and
- the foundation for setting the goals for practical outcomes and deciding on indicators by which to monitor those goals.

Indicators that monitor progress towards the creative goals (what could be) and the actual progress achieved by implementing the scoped program (what can be), and help in diagnosing the difference between them, all have the same requirements. They need to be:

- **s**ensitive to their task so they match the goals whose achievement they are supposed to indicate;
- **m**easurable so they can document progress trends forward or backward;
- **a**ccessible to all the parties involved in sustainability and health, including community, specialists and government agencies;
- **r**eliable over time and in parallel situations so they can be used for incorporating past experiences and other places; and
- **t**imely, so that they have immediate relevance, give early warning and can invoke the precautionary principle.

The program will by definition be about changing the biophysical environment in addition to introducing social change.

This chapter has explored the distinctive knowledges of the sectors involved in sustainability and health decision-making—individual change agents, local communities, specialist advisors, government agencies and holistic practitioners—and discusses methods for recruiting each of the knowledges. It applies the problem-solving process of the decision-making for participatory practice (D4P4) framework to scoping and monitoring the content of actual programs, incorporating all possible avenues of collaboration. The four-step cycle of place-based decision-making (developing principles, describing people and place, designing potential and doing in practice) provides the basis for scoping a program in a way that places the complexities of sustainability practice in a decision-making context. Since it is also an open-ended learning framework, it is particularly suited to planning and evaluating change-oriented sustainability and health programs.

The purpose of scoping, monitoring and evaluation is to advise decision-makers on the development of resources to meet sustainability and health goals. The dynamic nature of the environment and the health system remains a major hurdle for traditional statistical and experimental research to offer sound advice to public health sustainability practitioners. Epidemiology and environmental monitoring provide invaluable information that needs translation and interpretation before decision-makers (community, specialists and government) can apply it. Impact assessment and end-of-program evaluation have classically been based on reducing complex systems to simple factors that can be monitored by fixing them in time and by excluding confounding variables. This leads to interpretation of the changes in the object under assessment in isolation from its context. The results are accurate for that time and that place, but can be misleading if applied as projections to another time or place.

The scoping approach advocated here uses the tools referred to above in decision-making; for example, having established the principles by which the program will be managed, the indicators will be of behaviours consistent with those principles, as in the phrase 'walking your talk'. Reviews of major policy initiatives reveal that there are many more sustainability policy directives on the books than are implemented on the ground (MacDonald 1998). Evaluating environment and health issues for people and place draws on the experience of social and environmental impact assessment, epidemiology and state-of-the-environment monitoring, once some forecasting or visioning process has set the local goals. Progress toward local sustainability goals can be considered against the background of regional and national sets of data aggregated as genuine progress indicators, which amalgamate social, economic and ecological trends; or published as national and global state of the nation reports. The principles of adaptive management and GIS tools go beyond social and environmental impact assessments, giving the public health practitioner a way forward in this very difficult endeavour.

Setting goals for identifying and achieving the potential for change required for sustainability and health is one of the greatest challenges. What for some is a great leap forward is for others a mere step on the way to establishing sustainability and health for the long term. The dialogue between incremental and transformational change is a thread that continues throughout this book. Any indicators for adequacy of ways to achieve change will need to be placed in this perspective. A SWOT (strengths, weaknesses, opportunities and threats) analysis, a forecasting exercise and a scenario all attempt to estimate potential. SWOT tends to remain fixed in the status quo; forecasting can move beyond reality and scenarios give fixed expectations.

It is in planning, observing and recording practice and its outcomes that the bulk of evaluation occurs. Here the distinctions between the expected and the unexpected, the explicit and the implicit become of first importance. In areas as multifaceted and generally unpredictable as sustainability and health, all four dimensions need to be watched for and considered. The rapidly expanding field of sustainability indicators for every conceivable

The dynamic nature of the environment and the health system remains a major hurdle for traditional statistical and experimental research . . .

Setting goals for identifying and achieving the potential for change required for sustainability and health is one of the greatest challenges.

outcome can cause endless confusion and adds to the very fragmentation that working toward sustainability seeks to avoid. Chapters 1-4 offer a guide to scoping the issues, the ideas, the partners, the frameworks and the knowledge base for working with sustainability and health. The lesson from this chapter is that scoping the place-based decision-making cycle requires all the resources of the file (data collection and storage), the grid (cross-referencing data against possible causal factors), and the cycle (looking for directions).

For sustainability and health programs, all these are needed and more. The distinctive characteristic of the scoping process outlined here is that it is synoptic, that is, it includes objective and subjective, qualitative and quantitative data collection; inductive and deductive problem-solving processes; and the full range of knowledge cultures into which Western thinking has become divided. Moreover, these often divided dimensions are brought together in a single decision-making framework, which is in the form of a spiral of continuous learning and change. This synoptic scoping framework sets the foundation for sustainability and health acting, changing and managing, the rest of the chapters in this book.

Activity 5.3
Sharing ideas: brainstorming

Aim: for a working group to generate and accept creative ideas.

Time: one hour. Debrief 15 minutes.

Based on the notions that 'no idea is stupid' and that 'the best ideas come from left field', brainstorming is designed to get all possible ideas on the table, encourage all participants to contribute and stimulate their minds to generate creative options. This is particularly valuable if people are going to work together, since it allows everyone in the group to become familiar with other people's ideas before they fix their own.

Step 1. Appoint a facilitator and a recorder.

The facilitator explains the rules of dialogue and the purpose of brainstorming, then initiates the discussion by asking all present to identify an issue of universal concern about the project (it doesn't have to be the highest priority, just something everyone is concerned about). The recorder writes the issue at the head of a large sheet of paper or on a whiteboard.

Step 2. The facilitator encourages members of the group to contribute ideas on the issue in a 'rapid-fire' manner and sets these down as close to verbatim as possible; the recorder does not interpret in any way. Stop if necessary and ask the contributor to repeat that item. The recorder should group ideas as they come, and the facilitator checks with the group to see if it agrees with the grouping.

As facilitator, ensure all members of the group have the opportunity to contribute. Without naming individuals it is possible to pause at intervals and note aloud that some people have not contributed, and that now is their opportunity to have a say. Similarly, don't be shy of quietening participants who tend to dominate: 'Thanks; you've contributed a number of valuable suggestions. Could we now hear from others?' If anyone becomes dominant, introduce a rule that each participant can only speak once in the next round.

Step 3. As the momentum runs down, the facilitator leads discussion for group members to ask each other questions about their suggestions—questions of clarification only, not criticisms. This exercise is for learning from each other, not for arguing about who is right.

Step 4. Reflect on what is on the record and discuss what lessons have emerged for the joint project. Type up the material of the session and circulate to participants for comment.

Websites for indicator design

Compass, Alan AtKisson, sustainability consultant and author: http://www.AtKisson.com [20 February 2004]

Ecosystem indicators: http://www.heinzctr.org/ecosystems/ [20 February 2004]

Fondazione Eni Enrico Mattei research unit on sustainability indicators and environmental evaluation: http://www.feem.it/web/resun/sim1.html [20 February 2004]

Harvard forum for science and technology for sustainability: http://sustsci.harvard.edu/index.html [20 February 2004]

IISD Bellagio Principles on methods of assessment of sustainable development: http://www.iisd.org/pdf/bellagio.pdf [20 February 2004]

INFORM is an independent research organisation that examines the effects of business practices on the environment and on human health: http://www.informinc.org/ [20 February 2004]

International Center for Local Environment Initiatives monitoring systems: http://www.iclei.org/ [20 February 2004]

Joint Center for Sustainable Communities: http://www.usmayors.org/ USCM/sustainable/ [20 February 2004]

London sustainability exchange: http://www.lsx.org.uk/resources/ind-tk/ indics/index.shtml [20 February 2004]

National Center for Environmental Decision-Making Research: http:// iisd1.iisd.ca/measure/compindex.asp [20 February 2004]

National Strategies for Sustainable Development: http://www.nssd.net/ index1.html [20 February 2004]

Organisation for Economic Cooperation and Development environmental indicator reports: http://www.oecd.org/EN/home/0,,EN-home-567-nodirectorate-no-no-no-8,00.html [20 February 2004]

Southern California Studies Center: http://sc2.usc.edu/sg/index.html [20 February 2004]

United Nations Commission for Sustainable Development sustainability indicators http://www.un.org/esa/sustdev/isd.htm [20 February 2004]

Urban state of the environment reports worldwide: http://www.ceroi.net/ [20 February 2004]

Websites on integrated sustainability indicators:

http://www.sustainability.com/home.asp [20 February 2004]

http://www.sustainabilityindicators.org/resources/Resources.html [20 February 2004]

Dashboard: http://www.esl.jrc.it/envind/dashbrds.htm [20 February 2004]

Activity 5.4
Scoping and grounding: guided visioning exercise

Note: This exercise is best presented as a three-hour workshop.

Aim: to establish 'headline' sustainability goals and their progress indicators, shared by local change agents, local community interests, local specialist agencies and responsible government agencies.

Materials: a room with tables able to seat 6-12 around each table; a pack of stiff library cards, enough for three for each person; a whiteboard; marker pens and a roll of tape.

Time: two hours (three hours if there are more than 20 participants). Debriefing segment 30-60 minutes.

Participants: any number of people who have an interest in the region or place.

For the facilitator: settle the group in comfortable chairs in a circle around a table, close to a wall or whiteboard where you can pin up cards later. Spend 5-10 minutes discussing what it means to think 10 years into the future. Compare thinking forward to thinking back 10 years, with all the changes participants have experienced. (If there are people under 20 years of age, have them think forward into the unknown. If there are non-English speakers, be sure there is an interpreter. Both of these sets of contributions are especially valuable).

Key question for everyone to consider:

In the ********** region, what would people find if all the programs on social, economic and environmental sustainability they are designing now were actually working?

Make sure the group is in a quiet room with no interruptions. In a clear, slow, calm, deep voice, read the following script. Give time for people to develop the images in their minds. Some people will have greater difficulty visualising than others. This does not really matter; they can still contribute to the activity later. Pace the exercise yourself so you leave plenty of time for everyone to visualise the images, and move slowly from one set of images to the next.

*We are now going to take a trip to the future, to an ideal ********** region 20 years from now. This is not ********** as it is today, nor is it ********** as if everything had simply continued on as usual. This is ********** as we would like it to be if all of our work toward a more sustainable environment had been achieved. It is not pie in the sky, or an unrealistic Utopia, but what we can reasonably expect to achieve if we had a healthy, sustainable environment in which emergency risk management is fully implemented. All the problems of today have been solved.*

Make yourselves comfortable—you may find it useful to close your eyes so you can more easily imagine the landscape.

*I want you to come with me into our helicopter and first take it up high over **********, not ********** now, but in 20 years' time when all our efforts toward a sustainable environment have been established.*

Look at the landscape beneath you. What does it look like? What colours and shapes do you see? What time of year is it? What would it look like at a different time of year? Look out across the landscape at the cities, towns, buildings, spaces, farms, hills and valleys. What patterns do you see? What crops are growing? What stock is feeding? Where does water come from? How is the water distributed? How pure is the water?

What is it used for? Where does the waste water go? Where are the people? Can you see people and goods moving to and fro? How are they being moved? What sounds come up to you? What smells?

Now choose a place you want to visit, to see what it's like in 20 years' time. Take the helicopter to that place. Descend slowly, looking around you as you come down, at the patterns of buildings, of people, of spaces. Look at the shapes and structures of the buildings. Look at the spaces between them. As you get closer, listen to the sounds and smell the scents of the landscape.

Are there people around? Who is there? What ages are they? How do they react to you—and to each other? What activities are going on? Are there people working? Are there people relaxing? What else are they doing? Who is doing it? Now walk around and see what else there is.

Join one of the people as they move about. What are they doing? How do they look? Is this a good place to be? How are the people interacting with each other? Now join some other people. What is happening here and how does it feel?

Now imagine yourself in the open spaces. How is it different from the situation today? What is happening? What is happening in the neighbourhood and in the community? What are people happy about? What are they worried about?

Imagine that it is lunchtime. Where do people go for lunch? What do they talk about? What sort of food are they eating? Where did it come from? What do they do after lunch?

As the day comes to an end, go home with someone. How do they get home? Where is home? How far are they travelling? Go with them in their neighbourhood. Remember, this is a well-managed environment in which all your programs and changes are working. How does the neighbourhood feel? Do you feel secure about the future? How is the region being managed?

What are the decisions being made? What important changes have happened recently?

Now go into a house. Who is there? Is it a family? Who is in the family? Are they all receiving an income? What do they do? What about the others? Are there children? Do they go to school? What are they learning about their district and their environment?

When you feel that you know and understand how this place will be in 20 years' time, call up the helicopter and take it to a second place, somewhere in ********** you would like to visit. Again, look at the patterns and shapes as you descend. Walk around and explore the spaces. Listen to the people. Where are they? What are they doing? Ask them questions about what you want to know.

What work are they doing? Are they working together or separately?

Is it different on workdays and holidays? What do people do for time off?

Now call up the helicopter again and choose a third and last place where you'd like to find out what it's like 20 years from now. Take the helicopter over the top of the place, then slowly come down, exploring again like the last time. How does the country look? Who is in it? What are they doing? Do you see the very young and the very old? Where were they?

How was life for them? Did you call on the council office? What are people doing? What were their plans? Do the issues that worry you now seem to have been addressed?

What still needs to be done? Who is meeting the challenges?

Now climb back into your helicopter and take it once more out over the whole region, looking at the hills and valleys, rivers and towns. Bring it slowly back to [wherever you are] and come back to the present time, thinking about all you have seen. (Provide time here to return to the here and now.)

Now, before you forget what it was like, write down the 10 most noticeable things you saw, heard, smelled or touched.

Give the participants five minutes or so to write down the 10 things that stood out for them. If necessary, put some pressure on the participants to go to 10 items—the last two or three may be the most difficult, but often contain the most original ideas.

Next, ask people to rank their 10 ideas or issues in order of importance to them.

There will always be someone who is very practical, or not at all visual, or who has trouble doing the exercise; that's fine. They should be made to feel comfortable and asked to complete the 10 ideas from guesswork or their own experience rather than guided imagery.

Form groups of seven to 12 people around the tables, far enough apart not to disturb each other. Ask each person to write on three cards, in five words or fewer and in big letters people can read across the room, the three most important ideas among their 10. Each person is asked to stick his or her most important card of the three on the whiteboard or wall themselves (note: each participant does this, not the facilitator) and then read out the idea. Others may ask questions of clarification, but they may not offer comments or criticism. Each person should either put his or her card in a group with the others or start a new category. Don't let any of the participants be critical of anyone else's issues, but encourage each person to describe what their card means to them, and people to ask sympathetically what it means to them.

Then take a second round of cards, then the third. No criticism of any contribution is allowed. Short questions of clarification are permitted. Everyone puts their cards wherever they wish, and no one can move another person's card without permission.

When the cards have been collected into a minimum number of strands (probably about three, perhaps five or seven), each strand should be given an imaginative name/title encapsulating the central idea. This then gives the central themes for a sustainable and healthy environment in **********.

In a plenary session of all the groups involved, the themes are then reconciled into a minimum number of sustainability goals for the region (this is surprisingly easy, due to the process participants have shared).

After the themes have been agreed, take another half-hour for everyone to suggest how they would know whether the goals have been achieved. From the cluster of observations around each goal, select one primary indicator and a cluster of sub-indicators for the specific groups.

Outcome: 10-20 primary sustainability goals and their indicators recognisable by all decision-making interests in the region.

Postscript: The strength of the visioning method is that it is inclusive, not competitive: everyone's key goals can find a place. Negotiations can go on 'beyond win-win' to a third possibility that increases everyone's outcomes. The essential basis is that everyone undertaking the exercise belongs to or has an active interest in the place of the vision, and takes a positive view).

References

Abbott, D. 2002, 'Regaining our senses: Conceptual frameworks for environmental health' in *The New Public Health*, ed. F. Baum, Oxford University Press, Melbourne, p. 278

Aslin, H. and Brown, V. 2004, *Towards Whole of Community Engagement: A practical toolkit*, Murray-Darling Basin Commission, Canberra

AtKisson, A. 1999, *Believing Cassandra: An optimist looks at a pessimist's world*, Scribe Publications Pty Ltd, Melbourne

Briggs, D. and Wills, J. 1999, 'Presenting Decision-Makers with Their Choices: Environmental health indicators for NEHAPS' in *Environmental Health for All*, eds D.J. Briggs, R. Stern and T.L. Tinkler, Kluwer Academic Publishers, Dordrecht, pp. 187-201

Brown, V.A. 2001, 'Monitoring Changing Environments in Environmental Health' in *Environmental Health*, vol. 1, no. 1, pp. 21-34

Brown, V.A., Love, D., Griffith, R., Mossfield, A. and Benjamin, M. 2000, *Western Sydney Regional State of the Environment Report 2000* (Text, CD and Web-page), Western Sydney Regional Organisation of Councils, Blacktown www.wsroc.com.au/report/report/report.htm [20 February 2004]

Brown, V.A., Ritchie, J. and Rotem, A. 2001, 'Health Promotion and Environmental Management: A partnership for the future', *Health Promotion International*, vol. 7, no. 3, pp. 219-29

Checkland, P. 1993, *Systems Thinking, Systems Practice*, Wiley, Brisbane

Cole, D.C., Eyles, J. and Gibson, B.L. 1998, 'Indicators of Human Health in Ecosystems: What Do We Measure?', *The Science of the Total Environment*, vol. 224, no. 1, pp. 201-13

Deelstra, T. 1994, *Sustainable Cities for Europe*, International Institute for the Urban Environment, Delft

enHealth Council 1999, *The National Environmental Health Strategy*, Department of Health and Ageing, Canberra

Environment Canada 2002, *National State of the Environment Report*, Environment Canada, Ottowa

Ezzy, D. 2002, *Qualitative analysis: Practice and innovation*, Allen & Unwin, Crows Nest, New South Wales

Funtowicz, S. and Ravetz, J. 1990, *Uncertainty and Quality in Science for Policy*, Kluwer Academic Publishers, Dordrecht

Hamilton, C. 2002, *The Genuine Progress Indicator*, The Australia Institute, Canberra

Hancock, T. 1992, 'Promoting Health Environmentally' in *Supportive Environments for Health*, eds K. Deanard, T. Hancock, World Health Organisation, Copenhagen, p. 14

Harremoës, P., Gee, D., MacGarvin, M., Stirling, A., Keys, J., Wynne, B. and Guedes Vaz, S. eds 2002, *The Precautionary Principle in the 20th Century: Late lessons from early warnings*, Earthscan, London

Kant, E. translated by J.M.D. Meiklejohn 1995, *Critique of Pure Reason*, Alex Catalogue, NetLibrary, Boulder, Colorado

Kolb, D.A., Rubin, M. and McIntyre, J.M. 1974, *Organizational Psychology: An experiential approach*, Prentice Hall, New Jersey

MacDonald, M. 1998, *Agendas for Sustainability: Environment and development into the twenty-first century*, Routledge, London

National Research Council, 1999, *Our Common Journey: A transition towards sustainability*, National Academy Press, Washington

National State of the Environment Advisory Council 1994, *State of the Environment Australia*, Environment Australia, Canberra

Nix, H. 1993, In house seminar, Centre for Resource and Environmental Studies, Australian National University, Canberra

Organisation for Economic Cooperation and Development 1993a, *Core Set of Indicators for Environmental Performance Reviews*, OECD, Paris

—— 1993b, *The State of the Environment*, OECD, Paris

Pimental, D., Tort, M. and D'Anna, L. 1998, 'Ecology of Increasing Disease', *Bioscience*, October, vol. 48, no. 3, p. 10

Wackernagel, M. 2002, pers. comm, *International Sustainability Indicators Network*, www.ISIN.com [5 November 2002]

Wackernagel, M. and Rees, W. 1996, *Our Ecological Footprint: Reducing the human impact on the earth*, New Society Publishers, Gabriola Island, Canada

Western Sydney Regional Organisation of Councils and Brown,V.A., Love, D., Griffiths, R., Powell, J., Murphy, A. and Walmsley, A. 2000, *Western Sydney Regional State of the Environment Report 2000*, WSROC, Blacktown & Regional Integrated Monitoring Centre, University of Western Sydney www.wsroc.com.au/report/report/report.htm [20 February 2004]

World Commission on Environment and Development 1987, *Our Common Future: Report of the World Commission on Environment and Development*, Oxford University Press, New York

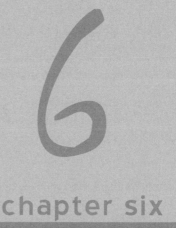

ACTING

chapter six

Practitioners as actors for sustainability and health

Glenda Verrinder, Rosemary Nicholson and Ron Pickett

Summary

Knowing is not enough; we must apply. Willing is not enough; we must do. Goethe

We need to strike a balance between sustaining the integrity of the environment and optimising the health of humans. What action do we need to take? To act for sustainability we need to engage in systems thinking. Acting for sustainability and health is having knowledge of the complexity of environmental, economic and social systems and their subsystems, understanding the interconnectedness of these systems and developing the capacity to interpret the connections. Respecting the diversity of viewpoints and differing interpretations of complex issues is also acting for sustainability and health. We need to understand the principles of sustainability and the processes and protocols to design for sustainability. This chapter continues the D4P4 model's process of 'what can be' and is about what sustainability of the environment and the health of the community mean as a social practice and a way of life. It is about acting for sustainability and health as individuals, as citizens and as public health practitioners and in partnership with others for now and for the future.

Chapter 6 Acting

Practitioners as actors for sustainability and health

Glenda Verrinder, Rosemary Nicholson and Ron Pickett

Key words

Systems thinking, interconnectedness, multiple perspectives, participation, partnerships, planning, acting

Learning outcomes

Public health practitioners and others will become lifelong learners and gain the knowledge and skills to be active participants in a sustainable society. This demands that all practitioners accept the challenge to position themselves at the individual and community level and become capable of enlightened personal action. After studying this chapter public health practitioners and students will be able to:

- identify their personal values in relation to sustainability and health;
- explore the process of thinking systematically in working with complex issues and multiple perspectives;
- demonstrate a capacity to understand the power of organising frameworks that guide action for sustainability and apply them to complex issues;
- demonstrate an understanding of the processes of establishing and working in partnerships;
- apply the principles of planning, implementing and evaluating their work;

- identify and prioritise issues where we can 'think future and act present' by acting locally, individually and collectively;
- engage enthusiastically with the subject material and develop in others a thirst for lifelong learning about sustainability.

Outline

6.1   Systems thinking
6.2   Planning the action
6.3   Acting together
6.4   Acting individually

Learning activities

6.1   Systems thinking: the futures wheel
6.2   Intersectoral action
6.3   Rich pictures or priority setting: nominal group process
6.4   Conflict resolution styles
6.5   Acting individually: do your ecological footprint

Readings

AtKisson, A. 1999, *Believing Cassandra: An Optimist Looks at a Pessimist's World*, Scribe Publications Pty Ltd, Melbourne, Chapter 1

Green Consumer Guide, http://www.thegreen consumerguide.com/ [13 January 2004]

Hancock, T. 2000, 'Healthy Communities Must Also Be Sustainable Communities', *Public Health Reports,* vol. 115, no. 3, pp. 151-6

Nicholson, R., Stephenson, P., Brown, V.A. and Mitchell, K. eds 2001, *Common Ground and Common Sense: Community-based environmental health planning*, Commonwealth of Australia, Canberra, Section 1

6.1 Systems thinking

We have evidence of the changes wrought by human activity and the consequences for the health of humans and other species (McMichael 2001). Globally there has been a call for change in the way we think about these problems and the way we do things (AtKisson 1999; Brown 2002; McMichael 2001; Suzuki 2002; Wilson 2002). We know that what we are doing is not sustainable, but people often feel powerless to do anything about it. Preceding chapters have provided us with a foundation from which we can act for sustainability; this chapter is about acting for sustainability and health as individuals, as citizens, as public health professionals, and in partnership with others.

What do we need to know? What skills do we need and how do we need to think to act individually and collectively, locally and globally now and for the future to achieve an environmentally sustainable, socially equitable, spiritually rich world? First, we need to understand the interconnections between environmental, social and economic systems and their subsystems. These systems are not only connected, but also interdependent. That means 'systems thinking' is required. There are multiple perspectives on what these systems and their interconnections look like, why they exist and how they are experienced. That means we need to understand that sustainability is seen through different lenses at different times by different people and in different places. As practitioners studying and working for sustainability, we have a responsibility to recognise and respect these multiple perspectives so we can identify the opportunities to optimise the health potential of members of the community.

We have evidence of the changes wrought by human activity and the consequences for the health of humans and other species.

Multiple perspectives

Everyone wants to change the world; no one wants to change their mind.

Tolstoy

Personal values

All professionals come to their jobs with a set of personal values that influences how they work. Given that we rarely work in isolation, there are a number of value positions among any workforce, including those arising from ecological and social justice perspectives. As professionals working for sustainability we need to be aware of the range of value positions and recognise that they will influence action. Multiple perspectives are covered in depth in Chapters 2 and 4, so this chapter will briefly discuss two important perspectives in acting for sustainability and health.

Ife (2002) provides a succinct discussion of ecological and social justice perspectives and the relationship between the two. He asserts that both perspectives need to be integrated to bring about a truly sustainable society, and that the ecological perspective does not of itself imply social justice principles.

A major focus for practitioners working for social justice is to challenge structural disadvantage. On one hand, without social justice principles an ecological perspective may reinforce structural disadvantage; on the other, one of the reasons a social justice perspective is inadequate without an ecological perspective is because of the conventional economic prescription for many social problems brought about through economic growth. Practitioners working for sustainability can challenge both the feasibility and desirability of continued growth, which Ife sees as contributing to the current ecological crisis. Both perspectives need to be understood in working toward sustainability.

We must examine our own value positions to incorporate ecological sustainability into our practice.

We must examine our own value positions to incorporate ecological sustainability into our practice. For practitioners, examining our values comes through the process of critical reflection. Ife (2002) refers to one of Marx's sayings, that it is through trying to change society that we come to understand it. The Marxist tradition uses 'praxis' to describe a cycle of doing, learning and critically reflecting. Through this process we achieve a deeper understanding from which we can inform practice and build theory; this in turn creates further understanding of practice, society, social change and values. The values line referred to in earlier chapters is a good example of a way of beginning to examine personal values. Some practitioners put time aside to reflect on their practice, others keep a diary or talk things through with colleagues or friends. Ife suggests that reading widely is also important (Ife 2002). Community values on particular issues will be reflected in policies, social commentaries and through the media. We can also learn a great deal about society, social change and our own values by reflecting on the work of painters, filmmakers, writers and artists of all descriptions.

To gain further insight into the many perspectives public health practitioners and others may encounter in acting for sustainability and health, it is useful to consider:

- cultural, ethnic, generational, historical, regional and national perspectives and philosophies concerning heritage, a sense of place and the influence on the environment;
- the relationship between personal, community and global visions for a sustainable future;
- the processes of planning, policymaking and action for sustainability by governments, businesses, non-government organisations and the community (Wheeler & Perraca Bijur 2000);
- the implications of the political, economic and socio-cultural changes needed to assure a more sustainable future; and that values change over time.

The Triple Bottom Line principle

The triple bottom line (TBL) principle already discussed in Chapters 2 and 5 has entered the language of policymakers. Benchmarks have been established, so action by practitioners will be affected and we need to speak the same language to communicate effectively in partnerships and in reports.

Advancing TBL requires decoupling the focus on resource use, business success and economic gain (or value) and adopting an integrated management system where value is added by sound performance in the immediate and long-term environmental and social (workplace and community) consequences of an operation. Integrating these three dimensions of TBL forms the foundation for effective governance for sustainability. For a corporate body, a government agency or other organisation these dimensions define the scope of their corporate citizenship by highlighting their commitment to long-term social and community issues, biodiversity and ecological integrity as well as economic issues without compromising the needs of future generations.

In systems thinking, these issues are combined not as single entities added to each other but as one entity, based on the thinking that the whole is greater than the sum of its parts—the single bottom line.

The precautionary principle

The precautionary principle ties together the ecological and social justice perspectives discussed earlier. It is one of the key principles of sustainable development, and arises from the notion that we should not have to live with the fear of harm to our health or environment. Further, it serves as

. . . we should not have to live with the fear of harm to our health or environment.

203

a basis for action when incomplete evidence is available. As practitioners working for sustainability we have a responsibility to introduce the concept of precaution and to develop techniques for its inclusion to promote change and to support other principles of sustainability and health.

Definitions of the precautionary principle include the following, from the Intergovernmental Agreement on the Environment (May 1992):

> *Where there are threats of serious or irreversible environmental damage, lack of full scientific certainty should not be used as a reason for postponing measures to prevent environmental degradation. In the application of the precautionary principle, public and private decisions should be guided by (i) careful evaluation to avoid, wherever practicable, serious or irreversible damage to the environment; and (ii) an assessment of the risk-weighted consequences of various options.* (Deville & Harding 1997, p. 13)

The precautionary principle ensures that decisions about new action are made thoughtfully and in the light of potential consequences. Instead of asking what level of harm is acceptable, a precautionary approach asks:

- is the activity, the technology or substance necessary?
- are there alternatives, and are they safer? and
- how much damage can be avoided? (Tickner et al. (nd))

The precautionary principle is beginning to seep into policy documents, legal agreements and economic thinking (Deville & Harding 1997). Bates (1995) proposes that the definition of the principle suggests a fundamental shift in the 'burden of proof' and while the implications of this are open to argument, the precautionary principle has been incorporated into the Intergovernmental Agreement on the Environment and various international agreements such as the Convention on Biological Diversity. Bates (1995) reports that it is being incorporated into statutes and 'may become a general principle of statutory interpretation to be applied to promote the objectives of environmental protection legislation, whether referred to in that legislation or not' (p. 34).

What yardstick do we need to determine whether we go ahead with the activity or the technology? Kirschenmann (1999) suggests we need to consider the magnitude, the geography, the biology and the social cost of the potential harm. The International Council for Local Environmental Initiatives (ICLEI) provides case studies from around the world that demonstrate the precautionary principle in action. These case studies

. . . we have a responsibility to introduce the concept of precaution and to develop techniques for its inclusion to promote change and to support other principles of sustainability and health.

demonstrate that precautionary principle needs to be applied across all sectors because decisions made in one sector will affect other sectors.

The way we think about systems

Implementing the precautionary principle has often meant tackling problems one at a time, but tackling problems in isolation or on an ad hoc basis has its limitations. For example, potential hazards such as pesticides are often addressed individually by agencies rather than as broader issues such as the need to promote sustainable agriculture, non-toxic products or to phase out dangerous chemicals. General systems theory provides a unifying framework where explanatory and analytical tools will help toward good decisions. As Senge says (1992, pp. 6-7):

... tackling problems in isolation or on an ad hoc basis has its limitations.

> *A cloud masses, the sky darkens, leaves twist upward and we know that it will rain. We also know that after the storm the runoff will feed the groundwater miles away, and the sky will grow clear by tomorrow. All these events are distant in time and space, and yet they are all connected within the same pattern. Each has an influence on the rest, an influence that is normally hidden from view. You can only understand the rainstorm by contemplating the whole, not any individual part of the pattern.*

In this chapter we present some of the ways of viewing systems. To act for sustainability and health we need to reflect on our perspectives and consider the human-planetary system and the relationships between its subsystems. The triple bottom line has already been discussed; Burrows et al. (1991) go further and outline social, cultural, belief, political, economic, educational, scientific, technical, biological and ecological subsystems. Box 6.1 shows how these authors separate the human-planetary system using these artificial subsystems. Compare this schema with the one presented in Box 6.2.

Box 6.1 Subsystems

- the *social* system is a complex open system with all people interacting with each other in some way;
- the *cultural* system establishes people's norms and values and is the basis of the social system;
- *belief* systems are linked to cultural systems and set the scene for behaviour patterns;

- the *political* system regulates personal power relationships in a system. For a healthy democracy it is important for a political system to remain open to allcomers with ideas, information and influences;
- the *economic* system regulates the use of human and material resources and the production and exchange of goods and services. Some people act primarily for economic reward;
- the *educational* system provides people with the knowledge, skills and wherewithal they need to live in the other systems and helps shape their belief system;
- the *scientific* system provides us with essential information about how the world works including the other systems within which we live. It helps shape our belief system;
- the *technical* system applies knowledge to the development of products and services. It is closely connected to the scientific and educational system and has an impact on the economic system and social systems, particularly in recent times;
- the *biological* system determines the operation of all living organisms as open systems, able to interact with each other and their environment; and
- the *ecological* system is the open system that includes organisms and their environment, in which there are interactions between individual organisms and their environment.

Source: Burrows et al. 1991, pp. 195-6

Box 6.2 The systemic nature of environmental health issues

Air is the aspect of physical environment that is most prone to global impact. Climate change threatens water supply, food production, spread of disease vectors and biodiversity. Locally, air spreads disease and emits noise. Air pollution affects health regionally and its management must deal with economic and social environments.

Shelter modifies physical environments at the local scale with most immediate links to air and land. Living and working spaces are critical environmental determinants of health. Global patterns of climate influence demand for shelter and regional economics determine the form it takes. Food, water and waste influence health in association with shelter across economic, regional and social environments.

Land use links most closely to local, economic and physical environments and planning separates shelter from waste to protect health. Land use also affects biodiversity regionally, while physical site works affect environments locally. Economic and social factors govern land use and in turn influence food, water and waste. Forestry affects greenhouse and global air quality, while the erosion it causes damages water quality regionally.

Waste affects land locally, water regionally and oceans globally. Cleaner production is an upstream way to manage waste. Waste must be well separated from food and shelter to control vectors and protect health. When mismanaged it affects local and regional air and water quality.

Water determines the distribution of population and influences social environments. Global phenomena determine climate, rainfall and evaporation. Water quality determines food safety and streams support regional migration of waste and agents of disease. Water resources influence land use in physical, local and economic environments; conversely, changes in land use and physical environments affect water quality.

Food is a major commodity. Clean water is critical in the production and processing of safe food and in minimising food-borne disease. Land influences food abundance and safety. Economic growth promotes food packaging and increases waste.

Source: Ireland 1999

The ecological or new public health view of health as 'the pattern that connects' (Kickbusch 1989, p. 50) is another living example of systems thinking, and one that is core to this chapter. Kickbusch described the systemic nature of contemporary public health in terms of:

- disease patterns linked to social inequities and ways of life in industrialised societies;
- health problems that are social rather than medical in nature; and
- health problems that tend to be cumulative, long term, chronic and not amenable to curative measures.

As systemic thinkers we have little interest in 'snapshots' of each component part; we seek instead to develop further our understanding of the inter-relatedness of the world to enable us to solve complex problems. In the words of Bawden (1997, pp. 1-6):

> No matter how much we study the parts of a system in isolation from each other—or even the way various parts are interconnected with each other—we cannot learn (nor therefore predict) the properties of any system as a whole, without studying it in its wholeness!
>
> No matter what you knew about my liver, my kidneys, my brain or whatever else about my body, you could never know about my sense of humour without experiencing 'me' as a whole person! Humour, like the mystery of life itself, is an emergent property.
>
> Whatever you knew about hydrogen and oxygen would not prepare you for the emergent property of 'wetness', which emerges when they combine to form water!

Another way of learning about systems and thinking of the interconnections has been put forward by Wheeler and Perraca Bijur (2000), who present sustainability from five perspectives. They believe that the TBL environmental, social and economic approach continues to promote sustainability as three discrete fields, making the integration into the whole more difficult. The first, 'thinking about and affecting the future', is about looking at a range of possible futures, how various systems might affect those futures and the skills required to affect the future positively. The second is called 'designing sustainable communities'. Communities were chosen because it is from them that people derive a sense of place—and, as the authors point out, a good focus where practitioners can move from reality to abstraction in environmental, social and economic systems. Good design can affect our lives positively. The third theme, 'stewardship of natural resources', is the cornerstone of acting for sustainability and health. It provides learners with an opportunity to learn about the natural world and the impact of activities in our social and economic systems. The fourth theme is 'sustainable economics'. Here, sustainable thinking revolves around economic, intellectual, natural, social and spiritual capitals, and the interaction and enhancement of these that is necessary for sustainable development. Finally, understanding the process of globalisation is necessary if we are to understand how our individual and collective actions can affect those beyond our own communities (Wheeler & Perraca Bijur 2000).

. . . we seek to develop further our understanding of the inter-relatedness of the world to enable us to solve complex problems.

Globalisation

While the negative impacts of globalisation on the environment, human health inequities and sustainability are well established, globalisation also brings a range of opportunities for positive international and collaborative action (Wise 2002). For example, new communication technologies have resulted in the 'democratisation of knowledge' and have opened up unprecedented channels for national and international networking. Already this has resulted in increased scrutiny of international organisations such as the World Bank and the World Trade Organisation. The Earth Dialogues Forum suggests that 'the promotion of universal access to the internet can contribute to knowledge sharing, development, and reducing the marginalisation of isolated communities' and calls for 'procuring IT for poverty alleviation' (Green Cross International 2002, p. 10).

While the negative impacts of globalisation on the environment, human health inequities and sustainability are well established . . .

Over recent years we have seen a strengthening of the environmental and women's movements, and the internationalisation of activism for indigenous and human rights (Wise 2002). We now have the capability to advocate collectively for greater government accountability and policy change, not only at the institutional level but also at national and international levels because it is at these levels that key decisions are made which affect the structural determinants of human health, equity and sustainability. Organisations such as the ICLEI and the International Union for Health Promotion and Education (IUHPE) operate to bring about positive changes toward sustainability and equity in health opportunities.

The themes presented here and those in previous chapters provide practitioners with entry points into multifaceted and complex issues and a way to realise their potential, define their role and think about systems and the connections between them.

Interconnections

Kidner (2000) suggests that the assumption that the human realm is increasingly separate from nature is taken for granted and a central tenet of science, economics, psychology, commonsense and almost every facet of the global commercial system. As humanity continues to remain predominantly disconnected from nature the results of our actions are becoming increasingly evident. On the other hand, Hancock (2000) suggests that somewhere around the middle of the last century a subtle but important shift in our perception of the environment began. He suggests that due to increased scientific and common understanding we came to realise that the environment was not something 'out there', but rather that we are but one species in the web of life. Drengson and Inoue (1995) support Hancock's view by suggesting that we know in our bones that we are not separated from nature, we are moved by its beauty, awed by its power and enchanted by its majesty. Indigenous people across the globe have known this for a long time. We do not wantonly destroy or pollute it, but there is patently a lack of respect for the planet, its creatures and the interactions between them. This has resulted in the destruction of ecosystems and extinction of species and the degradation of our heritage, and is a threat to our health and our existence.

This has resulted in the destruction of ecosystems and extinction of species . . .

The sewerage principle

Kickbusch (1989) attributes the apparently cavalier attitude of communities to their environment to the overwhelming success of the sewerage systems installed in the 19th century. These systems have served us so well that we have until very recently come to take for granted the seemingly limitless capacity of rivers and oceans to absorb as much waste as it suits us to flush away. Now that the system is under stress, Kickbusch (p. 16) laments the widespread belief that:

> *No matter what amount or type of side effect is produced through 'growth' there is an invisible hand and a working system there to receive it and get rid of it. All we do is flush it down and we private citizens as much as industry expect it to disappear and go away . . . Both 'the state' and 'nature' are expected to have an ever-expanding capacity to deal with the side effects of our forms of production, economic growth and ways of life.*

But she then notes (1989, p. 16):

> *There is no away in which to throw things any more. The problems we are faced with . . . have come upon us silently and cumulatively . . . And science has only limited answers. It is part of the problem.*

Science is not the problem, but we have invested in science at the expense of other knowledge such as local knowledge. We need to consider first, the interconnectedness of present and future political, economic, environmental and social issues; second, that there are limits to growth based on a finite supply of resources and the effects of these limits on our social and economic systems; third, the role and interconnection of sub-components (terrestrial, aquatic, marine and atmospheric) of the environmental systems that support life—and including the relationship between abundant, high quality water, soil and air); and fourth, the importance of biodiversity to sustainability of humankind (Wheeler & Perraca Bijur 2000).

WHO estimates that poor environmental quality contributes to 25 per cent of all preventable illnesses (Towards Earth Summit 2002). In an interview after the United Nations Conference on Environment and Development (UNCED) in Rio de Janeiro, Bruntland gave a baseline view of sustainable development: alleviating poverty should be priority number one. Very little else will matter if more than a billion people continue to live in absolute destitution. Only by educating people and giving them a fair chance to break out of poverty can we hope to find a sustainable relationship between population and resources. Otherwise we will be forced by default to continue over-using natural resources. This is what Indira Gandhi meant when she said that 'poverty is the greatest polluter' (Basch 1999, p. 53).

We know that eradicating poverty, changing consumption and production patterns would enable us to address critical sustainability issues and manage health better. We also know this is not new and that what is often lacking is the political will to make the necessary changes. The two questions are: what resources and strategies do we need to establish the change potential, and what systems and structures do we need to deliver change?

WHO estimates that poor environmental quality contributes to 25 per cent of all preventable illnesses . . .

Activity 6.1
Systems thinking: the futures wheel

Aims: by creating futures wheels we can diagnose how developments in one area will automatically lead to developments in other areas. We can begin to visualise how a predicted action or forecast in one area might affect another. Only if all the interacting elements are included in the problem-solving strategy will the solutions be long lasting.

Materials: large sheets of paper and coloured pens

Procedure: First agree as a management group on the issue or problem that is to be faced; for example, an acute rise in water costs, pollution of water supplies or oil dependency.

Brainstorm the impact this may have on other areas; for example, 'less pollution', 'alternative energy,' 'unemployment' and so on. Do a sample futures wheel to test the scope of the issue.

Decide on a forecast selected from the brainstormed list in the centre circle. Treat the forecasting as a creative, open-ended exercise, not a prediction of certainty.

Write down forecasts that will result directly from the initial forecast. Join the second ring of forecasts to the first with 'spokes'. Continue the forecasts out to a third, fourth, fifth ring and so on of forecasts.

When the system seems complete, identify which forecasts are related to each other and circle them in the same colour to identify them. This will demonstrate that the effects of change can be direct and indirect, but still related.

6.2 Planning the action

Having an understanding of the 'big picture' helps practitioners work at the local level. Thinking globally and acting locally has been the mantra for many. Today, the built environment is the principal environment with which people interact directly, and there are both direct and indirect impacts on our health as a result of our relationship with that environment. The built environment is described as part of the overall environment; it encompasses everything that is created or significantly modified by people—including settings such as homes, workplaces and playgrounds, overhead in the form of power lines, underground in the form of waste disposal sites and across the country in the form of highways (Health Canada, in Hancock 2000).

... that modifying the natural and built environments has been and remains a key strategy in the struggle to improve the health of the public.

Hancock reminds us that modifying the natural and built environments has been and remains a key strategy in the struggle to improve the health of the public. At the most basic level the provision of adequate shelter, potable water, air and food have a positive effect on health. However, the negative consequences include indoor air pollution, noise pollution and traffic hazards (Hancock 2000). The indirect health effects are those that come from the consequences of the impact of the built environment on the natural environment. They include diseases that result from the contamination of

Figure 6.1 Futures wheel using 'no oil' as an example

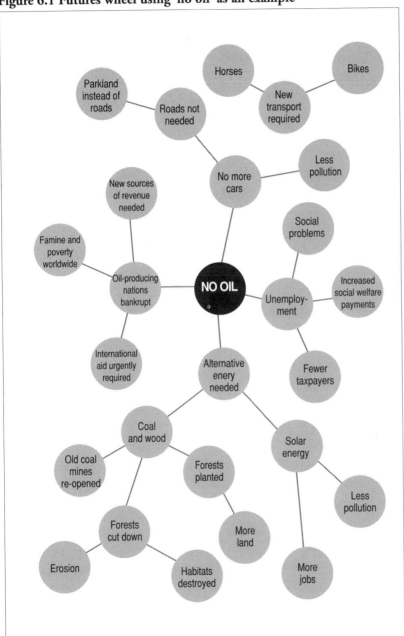

Source: Brown et al. 1995, pp. 206-8

air, food, food webs and water systems. For example, fallout from nuclear power plant disasters such as Chernobyl affected humans, stock and crops. Food web problems have also resulted in BSE in stock. Further the effects, including the health effects, of salinisation due to agricultural methods have yet to be fully felt.

The World Health Organisation (WHO) Healthy Cities project is a long-term international development project that aims to place health high on the agenda of decision-makers in cities throughout the world and to promote comprehensive local strategies for health and sustainable development based on the principles and objectives of the Alma-Ata Declaration and Agenda 21. Ultimately, the Healthy Cities project seeks to enhance the physical, mental, social and environmental wellbeing of people who live and work in cities.

When health is viewed beyond the disease and risk factor paradigm, a healthy community is a sustainable community and has been defined as a community that does not erode the natural capital of the Earth, and whose structure and function result in a harmonious relationship with local, regional and global ecosystems (Federation of Canadian Municipalities, in Hancock 2000).

This chapter encourages practitioners to examine their values and simultaneously develop their knowledge and skills to be active participants in a sustainable society. Each of the skills outlined here is a subject in its own right, so the following section will provide a few signposts public health practitioners can follow in their lifelong learning about acting for sustainability and health. The challenges include strengthening skills in planning, analysis, decision-making, communication, co-operation, conflict management, use of appropriate technologies and deep thinking.

Planning essentials for sustainability

Sound planning is part of a long-term transition to a sustainable future.

Sound planning is part of a long-term transition to a sustainable future. The fundamental tenet for any effective planning is an understanding of the systems involved. Practitioners use a number of planning frameworks in their work; here we outline some of the most common frameworks used for planning action in sustainability. Wheeler and Perraca Bijur (2000) suggest a number of essential planning skills:

- the ability to develop and use scenarios as a tool for strategic planning about sustainable development;

- the ability to create a 'what if' analysis and a systems approach to issues that influence the sustainability of systems of the environment, the economy and social equity; and
- the ability to apply strategic planning and total quality management techniques to actions to achieve sustainability.

A number of documents provide examples of strategic action plans for international, national, regional or local planning, and several have already been identified. The Ottawa Charter for Health Promotion and Agenda 21 discussed in Chapter 3 and the Bellagio Principles (Box 6.3) are all frameworks for action.

The Bellagio Principles serve as guidelines for the whole of the assessment process including the choice and design of indicators, their interpretation and communication of the result. They are inter-related and should be applied as a complete set. They are intended for use in starting and improving assessment activities of community groups, non-government organisations, corporations, national governments, and international institutions. For examples of the principles in action see Hardi and Zdan (1997), who present 10 case studies that demonstrate each principle.

Box 6.3 The Bellagio Principles

Guidelines for practical assessment of progress toward sustainable development

Assessment of progress toward sustainable development should:

Guiding vision and goals

- be guided by a clear vision of sustainable development and goals that define that vision

Holistic perspective

- include review of the whole system as well as its parts
- consider the wellbeing of social, ecological, and economic subsystems, their state as well as the direction and rate of change of that state, of their component parts, and the interaction between parts
- consider both positive and negative consequences of human activity, in a way that reflects the costs and benefits for human and ecological systems, in monetary and non-monetary terms

Essential elements

- consider equity and disparity within the current population and between present and future generations, dealing with such concerns as resource use, over-consumption and poverty, human rights, and access to services, as appropriate
- consider the ecological conditions on which life depends
- consider economic development and other, non-market activities that contribute to human/social wellbeing

Adequate scope

- adopt a time horizon long enough to capture both human and ecosystem time scales, thus responding to needs of future generations as well as those current to short-term decision-making
- define the space of study large enough to include not only local but also long distance impacts on people and ecosystems
- build on historic and current conditions to anticipate future conditions—where we want to go, where we could go

Practical focus

- use an explicit set of categories or an organising framework that links vision and goals to indicators and assessment criteria
- choose a limited number of key issues for analysis
- choose a limited number of indicators or indicator combinations to provide a clearer signal of progress
- use standardising measurement wherever possible to permit comparison, comparing indicator values to targets, reference values, ranges, thresholds, or direction of trends, as appropriate

Openness

- make the methods and data that are used accessible to all
- make explicit all judgments, assumptions and uncertainties in data and interpretations

Effective communication

- be designed to address the needs of the audience and set of users
- draw from indicators and other tools that are stimulating and serve to engage decision-makers

- aim, from the outset, for simplicity in structure and use of clear and plain language

Broad participation

- obtain broad representation of key grass-roots, professional, technical and social groups, including youth, women and indigenous people—to ensure recognition of diverse and changing values
- ensure the participation of decision-makers to secure a firm link to adopted policies and resulting action

Ongoing assessment

- develop a capacity for repeated measurement to determine trends
- be iterative, adaptive and responsive to change and uncertainty because systems are complex and change frequently
- adjust goals, frameworks and indicators as new insights are gained
- promote development of collective learning and feedback to decision-making

Institutional capacity

Continuity of assessing progress toward sustainable development should be assured by:

- clearly assigning responsibility and providing ongoing support in the decision-making process
- providing institutional capacity for data collection, maintenance and documentation
- supporting development of local assessment capacity.

Source: Hardi and Zdan 1997

Local Agenda 21

The 1992 Rio Earth Summit developed Agenda 21, a detailed guide for governments on establishing environmental policies for sustainable development into the 21st century. Agenda 21 identifies 39 action areas, each with an associated set of objectives and activities. Chapter 28 of the document calls on local governments around the world to initiate a Local Agenda 21 based on:

- *consultation and consensus building* with citizens, local, civic, community, business and industrial organisations: Local Agenda 21 requires that local councils create conditions and mechanisms for inputs into policy formulation from a range of local interest groups, and in particular those generally excluded from the decision-making process (such as women and youth);

- *stakeholder dialogues:* local authorities need to enter into dialogue with citizens, local organisations and private enterprise to develop shared perceptions and negotiated agreements on prioritised action programs for problem solving;

- the use of *shared knowledge* to analyse problems and design policy options; this may involve workshops, meetings, focus groups, surveys and so on. Creation of this shared knowledge is inevitably resource-intensive;

- *comprehensiveness:* in terms of issues to be tackled in different economic and social sectors, and timelines for action plans on different issues;

- *joint implementation:* this requires participating groups to play more than just an advocacy role. There is also an expectation that they commit resources towards the implementation of agreed solutions; and

- *cross-border networking:* networking at national, regional and international levels facilitates the reframing of local interests to globally sharable long-term objectives. Adapted from Barrett and Usui (2002), Local Agenda 21 is promoted internationally by ICLEI, who provide case studies to demonstrate these action areas. To view these studies go to http://www.iclei.org/.

The WHO Healthy Cities project

A healthy city is . . . one that improves its environment and expands its resources so people can support each other in achieving their highest potential.

The WHO Healthy Cities project began in Europe in 1987. Whereas Local Agenda 21 provides a framework for local action toward sustainability, the primary concern of Healthy Cities is human health. A healthy city is described by WHO (1992, in Chu & Simpson 1994) as one that improves its environment and expands its resources so people can support each other in achieving their highest potential. While each project will necessarily differ according to the cultural norms, needs and characteristics of the locality, all share the six process characteristics of commitment to health, political decision-making, intersectoral action, community participation, innovation and healthy public policy (Chu & Simpson 1994).

WHO (Chu & Simpson 1994) specifies 11 outcomes for which a healthy city should strive:

1. A clean, safe physical environment.

2. An ecosystem that is stable now and sustainable in the long term.

3. A strong, mutually supportive and non-exploitative community.

4. A high degree of participation and control by the public over the decisions affecting their lives, health and wellbeing.

5. The meeting of basic needs (food, water, income, safety and work).

6. Access to a wide variety of experience and resources, with the chance for a wide variety of contact, interactions and communication.

7. A diverse, vital and innovative city economy.

8. The encouragement of connectedness with the past, with the cultural and biological heritage of city dwellers and with other groups and individuals.

9. A form that is compatible with and enhances the preceding characteristics.

10. An optimum level of appropriate public health and sick care services accessible to all.

11. High health status.

For a recent update of healthy cities in action internationally visit the website of the World Health Organisation Regional Office for Europe http://www.euro.who.int/healthy-cities.

Local Agenda 21 and the WHO Healthy Cities project, while differing in focus, share similar process elements in that both:

- focus on local government;
- are predicated on community participation; and
- involve planning frameworks that integrate technical and scientific data with qualitative measures of, for example, community perception of health and environmental issues.

The following case study provides an example of how action for sustainability and health can be taken in a city.

Box 6.4 Rural City Farm: cultivating a vital urban community

City Farm is a youth project run under the auspices of Men in Trees and promotes healthy urban communities and environments. City Farm is a non-profit organisation that is involved in a range of sustainability issues including community development, land reclamation, organic food production and waste management.

City Farm transformed a derelict scrap metal yard into a thriving community garden a 15-minute walk from the central business district. There is a strong focus on social issues, providing a positive space for many of Perth's youth, and the farm adopts permaculture principles. It began as a youth centre that promoted environmental awareness through information, education, networking and action. Now staff and volunteers take responsibility for the day-to-day tasks of feeding the animals and watering the gardens. This egalitarian ethic can be observed in its democratic approach to decision-making, with all volunteers having a voice on management issues.

Source: Strange 2002

There are planning principles in which people can work at any level. Each planning framework speaks to practitioners in different ways depending on the circumstances. It is useful to know not only what the processes are but also what the documents look like at each of the local, regional or provincial, national and global planning levels. We need go no further than *Grass Roots and Common Ground* (Brown et al. 2001) and the *Planning and Evaluation Wizard* (South Australian Community Health Research Unit nd) for excellent resources for planning at the local level. For regional or provincial planning see *Hope for the Future: The Western Australia State Sustainability Strategy* (Government of Western Australia 2003) as an example. The WHO Healthy Cities website gives practitioners step-by-step assistance in planning a healthy city as well as providing excellent examples from around the world.

Activity 6.2

Intersectoral action

You are a public health practitioner who has been asked by the local government manager of health services at the municipality in which you work to help gather a team of people together to develop a municipal public health plan. Imagine the people sitting around the table in the boardroom at the municipal offices. Write down which sectors need to be represented and why.

Analysis

An integrated approach to the planning process requires that practitioners have analysis skills for planning, evaluation, research and other organising activities. Wheeler and Perraca Bijur (2000) suggest these include skills where practitioners are able first to frame appropriate questions for research; and second, to use and create models that define and describe the interactions in and between environmental, social and economic systems and predict probable interactions and outcomes.

Frame appropriate questions for research

The research question has been likened to a door to the research field under study. It serves to circumscribe an essential area of a more complex field (Flick 1998). Careful formulation of the question is fundamental to sound research design. The research question essentially gives purpose to the research. It determines the focus of the study; for example, knowledge, attitudes, awareness, behaviour change or longer-term changes to the environment or to human health. The question also influences the choice of method, ensures the appropriateness and meaningful interpretation of data and serves as a basis for determining what to leave out and what to include in a study. The proficient researcher sets precise and clearly stated questions while remaining open to new or surprising results.

Models that define and describe the interactions in and between environmental, social and economic systems

The following model represents a framework for environment and health by overlaying the scales of health impact over the social, physical and economic aspects of the environment (Figure 6.2). Six focal areas of environmental health (air, shelter, land, waste, water and food) are then introduced as a way of grounding the framework in real world issues; what emerges is an integrated whole (Figure 6.3).

A chequerboard model (Figure 6.4) is a useful organisational tool with which to represent integrated action for sustainability. The model places experience on the outer rim then links this to practice at the next level in, introducing policy to guide practice. Finally it focuses on action, placing problem-solving at the centre of learning. Sometimes there are no precedents to follow, so learning becomes a core skill in addressing problems of sustainability.

Figure 6.2 Windows on environment and health

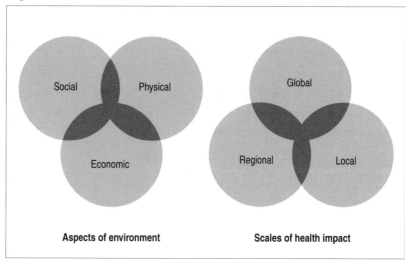

Source: Ireland 1999

Figure 6.3 Grounding the environment for health

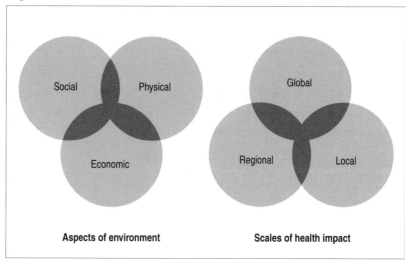

Source: Ireland 1999

Interventions dealing with any one of the six focal areas illustrated in Figures 6.3 and 6.4 begin with an experience that gives rise to concern. Current best practice points to a way forward, policy guides choice of alternatives and action follows. Ultimately the actor for sustainability must

Figure 6.4 A chequerboard model of integrated action for sustainability

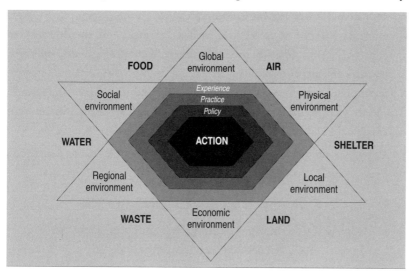

Source: Ireland 1999

find balance in the integrated whole. Finding this balance is where problem-based learning becomes a way of working together. It proceeds in repeating cycles of plan-act-reflect-learn (introduced by Kolb in the 1970s).

Other skills that may be needed by practitioners include being able to:

- map systems (environmental, economic and social) behaviour focusing on cause and effect and change over time;
- create concept maps and timelines describing environmental, social and economic systems;
- observe and identify patterns occurring in the natural (environmental), human built (social) and abstract (economic) realms;
- identify data needs and develop appropriate data acquisition protocols; and
- analyse, interpret, map and summarise common and disparate sets of data. (Wheeler & Perraca Bijur 2000)

Use of appropriate technology

A range of technological skills will be needed in relation to these last five points to act for sustainability. Working collaboratively is an excellent way of pooling expertise and maximising the potential of the team. In a mutually supportive environment the team will be able to use:

- a range of resources and technologies to gather and analyse information, address and define driving questions;
- a wide range of technologies, including email and the Internet to effectively communicate and co-ordinate with peer groups, mentors, teachers and the community;
- appropriate mapping technologies (such as GIS or remote sensing) and visualisation techniques (such as inspiration and strategic questioning); and
- software tools such as the Ecological Footprint Calculator (Redefining Progress nd).

Activity 6.3

Rich pictures or priority-setting: nominal group process
http://allenandunwin.com/sustainhealth

The nominal group process is a means of decision-making that enables all group members to have an equal voice.

The nominal group process is a means of decision-making that enables all group members to have an equal voice. 'Nominal' refers to a set of items listed in order of preference and 'group' to the use of group members to agree on the order. The method consists of a series of small-group procedures designed to compensate for the usual inequalities of social power that emerge in most planned meetings. Those who use the method should keep in mind that its purpose is to identify and rank problems, not to solve them.

The method is effective for generating ideas and gaining equal participation from group members. It is not a means of clarifying values, nor is it a decision-making strategy; it is a method for arriving at informed agreement as to priorities. The method works as follows.

Arrange the participants into groups of six to seven members: it is important that the size does not exceed seven, to allow for appropriate interaction. Participants should be representative of and knowledgeable about the community or task in question.

Pose a single question to the group, summarising the issue: it is best if the question can be in writing on a black/whiteboard, flip chart or handout sheet. The question should be generated following consideration of:

- the objective of the meeting;
- examples of the type of items sought;

- the development of alternative questions; and
- the pilot testing of alternative questions with a sample group.

Examples of the type of question are: 'of all the topics we could include in this program, which do you consider the most central?' or 'of all possible avenues for action on environmental health management, which do you consider is the most valuable?'

Have the participants of each small group write down their responses: sheets of paper with the question written at the top can be given out; this provides an easy reference point for the group members. If this is not possible, display the question on a blackboard, flip chart or using an overhead projector. Although the actual amount of time necessary to complete this assignment will vary depending on the question posed, it should take about 15 minutes. It is important that the group proceed in silence (this is the responsibility of the facilitator), to enable the group to reflect carefully on its ideas and to be involved in a competition-free atmosphere.

The facilitator elicits individual responses: first, one participant is asked to give his or her most important single response; this continues until each participant has contributed a single response. As the responses are stated they are written down by the facilitator on a blackboard or flip chart, each item being given a number. The same process is repeated until all contributions have been recorded. This procedure enables each group member to play a truly participating role. Discussion is only permitted for points of clarification, and not on the form, format or meaning or value of a participant's response.

Clarify the meaning of the responses: take time to ask if each response is clearly understood. Allow participants time to discuss what they meant by a particular response, the logic behind it, even its relative importance. This is not the time for debate or lobbying; the facilitator must direct proceedings so only clarification takes place.

Conduct a preliminary vote: from the original listing of responses on the blackboard or flip chart, participants are directed to select a stated number of the items they consider are the most important (for example, out of the summary of 20 individual responses, each participant is to select and rank seven). This is accomplished by asking each participant to write each of the statements on a separate card first, then rank-ordering them. The topics can be pulled together by group agreement on priorities or numerically (seven points would be assigned to the most important). As a rule of thumb, group members can prioritise only five to nine items with some degree of reliability. The item with the largest numerical total represents the top priority issue.

Confirm the vote: it is important to discuss the various explanations related to choosing. Discussion regarding the high and low vote-getters may be of value, and it may be useful to redefine the meaning of selected items to be sure all group members are clear on their meaning. Identify and value the various perspectives and discuss how they can be illuminated in a review.

Source: Nicholson et al. 2001

6.3 Acting together

Decision-making processes

'Participation is a keystone of the new public health, but achieving increased participation in public decision-making and in public health endeavors is difficult in complex societies.'

'Participation is a keystone of the new public health, but achieving increased participation in public decision-making and in public health endeavors is difficult in complex societies' (Baum 2002, p. 342). The positive impact of participation on health has been acknowledged in WHO documents such as the Ottawa Charter for Health Promotion. Researchers across the globe (Putnam in the United States, Veenstra and Lomos in Canada, Cox in Australia and Gillies in the United Kingdom) are among many who argue that investment in the social fabric of society is as important as other forms of capital investment and that participation in decision-making processes is a critical part of developing social capital. There are two beliefs that connect the importance of participation and health. First, participation overcomes individual and collective powerlessness, which contributes to health; and second, participation in health initiatives improves their relevance, effectiveness and quality (Baum 2002, pp. 342-9).

Participatory democracy

Democracy means rule by the people, and in participatory democracy 'the people' participate directly in decision-making in contrast to representative democracy, where 'the people' elect representatives to participate in decision-making on their behalf. The key characteristics of participatory democracy include decentralisation, accountability, education and obligation (Ife 2002). This means:

- opportunities must be created so 'bottom up' decisions are made;
- the people are not only responsible for making decisions but also for those decisions being carried out;
- the people must be adequately equipped to make informed decisions; and
- participation is an obligation, not just a right (Ife 2002).

Participatory democracy is also known as community participation, empowerment, community development or capacity building. There are many models, schemas and typologies that outline the principles necessary for healthy participation and others that describe the types and approaches. The International Association of Public Participation (nd) (Box 6.5) developed a spectrum of participation and Arnstein (1969) addresses the important issue of power sharing in her schema in Box 6.6.

Participatory democracy is also known as community participation, empowerment, community development or capacity building.

Power sharing is the key issue. It is important to recognise and be transparent about what type of participation is being sought so that expectations are understood. People will participate in decision-making under the right conditions. Ife (2002) submits that people will participate if they feel the issue or activity is important; they will be more likely to act if they have identified the issue or activity of importance, using a bottom-up approach to decision-making. Consciousness raising may need to take place, and people must also feel their individual and collective contributions will make a difference. Achievable goals are also necessary, as are different forms of participation, resources such as transport and consideration of things such as time and location. Finally, structures and processes must not be alienating. Knowledge, skills and confidence in participating may need to be developed over time.

People need to be involved in identifying needs, planning action, implementing the plans and evaluating the processes. Bierle (1999) proposes a framework that evaluates the outcomes of participatory processes using a set of 'social' goals. These goals are: educating the public; incorporating public values, assumptions and preferences into decision-making; increasing the substantive quality of decisions; fostering trust in institutions; reducing conflict; and making decisions cost effectively.

Box 6.5 Spectrum of participation

INFORM	CONSULT	INVOLVE	COLLABORATE	EMPOWER
Public participation goal	**Public participation goal**	**Public participation goal**	**Public participation goal**	**Public participation goal**
To provide the public with balanced and objective information to assist them in understanding the problems, alternatives and/or solutions.	To obtain public feedback on analysis, alternatives and/ or decisions.	To work directly with the public throughout the process to ensure that public issues and concerns are consistently understood and considered.	To partner with the public in each aspect of the decision, including the development of alternatives and the identification of the preferred solution.	To place final decision-making in the hands of the public.
Promise to the public	**Promise to the public**	**Promise to the public**	**Promise to the public**	**Promise to the public**
We will keep you informed.	We will keep you informed, listen to and acknowledge concerns and provide feedback on how public input influenced the decision.	We will work with you to ensure that your concerns and issues are directly reflected in the alternatives developed and provide feedback on how public input influenced the decision.	We will look to you for direct advice and innovation in formulating solutions and incorporate your advice and recommendations into the decisions to the maximum extent possible.	We will implement what you decide.
Example tools	**Example tools**	**Example tools**	**Example tools**	**Example tools**
• fact sheets • websites • open houses	• public comment • focus groups • surveys • public meetings	• workshops • deliberate polling	• citizen advisory committees • consensus building	• citizen juries • ballots • delegated decisions

Source: International Association of Public Participation (nd)

Box 6.6 Approaches to participation

	Citizen control	Citizens have absolute control over programs—but do they have the resources for their project to succeed?
Degrees of citizen power	Delegated power	Citizens have the majority of decision-making power
	Partnership	Power sharing between citizens and power-holders
	Placation	Giving a few people power, but they can be outvoted because they are outnumbered on committees and so on
Degrees of tokenism	Consultation	Asking people's opinions, but no responsibility to act on what they say
	Informing	People are told about changes
Non-participation	Therapy	People are involved in group activities to change their behaviour
	Manipulation	people are placed on committees to enlist their support

Source: Arnstein 1969

People need to be involved in identifying needs, planning action, implementing the plans and evaluating the processes.

The Cs in participation

Constructs, collaboration and co-operation skills

In the preceding chapters we examined the different perspectives practitioners encounter in working towards sustainability and health. These perspectives shape the successes and challenges of participation in decision-making.

Collaboration and co-operation are the norm in some cultures, while in others competition appears to be the norm. Capitalism fosters competition and the institutions in capitalist society assume a competitive ethic. There is competition in employment and education; graded examinations in subjects from music to mathematics, and competitions in everything from rock climbing to chess.

There can be no community without some level of commitment to co-operation, however, and research on animal behaviour and human evolution (Kropotkin 1972, in Ife 2002) suggests that co-operation is the norm and the dynamic that has led to progress and success for human and animal societies (Ife 2002). Practitioners should therefore seek to challenge the dominance of the competitive ethic. They need to be able to develop co-operative strategies for action and develop shared visions about the future. Some of the strategies include building trust, building teams and building community competence. Box 6.7 provides examples of how practitioners can encourage participation in planning. Some of these techniques such as questionnaire development, conducting focus groups and the analysis of the information derived from these are part of qualitative research methods, and social scientists, who are familiar with them, would be valuable members of the planning team.

Box 6.7 Twenty participatory techniques in participatory evaluation

Rich pictures: a pictorial representation of all of the things that need to be considered

Brainstorming: gain a lot of ideas quickly without getting bogged down in detail

Visualising: a shared vision of the outcome

Questionnaires: gain information from a large number of people in a structured way

Mind-mapping: see links between clusters of ideas to consider all aspects

Cause and effect mapping: separate root causes of problems from symptoms

Historical analysis: maps change and provides a context for the current situation

Locality mapping: draws on local knowledge about the area

Focus groups: general information on an issue is obtained from specific group/s

Semi-structured interviewing: guided conversations on broad issues

Flow diagrams: illustrates and analyses consequences of certain issues and/or actions

SWOT analysis: identifies strengths, weaknesses, opportunities and threats

Institutional linkage diagrams: interactions between organisations on particular issues

Information tabulation and graphing: for comprehension and easy analysis

Matrix analysis: ranking the value of a particular activity according to a set of criteria

Issue analysis: thematic analysis of information from a range of sources

Delphi technique: cluster, organise, rank information

Inter-relationship diagrams: what causes are the most important and how do they relate

Nominal group technique: rank a list of problems, issues or actions

Action planning: identify specific responsibilities and resources to achieve an objective

Source: Woodhill and Robins 1998, pp. 45-53

Consensus

Consensus is built differently in different cultures: in some cultures it is the norm; in others it is not. It is 'the most acceptable solution for all' (Heron 1999, p. 89). That is, to reach a consensus, groups need to agree on a course of action that best meets the needs of the whole group. The decision may not be the preferred option of some, but diversity is respected and commitments are made to the action. It is a time-consuming commitment and it is likely to be difficult. Expertise is needed in the process of talking the issues through and so practitioners need skills in listening, empathising, reframing and communication (Ife 2002).

Communication skills

Fundamentally, a practitioner acting for sustainability and health needs to be able to:

- communicate information and viewpoints effectively; and
- be fluent in the language of systems to describe the various constructs and processes to others who have different perspectives (Wheeler & Perraca Bijur 2000).

Effective verbal and non-verbal communication requires highly developed interpersonal skills as well as knowledge about communication patterns in and between communities, speaking to varied audiences and writing for different purposes. Practitioners need to be able to apply the overall principles and processes to local and regional issues to establish a sense of ownership, involvement and a sense of place. *Common Ground and Common Sense* (Nicholson et al. 2001) provides practitioners with excellent guidelines for communicating in communities. The personal skills required include the ability to:

We need to be able to work toward negotiated consensus and co-operative resolution of conflict . . .

- ensure that the conversation is one of genuine dialogue and not a game of power and control;
- create and maintain an atmosphere of mutual trust and acceptance;
- be aware of cultural differences and sensitivities in communication;
- listen carefully;
- state one's message clearly using language that is readily understood;
- keep a conversation focused and directed where necessary;
- be aware of the other person's time constraints and priorities;
- be aware of the importance of the physical environment; and
- encourage the other to reflect on the implications of what is being discussed (Ife 2002, p. 240).

Conflict management

We need to be able to work toward negotiated consensus and co-operative resolution of conflict, so it is advisable to explore causes of conflict and forms of conflict resolution. At various times there may be tension due to unclear expectations, broken agreements, irrational outbursts, conflicting agendas and so on. Classic conflict resolution techniques include controlled discussion, role reversal, hidden agenda counselling and co-operative problem solving (Heron 1999):

- Controlled discussion is designed to get combatants listening to each other. The facilitator umpires an exchange of views. There are two rules: each person makes only one point at a time, and each person restates the point to the other's satisfaction before replying.
- Role reversal: the facilitator umpires an exchange of views with each person taking the other person's position.
- Hidden agenda counselling: ask each person to state what he or she needs from the other by addressing an empty chair: this can uncover a hidden agenda that has nothing to do with the current situation.
- Co-operative problem solving: the facilitator takes people through the diagnosis, treatment and follow-up problem-solving cycle. Each person must state clearly what the problem is, to what degree each is responsible and if there are any other causes. Possible solutions are identified and an appropriate action plan including an evaluation of the plan is agreed on.

It is useful for practitioners to be aware of their preferred style of conflict resolution and what works best in different contexts.

It is useful for practitioners to be aware of their preferred style of conflict resolution and what works best in different contexts. *Common Ground and Common Sense* (Nicholson et al. 2001) provides excellent guidelines and activities, recreated in this book.

> **Activity 6.4**
> **Conflict resolution styles**
> http://www.allenandunwin.com/sustainandhealth

AtKisson's action guide

A strong argument for reconnecting ourselves to the web of life and acting for sustainability and health is provided by AtKisson (1999). He offers some pathways for examining and acting on changes at local, national and global scales and has developed a prototype city monitoring system for progress toward sustainable development, Sustainable Seattle, which has become a classic tool; established COMPASS, a monitoring system; and his book *Believing Cassandra* (1999) provides case studies of individual approaches to change. The following is one of these.

> **Box 6.8 The transformation of Curitiba, Brazil: a story from**
> *Believing Cassandra*
>
> Curitiba transformed itself into one of the most liveable cities in the
> world. The transformation began one weekend when the road in a major
> city shopping block was removed and became a car free zone, pedestrian
> mall and garden. It was such a popular move that Curitiba citizens wanted
> to extend this space. Since then a space-age-looking bus system transports
> people around the city on dedicated avenues. The old buses are used as
> mobile schools that visit poor neighbourhoods. In return for sacks of
> garbage, the citizens in these neighbourhoods receive food and vocational
> training and also advice from experts about how to improve and beautify
> their houses and surroundings. Bus routes are also connecting poorer
> neighbourhoods to new industrial estates that have been designed to have
> green space. Children are hired as gardeners in the newly created parks.
> The ideas are generated by citizens from different disciplines in charettes
> (brainstorming sessions). The transformation has been done on a low
> budget and made possible through creativity, ingenuity and passion. The
> city is less polluted, more convenient, more efficient, more prosperous and
> more humane.
> *Source:* AtKisson 1999, p. 159

In Chapter 1 AtKisson gives three conditions for the physical survival of the
human species. The underlying principles from that natural step process are:

- not using up renewable natural resources faster than they can replenish
  themselves;
- investing ahead to develop replacements for depleted non-renewable
  resources while we still have the wealth from using the resources; and
- not producing wastes faster than natural processes can absorb them.

AtKisson points out that mere physical survival is not enough; humanely
governed sustainable development is required for survival to be worthwhile.
He recommends we need to:

- redesign, rebuild and rethink our cities, industries, transport systems and
  educational programs — this will require transformational thinking;
- decouple development from production, consumption and pollution
  and link it to learning, improving, rebuilding and reorganising; and
- incorporate sustainable practices in living, in business and as a community.

These actions fit well with the frameworks for action discussed in this and previous chapters. For public health professionals the Ottawa Charter for Health Promotion outlined in Chapter 3 will be more familiar. This charter has five action areas that have helped practitioners to plan for change and are consonant with the messages of AtKisson. Building healthy public policy and providing supportive environments means that policies must be developed that protect the natural and built environment; developing personal skills means turning change into routine behaviour; reorienting health services means that protecting the environment and promoting health is everybody's business; and nothing will be sustainable without strengthening community action. We have already seen, for example, a reduction in the use of chlorofluorocarbons and other ozone-depleting substances with commensurate structural and individual change to reduce exposure to ultraviolet radiation. The major ozone-depleting substances include chlorofluorocarbons, halons and methyl bromide, used in many industries. Global consumption of these substances is now limited by the Montreal Protocol on Substances that Deplete the Ozone Layer. Accumulation of ozone-depleting substances is now declining slowly.

There are key issues for people who want to and have the opportunity to be responsible consumers.

6.4 Acting individually

Acting collectively may help us also to act individually. We can become active and work in the ways described and we can make changes in our own lives, the lives of those around us and those that may follow us. Population and consumption are the key global threats in the developed world at least, where the economic imperative threatens ecological sustainability. As Carlyle says:

> *Each of us, every day, makes decisions that affect how the future will look back at us. A collection of small decisions like pebbles that build in number until they gather the momentum of an avalanche. Starting from when we get out of bed, we decide whether to put the heater or air conditioner on, what to wear, what to have for breakfast, how to get to work, how to spend lunchtime, what to shop for . . . these small decisions made by more than a billion people all over the developed world have ramifications that can affect the world economic order, the state of Third World debt, the future of ecosystems and the global climate.* (Carlyle, in Heycox 1991, p. 126)

There are key issues for people who want to and have the opportunity to be responsible consumers. Elkington and Hailes (1988) provide some useful tips. They suggest avoiding products likely to endanger a person's health; cause significant damage to the environment or use a disproportionate amount of energy at any stage of manufacture, use or disposal; cause unnecessary waste; use materials from threatened species or environments; or adversely affect other species or people in other countries. We need to become informed consumers. As John Stuart Mill said:

> *I do not know why it should be a matter for congratulation that persons who are already richer than anyone else needs to be should have doubled their means of consuming things which give little or no pleasure except as representation of wealth.* (Mill 1857, in Burrows et al. 1991, p. 5)

Ultimately, each practitioner may need to strike a balance between his or her principles and those of others. Ethics, it has been said, 'are the foundation upon which legal, institutional and other facets of sustainable development should be built' (Green Cross International 2002, p. 6). In Box 6.9, Soskolne and Light (1996) provide environmental epidemiologists with ethical guidelines for practice. Other practitioners may find some or all of these useful as well.

Box 6.9 Ethical guidelines for practice

Obligations to research participants

- Respect the rights and personal autonomy of all
- Advise of both individual and collective benefits and harms from proposed research
- Protect their welfare
- Obtain informed consent whenever feasible
- Protect privacy/maintain confidentiality
- Use data and specimens for only the purpose(s) for which consent was provided

Obligations to society

- Avoid partiality
- Distinguish one's role as a scientist from that of an advocate
- The public interest always takes precedence over any other interest

- Be objective in disseminating research findings and be understandable in public discussions
- Involve communities being proposed for study throughout all stages of research and its reporting
- Engage with other disciplines to advance and maximise the public utility of environmental epidemiology• Consider the broader social consequences, including psychosocial and physical health outcomes
- Consider equity and remediation in the allocation of resources applied to environmental epidemiology research across the different areas of research, social strata and jurisdictions
- Environmental epidemiology findings are based on uncertainty and must be used appropriately in their application to, for example, the development of risk analysis, policy and interventions
- Be diligent in executing professional responsibilities

Obligations to sponsors and employers
- Ensure both researcher and sponsor/employer are apprised of each other's respective responsibilities and expectations
- Emphasise obligations to other parties
- Protect privileged information, but release research methods, procedures and results

Obligations to colleagues
- Promote rigour in research design and neutrality in the execution of research
- Report and publish methods and results in the peer-reviewed literature of all studies, regardless of whether the findings are positive, negative or have no effect
- Confront unacceptable behaviour and conditions
- Communicate ethical requirements

Obligations across all the above-named groups
- Consult with stakeholders, including community members
- Avoid conflicting interests and partiality
- Pursue responsibilities with due diligence
- Communicate findings in publicly understandable ways

Source: Soskolne and Light 1996

Deep thinking

This chapter encourages practitioners to improve their knowledge of multiple perspectives and systems thinking and strengthen a number of skills, including their deep thinking skills. Chapter 2 explored a number of philosophical frameworks that provide us with information about the value positions people may bring, and there are plenty of conceptual frameworks from which we can draw inspiration for action. This brings us back to the beginning. Deep ecology, for example, is one way of rethinking sustainability. The principles from deep ecology may be a platform from which we take action. Drengson (Drengson & Inoue 1995, p. 157) suggests there are three purposes to this rethinking:

- it can provide a firm philosophical grounding for activism;
- it can encourage decision-makers to connect philosophical and religious assertion with concrete policy; and
- it can be used to get as many people as possible to think about themselves and nature in a new way. Philosopher, ecologist and founding father of the deep ecology movement, Naess is reported as talking about the tendencies among the supporters of deep ecology to:

Using simple means; anti consumerism; appreciation of ethnic and cultural differences; efforts to satisfy vital needs rather than desires; going for depth and richness of experience rather than intensity; attempts to live in nature and promote community rather than society; appreciating all life forms; efforts to protect local ecosystems; protecting wild species in conflicts with domestic animals; acting non violently . . . concern about the situation of the third and fourth world and the attempt to avoid a standard of living too much different from and higher than the needy. Global solidarity lifestyles; appreciation of lifestyles, which are universable, which are not blatantly impossible to sustain without injustice towards fellow humans or other species

(Naess, in Sessions 1995, p. 61)

This requires a different approach from the way we do business now. These actions spell out the principles that underpin the social and ecological perspectives discussed earlier in the chapter and that provide the foundation from which we can act for sustainability and health.

Dauncey in *Stormy Weather* (2001) provides us with solutions for individuals, citizens' organisations, cities and towns, businesses, energy companies, automobile companies, state and national governments, developing countries and for the planet as a whole. Box 6.10 provides us with ten solutions for individuals as an example.

Box 6.10 Climate change: ten solutions for individuals

- grasp the big picture
- travel more sustainably
- if you must use a car, switch to the most fuel-efficient model
- choose energy efficient appliances
- make your home more efficient
- use the sun's energy
- buy green power
- switch to a more organic vegetarian diet
- invest in solar funds
- live more sustainably

Source: Dauncey 2001

**Activity 6.5
Acting individually: measure your ecological footprint
http://www.allenandunwin/sustainhealth**

Conclusion

In this chapter we have suggested that because we live in a complex world, practitioners will need to understand the importance of systems thinking to act for sustainability and health. In a complex world there will be multiple perspectives and the first perspective to identify is our own. Practitioners may have responsibility working in partnerships to guide action and therefore an understanding of organising frameworks that can be applied to complex issues is needed. Regardless of the place, the people and the time, the values, principles and action frameworks outlined in this chapter can support relevant and achievable action for sustainability.

References

Arnstein, S.R. 1969, 'A Ladder of Citizen Participation', *Journal of the American Institute of Planners,* vol. 35, no. 1, pp. 216-24

AtKisson, A. 1999, *Believing Cassandra: An optimist looks at a pessimist's world,* Scribe Publications Pty Ltd, Melbourne

Barrett, B. and Usui, M. 2002, 'Local Agenda 21 in Japan: Transforming local environmental governance', *Local Environment,* vol. 7, no. 1, pp. 49-67

Basch, P.F. 1999, *Textbook of International Health,* Oxford University Press, New York

Bates, G.M. 1995, *Environmental Law in Australia,* Butterworths, Sydney

Baum, F. 2002, *The New Public Health: An Australian perspective,* Oxford University Press, South Melbourne

Bawden, R. 1997, 'Systems Thinking for the Systemic Age', *ABN Newsletter,* pp. 1-6

Bierle, T. 1999, 'Using Social Goals to Evaluate Public Participation', *Policy Studies Review,* vol. 16, no. 3/4, pp. 76-103

Brown, L. 2002, *Eco-Economy: Building an economy for the earth,* W.W. Norton and Co., New York

Brown, V., Ingle Smith, D., Wiseman, R. and Handmer, J. 1995, *Risks and Opportunities,* Earthscan, London

Brown, V.A., Stephenson, P.H., Nicholson, R., Bennet, K.A. and Smith, J. 2001, *Grass Roots and Common Ground,* University of Western Sydney, Richmond, New South Wales

Burrows, B.C., Mayne, A.J. and Newbury, P. 1991, *Into the 21st Century: A handbook for a sustainable future,* Adamantine Press, Twickenham

Chu, C. and Simpson, R. 1994, *Ecological Public Health: From vision to practice,* Joint Publication of Centre for Health Promotion, University of Toronto and Institute of Applied Environmental Research, Griffith University, Brisbane

Dauncey, G. 2001, *Stormy Weather: 101 solutions to global climate change,* New Society: Jon Carpenter, Philadelphia

Deville, A. and Harding, R. 1997, *Applying the Precautionary Principle,* Federation Press, Annandale, New South Wales

Drengson, A. and Inoue, Y. eds 1995, *The Deep Ecology Movement: An introductory anthology,* North Atlantic Books, Berkeley, California

Elkington, J. and Hailes, J. 1988, *The Green Consumer Guide,* Victor Gollancz Ltd, London

Flick, U. 1998, *An Introduction to Qualitative Research,* Sage, London

Government of Western Australia 2003, *Hope for the Future: The Western Australia state sustainability strategy,* http://www.sustainability.dpc.wa.gov.au/docs/Strategy.htm [7 February 2004]

Green Consumer Guide, http://www.thegreenconsumerguide.com/ [13 January 2004]

Green Cross International 2002, 'Globalisation and Sustainable Development: Is ethics the missing link? Synthesis report', *Earth Dialogues Forum,* Lyon, 21-23 February 2002

Hancock, T. 2000, 'Healthy Communities Must Also Be Sustainable Communities', *Public Health Reports,* vol. 115, no. 3, pp. 151-6

Hardi, P. and Zdan, T. 1997, *Assessing Sustainable Development: Principals in practice,* International Institute for Sustainable Development, Winnipeg

Healthy Cities/Healthy Communites, http://www.well.com/user/bbear/hc_articles.html [13 January 2004]

Heron, J. 1999, *The Complete Facilitators Handbook,* Kogan Page Ltd, London

Heycox, K. 1991, *A Question of Survival,* ABC Enterprises, Crows Nest, New South Wales

Ife, J. 2002, *Community Development: Community-based alternatives in an age of globalisation,* Pearson Education, Frenchs Forest, New South Wales

International Association of Public Participation, http://www.iap2.org/ [7 February 2004]

International Council for Local Environmental Initiatives, http://www.iclei.org/ [13 January 2004]

International Union for Health Promotion and Education, http://www.iuhpe.org [7 February 2004]

Ireland, J. 1999, *Environmental Management for Health: Community based approaches for healthy islands,* Short Course Program for Environmental Health Officers of the Pacific, Suva, Fiji, WHO Collaborating Centre for Environmental Health, University of Western Sydney

Kickbusch, I. 1989, 'Good Planets Are Hard to Find: Approaches for an ecological base for public health', *A Sustainable Health Future Towards an Ecology of Health: Proceedings of a national workshop,* Melbourne

Kidner, D.W. 2000, 'Fabricating Nature: A critique of the social construction of nature', *Environmental Ethics,* vol. 22, no. 4, pp. 339-58

Kirschenmann, F. 1999, 'Can We Say "Yes" to Agriculture Using the Precautionary Principle: A farmer's perspective', *Protecting Public Health and the Environment: Implementing the precautionary principle,* eds C. Raffensperger and J.A. Tickner, Island Press, Washington DC, pp. 279-93

Naess, A. 1995, 'Platform Principles of the Deep Ecology Movement' in *The Deep Ecology Movement: An introductory anthology,* eds A. Drengson and Y. Inoue, North Atlantic Books, Berkeley, California

New Scientist Online 2001, www.newscientist.com/hottopics/environment/quiz2.jsp [13 January 2004]

Nicholson, R., Stephenson, P., Brown, V.A. and Mitchell, K. eds 2001, *Common Ground and Common Sense: Community-based environmental health planning,* Commonwealth of Australia, Canberra

Redefining Progress nd, *Ecological Footprint Calculator,* http://www.redefiningprogress.org/programs/sustainability/ef/ [13 January 2004]

Senge, P.M. 1992, *The Fifth Discipline: The art and practice of the learning organization,* Century Business, London

Sessions, G. 1995, 'Arne Naess and the Union of Theory and Practice', *The Deep Ecology Movement: An introductory anthology,* eds A. Drengson and Y. Inoue, North Atlantic Books, Berkeley, California

Soskolne, C.L. and Light, A. 1996, 'Towards Ethics: Guidelines for environmental epidemiologists', *Science of Total Environment,* pp. 137-47

South Australian Community Health Research Unit nd, *Planning and Evaluation Wizard,* http://www.sachru.sa.gov.au/PEW/index.htm [7 February 2004]

Strange, L. 2002, *Perth City Farm: Cultivating a Vital Urban Community: Sustainability case study*, Student Project, Department of Premier and Cabinet, Government of Western Australia, Perth

Suzuki, D. 2002, *Healthy Ecosystems, Healthy People: Linkages between biodiversity, ecosystem health and human health*, Keynote Address, International Society for Ecosystem Health, 6-11 June 2002, Washington DC

Tickner, J., Raffensperger, C. and Myers, N. (nd), *The Precautionary Principle in Action: A handbook*, Science and Environmental Health Network, New York

Towards Earth Summit 2002, 'Earth Summit 2002, Building Partnerships for Sustainable Development', Briefing Paper on Health and Environment, *Social Briefing No 3*, http://www.earthsummit2002.org/es/issues/health/health.htm [11 February 2004]

Wheeler, K.A. and Perraca Bijur, A. eds 2000, *Education for a Sustainable Future: A paradigm of hope for the 21st century*, Innovations in Science Education and Technology, Kluwer Academic/Plenum Publishers, New York

Wilson, E.O. 2002, 'The Bottleneck', *Scientific American*, February

Wise, M. 2002, 'Global Health Promotion: How can Australia contribute?', *Health Promotion Journal of Australia*, vol. 13, no. 1

Woodhill, J. and Robins, L. 1998, *Participatory Evaluation for Landcare and Catchment Groups: A guide for facilitators*, Greening Australia, Yarralumla, ACT

World Health Organisation Regional Office for Europe 1997, *Twenty Steps for Developing a Healthy Cities Project*, 3rd edn, WHO, Geneva

—— http://www.euro.who.int/healthy-cities [8 February 2004]

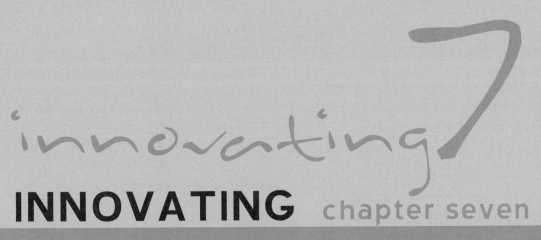

INNOVATING chapter seven

Practitioners as innovators for sustainability and health

Glenda Verrinder

Summary

Become the change you seek in the world. Mahatma Gandhi

This chapter is about changing our way of living for sustainability and health, locally and globally, individually and collectively, now and for the future. In particular it is about how practitioners can develop into innovators and change agents to work with individuals, groups, organisations and communities, to build capacity and to create and embrace innovation in working toward sustainability and health. We have known about the need for changing the way we do things for some time, but in our role as innovators and change agents we need to understand the dynamics of change in communities and our specific role in facilitating change. As public health practitioners we are often involved in structural change from the bottom up, so we need skills in consciousness raising, social animation, imagining, networking, learning, advocating, teaching and researching.

Chapter 7 Innovating

Practitioners as innovators for sustainability and health

Glenda Verrinder

Key words

Innovation, change agent, structural change, barriers to change, learning communities, capacity building, empowerment, consciousness raising, advocacy, imagination, education, research

Goal

To help public health practitioners and others embrace innovation and become change agents to work with communities to build community capacity and challenge the norms when needed in working toward sustainability and health.

Learning outcomes

After studying this chapter, the public health practitioner and students will be able to:

- demonstrate an understanding of the nature and dynamics of change and of being an innovator and change agent in public health practice;
- demonstrate an understanding of the roles of public health practitioners and colleagues in capacity building in groups, organisations and communities;
- demonstrate an understanding of the principles of promoting sustainability to individuals, organisations and communities;
- demonstrate a capacity to understand the importance of empowerment and the effectiveness of imagination in working with communities; and

- demonstrate a capacity to understand the importance of consciousness raising and initiating learning communities.

Outline

7.1 Structural change for sustainability
7.2 Capacity building for structural change
7.3 Education for sustainability
7.4 Research for sustainability

Learning activities

7.1 Reflection
7.2 Diffusion of innovation game
7.3 Imagining, settings for innovation
7.4 Writing a media release

Readings

AtKisson, A. 1999, *Believing Cassandra: An optimist looks at a pessimist's world*, Scribe Publications Pty Ltd, Melbourne

Kelly, P. and Carmody, K. 1991, 'From Little Things Big Things Grow' [CD], *Comedy*, Mushroom/Larrikin, Sydney

Wallerstein, N. and Bernstein, E. 1998, 'Empowerment Education: Friere's ideas adapted to health education', *Health Education Quarterly*, vol. 15, no. 4, pp. 379-94

7.1 Structural change for sustainability

The more clearly we can focus our attention on the wonders and realities of the universe about us, the less taste we shall have for destruction. Rachel Carson

We have known about the need for changing our ways for some time. Rachel Carson's landmark *Silent Spring* (1962) 'blew the whistle' on the harmful environmental effects of pesticide use. Since *The Limits to Growth* (Meadows et al.) was published in 1972, we have developed our understanding of the cumulative and interactive effects of population growth, energy use and industrial pollution on the self-renewing capacity of the environment. The predictions of ozone depletion, global warming and water depletion date from this time.

We have known about the need for changing our ways for some time.

Rachel Carson may not have considered herself an innovator or change agent, but her work inspired changes in environment policy and gave rise to a new ecological consciousness. In the ensuing years an ever-increasing rate of environmental decline led to recognition that some form of global intervention and change in our attitudes to growth and development was required. In 1986 the United Nations World Conference on Environment and Development used the term sustainable development to articulate its concern for the breaching of global life-support systems, and proposed that considerable reorientation of professions and industries was needed to halt and reverse degradation. That degradation continues, with serious implications for people and their health, means practitioners need to reflect on their roles if they are to play a part in stemming environmental destruction and improving the health of the public.

What will it take to come to terms with the effects of the burden of humans and their activities on Earth and its life-supporting capacity? What will it take to control population, develop new economic paradigms, reduce consumption, reduce the gap between rich and poor, develop sustainable agriculture, control pollution, apply new technology for renewable energy and conserve natural resources?

Changes in these areas need to happen, but there have obviously been barriers to effective action and those barriers need to be identified. Some would say the problems we face are due to fundamental aspects of human nature: selfishness, greed, intolerance and complacency. Other major causes include ignorance, lack of awareness and imprisonment by outdated dogmas and inadequate conceptual frameworks (Burrows et al. 1991). Different cultures have different opinions about the problems, the causes and the solutions for unsustainable development, but it is clear we do not have much more time to debate the issues (Yassi et al. 2001). For this reason practitioners must act positively on new ways of doing things; as innovators and agents of change, and as people who actively and effectively promote new ideas (AtKisson 1999).

Public health practitioners and others have been asked to think globally and act locally. This means acting individually and collectively. We know that for individuals to act, the concept of empowerment is particularly important. To feel empowered is to feel in control of one's life and to participate in decision-making about the things that affect us. To act collectively, there must be networks between people that lead to co-operation and beneficial outcomes. That is, social capital is a prerequisite to facilitate change in the community. 'The term "social capital", has been used as shorthand for a measure of the level of trust, positive social networks and extent of cooperative relationships . . . that exist in society' (Baum 2002, p. 241). With these prerequisites in mind an assessment of barriers at the community level may be needed.

To feel empowered is to feel in control of one's life and to participate in decision-making about the things that affect us.

Barriers to change

Clearly there are barriers to acting for sustainability and health, and it would be useful to review the constructions of knowledge defined earlier in Chapter 4. At the second EcoSummit in Halifax, Nova Scotia (2000) a number of barriers to effective action to curb the effects humans are having on the planet were identified (Costanza & Jorgensen 2002), including:

- *sustenance needs:* if basic, short-term needs of food, water and shelter are not being met, education about the importance of ecosystem health for human health in the long term will be a low priority;
- *little connection to the land:* as life in industrialised countries becomes more urbanised and professions more specialised, people have forgotten they are reliant on and part of nature;
- *resistance to change:* some people cling to the idea that there will always be some new resources or reserves to tap;
- *ignorance:* many people are simply not aware of the state of the environment and the impact that this will have on their health; and

- *low critical mass:* new ideas require some level of general acceptance before they gain sufficient critical mass to demonstrably influence public opinion and policy (Costanza & Jorgensen 2002).

It is not only the numbers that count but also who embraces the ideas. Rapport (2001) offers further insight into major barriers to effective action. He suggests these include the dominance of the global economy by high-income countries and inadequate governance and governing systems, and talks not about ignorance *per se* but severance of fields of knowledge (disciplines). There are many more barriers that permeate different cultures such as racism and sexism that inhibit change.

It is not only the numbers that count but also who embraces the ideas.

To identify the barriers, the people affected and what contributes to a problem, we can use models such as PRECEDE (predisposing, reinforcing, enabling causes in educational diagnosis and evaluation) for analysis (Green & Kreuter 1999). This provides a causal pathway of factors that contribute to a particular problem. Understanding this helps us to take action in a comprehensive way. There are three levels in the causal pathway: risk markers, risk factors and contributing factors. Contributing factors can be divided into predisposing, enabling and reinforcing factors (Green & Kreuter 1999).

For example, if our problem is that the burden of humans and their activities is overpowering the Earth and its capacity, risk markers signal where the problem is occurring and with or to whom. These are associated with the occurrence of the problem but do not necessarily contribute to it. Risk factors account for why the problem is occurring; the dominant risk factor might be that we have not developed an ecocentric or environmental perspective. The third category is the contributing factors; the things that contribute to our anthropocentrism. These can be divided into predisposing, enabling and reinforcing factors which can include, for example, the belief in the importance of the economy above all else, the availability of consumer goods and the reinforcement of conspicuous consumption. To bring about change we need to work on all these areas. Further, we can also take any one of these contributing factors and ask what contributes to it; this can provide individuals or communities with a basis for effective action. Box 7.1 provides some seeds for thought in acting collectively to overcome barriers to action.

> **Box 7.1 Overcoming barriers to change**
>
> - encouraging community empowerment;
> - responsive governance;
> - building transdisciplinary education;
> - accelerating government and intergovernment mandates for credible information on regional trends in ecosystem health;
> - communicating the science of the total environment;
> - developing the use of economic instruments to effect fundamental structural change in economic activity;
> - making the 'invisible hand' visible; and
> - encouraging diversity of views.
>
> *Source:* Rapport 2001, pp. 189-90

Diffusion of innovation

Understanding universal barriers to change and using processes to identify local barriers are part of the action needed in working for sustainability and health.

Understanding universal barriers to change and using processes to identify local barriers are part of the action needed in working for sustainability and health. We also need to understand how new ideas may be taken up.

The diffusion of innovations theory (Rogers 1995) provides us with a way of understanding how new ideas are taken up (or not); that is, how change takes place in a community. Diffusion theory has also been associated with marketing strategies, which will be discussed later. AtKisson has used diffusion theory extensively and devotes a chapter to it in *Believing Cassandra* (1999). Diffusion is defined as the process by which an innovation is communicated through certain channels over time among members of a social system. An innovation is defined as an idea, practice or object perceived as new by an individual or other 'unit of adoption', that is, a group, an organisation or community (Rogers 1995, pp. 10-11). The process works in this unit as clarity to a few, then gradual and later rapid uptake by the rest of the group, organisation or community. Five general factors that influence the speed and success with which new ideas are taken up have been identified: relative advantage, compatibility, complexity, trialability and observability (Rogers 1995).

In theory, the success or otherwise of innovation depends on how it is seen by various groups; for example, whether the innovation is seen as compatible with the established culture, or how the relative advantage of the innovation is perceived. The simplicity and flexibility of innovation together with its reversibility and the perceived risk of its adoption will also affect the extent to which innovation is taken up by the community. Further, the observability of results will influence whether others take up the change (AtKisson 1999). An in-depth study of these factors and other theories may provide useful information for agents of change. The important thing is to know the community and what is likely to influence its response.

AtKisson (1999) classifies several kinds of adopters: innovators, change agents, transformers, mainstreamers, unwilling laggards, reactionaries; there are also iconoclasts, spiritual recluses and curmudgeons. Innovators are the progenitors of new ideas; they may be considered 'fringe', eccentric or unpredictable by the rest of the community and so may not be trusted. Change agents are the 'ideas brokers' for the innovator. Transformers or early adopters in the mainstream are open to new ideas and want to promote change. Mainstreamers can be persuaded that the innovation is a good idea and will change when they see the majority changing, but unwilling laggards (who are the late majority and who constitute about the same number as the mainstreamers) are the sceptics who need to be convinced of the benefits before they adopt a change. Reactionaries have a vested interest in keeping things as they are. Iconoclasts highlight problems but do not generate ideas; they may be silent partners of innovators. Spiritual recluses may proffer the philosophical underpinning and influence the atmosphere for change, while curmudgeons see change efforts as useless. AtKisson (1999) suggests we all play all of those roles in different contexts.

The important thing is to know the community and what is likely to influence its response.

Activity 7.1
Reflection

Aim: to check out your own position.

Think of a situation where someone other than you was proposing a change (innovation) in your community. Which characteristic of those described above do you identify with most in this particular situation? Were you a change agent? A mainstreamer? A laggard?

> ### Box 7.2 The innovation diffusion game from *Believing Cassandra*
>
> I present the fictional situation (involving the promotion of a river clean-up project), and at random everyone draws a role card from a hat. There's one innovator, a few change agents, a handful of transformers and reactionaries.
>
> The rest of the participants are mostly divided between mainstreamers and laggards, but there's a spiritual recluse and a curmudgeon thrown in there just for fun. Nobody knows who's playing what role; only each person's behaviour, as directed by the role cards, provides other players with a clue . . . At first it's the usual confusing babble of activity—fun to be a spectator, because these folks are really getting into their roles. Then a remarkable thing happens. The fictional innovation sweeps through the crowd like wildfire, becoming almost universally adopted by this simulated culture in a matter of minutes . . . I've done this game a lot, but I've never seen anything like this rapid transformation. What happened? I asked the group . . . Something about what the change agents did, some way they effectively boxed out the original innovator (who can sometimes be a pain in the neck, hurting the cause more than helping with his insistence on intellectual purity) and identified the transformers quickly, while the iconoclasts kept the reactionaries busy (AtKisson 1999).

Activity 7.2
Diffusion of innovation game
http://allenandunwin.com/sustainhealth

Structuration theory

Another theory relating to the continuation and/or transformation of social systems is structuration theory, developed by Giddens (1984). According to Giddens, social structures and social action ('agency') are interdependent aspects of the same phenomenon. The continuation or reproduction of social systems or structures occurs through the actions of individuals applying shared knowledge or rules for behaviour; the transformation of social systems or structures, on the other hand, occurs as a result of what Giddens describes as 'reflexive monitoring of actions'. Through this process, humans monitor their own and others' conduct to determine whether intended outcomes have been achieved. New patterns of behaviour may be initiated where objectives are not being achieved.

In a study of the motivations for the 'greening' of the manufacturing industry (clearly a transformation from the norm), Townsend (1998) highlighted the importance of structural factors such as regulatory pressures and choice or agency, particularly relating to the environmental awareness or concern of the chief executive officer or other key individual, in prompting the move toward 'greening'.

Innovators are essential for structural change. The Balaton Group, for example, is an international network of innovators who work in a variety of occupations and organisations around the globe. These activists are 'dedicated to communicating, negotiating, inspiring, and getting things done' (Balaton Group). The purpose of the network is to find, train, link and support people who are active in promoting sustainability; make them more effective by helping them gain access to resources of all kinds; and create opportunities for them to act in concert as a multinational community (Balaton Group). That is, this group works to build the capacity of individuals and organisations to act for sustainability.

7.2 Capacity building for structural change

If you think you are too small to be effective you've never been in bed with a mosquito! Anita Roddick

In 'walking the walk' there are a number of roles practitioners might take on in working toward change for sustainability and health. These roles may take practitioners to the international, national, provincial or local level. Practitioners who work from ecological and social justice perspectives think of their role as including everything from consciousness raising to visualising and advocacy. Practitioners may need to play those roles at all or one of those levels.

Ife (2002, pp. 226-8) provides a critique of the 'cookbook approach' to working in communities. This critique is useful for practitioners who work in any setting. The way the cookbook approach is presented tends to make the process of working in a community appear that it can be ordered and linear. In fact, working in communities is rarely like that and working toward change for sustainability would be no different. Another limitation of this approach is that each setting is different, so each approach needs to be different. The culture, the resources and the reason for its existence need to be considered.

In 'walking the walk' there are a number of roles practitioners might take on in working toward change for sustainability and health.

Furthermore, each practitioner is different. In Chapter 6 we discussed how personal values and experiences influence the way people work.

Finally, while some practitioners specialise in, for example, advocacy, there are some roles we have selected for this chapter that practitioners working within an ecological and social justice framework will probably take on as a matter of course in working for change in sustainability and health.

Empowerment

Empowerment seeks to increase the power of the disadvantaged (Ife 2002) and is central to social justice, yet the process is often misunderstood. This may be because the concept of power is complex and vigorously contested. Practitioners working for change in sustainability and health need to become familiar with empowerment discourse. Empowerment has been defined as:

> *A social action process that promotes participation of people, organisations, and communities towards the goals of increased individual and community control, political efficacy, improved quality of community life, and social justice.* (Wallerstein 1992, p. 198)

Empowerment can be achieved through policy and planning . . .

A number of strategies has been proposed to achieve empowerment, including policy and planning, social and political action, and education and consciousness raising (Ife 2002).

Empowerment can be achieved through policy and planning when strategies (discussed in Chapter 6) of affirmative action, participatory democracy and genuine partnering are embedded in the policy and planning processes. Empowerment through social and political action is often achieved through consciousness raising, which is part of the education process. Empowered individuals and communities then actively participate in the decisions that affect their lives. Ideally, this may be changing the structures in society that disadvantaged them in the first place (Ife 2002). Consciousness raising is the first step along the road to empowerment.

Consciousness raising

Consciousness raising is part of an innovator's or change agent's everyday practice. People who are involved in consciousness raising are engaged in examining the social structures in which they live and in implementing social change strategies that challenge oppression and foster empowerment. The aim is for people to move from passivism to activism. Consciousness raising is not a separate activity but rather embedded in the context of everyday life. It is about the sharing of experiences. Ife (2002) suggests that there are four aspects to this sharing: linking the personal and the political, the development of a dialogical relationship, the sharing of experiences of oppression and the opening up of possibilities for action. Consciousness-raising processes develop community connectedness, build social capital and increase the capacity of individuals and communities to act.

There is abundant information about community connectedness, social capital and capacity building that will not be covered here. However, there are roles that practitioners can take as change agents within communities that will contribute to building social capital in communities. Using imagination is one of them.

Imagination as a social movement

Imagination is the realm of the future, utterly democratic, not determined by current arrangements. As a movement, imagination draws upon people's deepest urge to be connected and to contribute to a larger purpose. It brings people together meaningfully to talk and listen with one another, to share their personal and collective aspirations. (Browne & Jain 2002, p. 2)

Imagination is another and very positive way of thinking about how changes might take place. Browne and Jain (2002) offer valuable advice in this respect. Imagination is not in short supply. Bringing people together under this umbrella is a way of generating the energy and commitment needed to transform dreams into realities. The movement relies on the strength of collective imagination (Browne & Jain 2002). 'Imagine Chicago' began in the early 1990s with the aim of transforming the city into a citywide community. Since then the ideas emanating from that movement have travelled the world. The ideas of this movement could be used in any context. Browne and Jain (2002) have now told the story of the collective experiences of this movement in *Imagine Chicago: Ten years of imagination in action.*

Imagine Chicago identified change agents in organisations, institutions and communities and gave them development tools and opportunities to make a difference. Imagine Chicago created personal development opportunities that inspired and informed to sustain lasting institutional, community and systemic change. Through its many collaborations, Imagine Chicago builds intergenerational and intercultural networks of individuals and organisations committed to developing a vital citywide community (Imagine Chicago, http://www.imaginechicago.org).

Imagination is another and very positive way of thinking about how changes might take place.

253

The core assumptions on which Imagine Chicago is built are:

- everyone has a unique contribution to make that must be shared for the common good;
- organisations can be created that make productive use of those unique contributions and that are in harmony with our beliefs;
- the sum of the whole is greater than the parts;
- friendship provides a good working model for the kind of relationships necessary to develop a vibrant city; and
- we need to connect people, organisations and places to work collectively. (Browne & Jain 2002)

Appreciative inquiry questions are always positive questions around affirmative topics.

Using imagination as described above and creating intergenerational learning communities is one way of building capacity in individuals, organisations and communities. Browne and Jain (2002) put forward the idea that words can shape people's thoughts and actions. They believe that they can be positive and expand people's thoughts to realise their full potential or, conversely, make people feel inadequate and incapable of realising that potential. The use of appreciative inquiry to discover, understand and foster innovations through the gathering of positive stories and images and the construction of positive interactions has been used worldwide. It seeks out the very best of what is to help ignite the collective imagination of what could be. The aim is to generate new knowledge that expands the realm of the possible, helps members of an organisation or community envisage a collectively desired future and work together to create it. Appreciative inquiry questions are always positive questions around affirmative topics. Box 7.3 demonstrates the style of these questions (Browne & Jain 2002).

Box 7.3 Appreciative inquiry

To design good appreciative inquiry questions, remember to:

- allow questions to evoke ultimate concerns: ask about high point stories, most valued qualities and so on;
- use positive questions that build on positive assumptions: what is it about this organisation/town that makes you glad you are a part of it?;
- give a thought-provoking, appealing definition of the topic: for example, 'a leader is anyone who wants to help at this time';

- present questions as an invitation: use expansive positive feeling, experiential words;
- enhance the possibilities of storytelling by asking questions that focus on personal experiences;
- phrase questions in a conversational and friendly tone and listen eagerly as you would to a close friend;
- ask open questions to which you do not know the answer, expecting to learn something surprising and wonderful; and
- value the experience of the person being interviewed.

Source: Browne & Jain 2002, p. 12

Visioning

A vision for sustainability and health reflects the values, concerns and hopes of that community; it is easily understood and inspirational, creating clarification, connection and a desire for excellence. Visualising can be very similar to imagining in that the process generates creative thinking. It is often suggested as a strategy in participatory planning processes, which were discussed in the previous chapter. However, it is mentioned here because groups, organisations and communities that have a shared vision of the direction in which they are heading are in a better position to make the changes they want rather than reacting to change forced on them by outside forces. In visualising the process is probably more important than the outcome. The more people who are involved the better, because the more people who contribute to the vision the greater the chance of it being successful. Present realities should not inhibit creativity and, as in the case of imagining, the language should be positive. The emerging vision needs to be regularly validated by the people involved so anxieties are aired and the vision is a shared one. The new vision needs to be announced and celebrated and finally, in the words of Wheeler and Perraca Bijur (2000), beyond talking the talk, you must walk the walk with full integrity (p. 220) (Activity 5.4).

A vision for sustainability and health reflects the values, concerns and hopes of that community.

Activity 7.3
Imagining, settings for innovation

Managing for sustainability and health is discussed in detail in Chapter 8; however, some of the options for public health practitioners and colleagues to facilitate structural change at the community level are discussed here. Community groups will be created, sustained and facilitated in different ways, 'but all have to be conscious in the exercise of decision-making and finding a good balance between autonomy, co-operation and hierarchy' (Heron 1999, p. 329). Social change theory seminars, community action groups, occupational action groups, organisational action groups and new institutions are five approaches outlined below that may be useful for practitioners in facilitating change (Heron 1999).

Social change theory seminars: these study groups are consciousness-raising groups that explore issues of change. There is a critique of personal, transpersonal and social issues. The research, reflection and dialogue that occur during this process are likely to produce more perceptive and effective action than if this had not been done. Relevant research data is collected to assist in the analysis of the current social structure and support the vision developed by the group.

Community action groups: these groups come together to engage in direct action for social change on issues of concern to them. The groups are communities of interest who perhaps share the same occupation, beliefs or concerns and who meet regularly to take action. These groups include: community development, mutual aid, peer self-help and new society education and action.

Mutual aid: this is an exercise in reciprocity where people set up a network and agree on a system of exchange of labour. There are numerous examples worldwide such as the local exchange and trading systems in the United Kingdom (Heron 1999); Barteryourservices in the United States (http://www .barteryourservices.com/cgi-bin/free_search.pl) or labour exchange trading systems (LETS) where expertise, goods or labour are exchanged.

Peer self-help: mutual support is given to group members with similar problems of a personal nature that affect them directly. The members share experiences and identify common needs and areas for social action for themselves or on behalf of others in similar situations. The problems may be anything from a particular disease affecting individuals such as asthma, to psychosocial issues such as drug dependency, or life stage issues such as retirement and so on.

New society education and action: this is a consciousness-raising group where cultural and ecological issues for social action are identified. The issues may be global or local. But thinking globally/acting locally may be the thrust of their action. Heron (1999) cites many examples such as green consumerism, pollution, renewable energy, work co-operatives and so on.

Occupational action groups: occupational ties alone connect the group, which works collectively for the profession. Trade unions are the best example.

Organisational action groups: these groups work for organisational change. They may or may not have similar occupations but their aim is often for a better balance of hierarchy, co-operation and autonomy within an organisation.

Community development: community development groups are local groups that work at the local level on local issues with or without the support of local government. This will be discussed in more depth later.

New institutions: all the previous activities converge on the creation of new institutions, the social structures of a new society (Heron 1999). Change agents may need to create, facilitate and help sustain any of these groups and so an understanding of group dynamics and facilitation skills is required. Facilitation for structural change in a group requires:

- *Emotion:* the group must have ways of working through situations where distress is evident. Past hurts and current realities must be clarified.
- *Power:* a working balance between autonomy, co-operation and hierarchy needs to be established.
- *Inquiry:* a cycle of research, experience and reflection that sits within the goals of the group is the process.
- *Co-operation:* establishing mutual aid is helpful.
- *Conflict:* strategies for conflict resolution need to be developed.
- *Affirmation:* time should be taken to appreciate group member qualities, skills and action.
- *Celebration:* time should be taken to have fun and to celebrate achievements and differences. (Heron 1999)

Techniques for soft revolution

Heron (1999) suggests that for those wanting to introduce change in rigid institutions it may be useful to:

- appeal to the stated values of the institution;
- appeal to a precedent set by another division in the same institution;
- confront the person who is undermining the initiatives for change face-to-face; or
- launch innovations in the open spaces between the gridlines of the closed system of the institution.

Social animation

Facilitating change means working to enable others to become actively involved in the change process.

Facilitating change means working to enable others to become actively involved in the change process. Ife (2002) suggests that the change agent's ability to inspire, enthuse, stimulate, energise and motivate others into action forms a part of that work and terms it 'social animation'. According to Ife there are six aspects of successful animation: enthusiasm, commitment, integrity, communication, understanding and analysis, and personality. The enthusiasm needs to be genuine and the source of the commitment needs to be firmly rooted in the aims of sustainability and social justice. These two characteristics (together with being seen to be trustworthy and non-manipulative) will send a message of integrity to the community.

Box 7.4 The shared action story

St Luke's Anglicare received funding from the Ian Potter Foundation to work in two suburbs identified by various health, justice and other agencies as having significant numbers of vulnerable families. Two community development workers were employed to work in partnership with residents to develop and evaluate a program designed to enhance the safety and wellbeing of families in the area. The initial discussions of Shared Action centred on the residents' vision of a healthy, safe and pleasant community; what affected residents' wellbeing, and what projects would achieve the vision. A reference group from the suburbs and agencies working in the areas was formed. This group talked about some of the problems that had been identified and whether people could change.

Community engagement really began with community barbecues and shared action parties where people invited their neighbours. The vision that emerged was that the communication and relationships in the community needed to be enhanced and that a better physical environment would go some way to helping this process. Over a three-year period a sport and recreation club and a family park were planned, built and used by the community. People participated on the basis of what they had to offer to ensure sustainability and community ownership.

The project continues under community ownership. Community members have participated in presentations at local, national and international community development conferences, in the planning and redevelopment of housing, and in a range of local employment projects. In the evaluation, community members report they now have confidence to take action to create a safe and healthy community, are proud of the progress that has been made and proud of where they live.

Source: Beilharz 2002

The communication skills discussed in Chapter 6 are clearly important for successful animation, as is the practitioner's ability to understand and analyse the situation as part of their reflective practice. Finally, it is useful to develop an awareness of one's own personality and how to use that to best effect (Ife 2002). However, the practitioner as innovator or change agent is only one half of the equation. The community is the other half, and the prerequisites for change include empowered individuals and social capital. Social capital is dependent upon social connectedness.

Social capital is dependent upon social connectedness.

Networking

Networking is one of the most important change strategies. It is necessary to network with a wide variety of people and groups in and outside one's usual context. Networks need to remain open and to involve people from the grass roots. This prevents the possibility of unofficial network elites forming (Ife 2002). In the next chapter on managing for sustainability, action networks will be discussed. The Balaton Group mentioned previously, and the groups in the following box, are good examples of how networks can work.

> **Box 7.5** *Local Heroes*
>
> *Local Heroes* (McPhillips 2002) is a collection of stories about individuals and groups who became change agents to achieve justice and make their communities safer and cleaner. The issues they addressed ranged from lead contamination to smog and chemical poisoning. The LEAD Group, for example, aimed to eliminate childhood lead poisoning. Three young mothers founded the group and a submission from one of its members resulted in a blood lead survey of their area, the results of which became critical in the setting up of a lead taskforce. The LEAD group created a network by working with other groups (NO-LEAD and Greenpeace) and together lobbied politicians to reduce the amount of lead in leaded petrol. Information about lead poisoning has been disseminated by various means including a national advisory service called LEADLINE, a quarterly journal called *LEAD Action News* and fact sheets. These publications, together with information stalls at expos and workshops for parents, have helped solve the lead problems of thousands of families.
>
> *Source:* O'Brien 2002

Advocacy

Working out which elected official you need to lobby is a skill in itself.

Public health practitioners can be called on by groups, communities or organisations to act on their behalf. This raises issues of empowerment because it assumes that the advocate can be a better representative of the views of those they represent. An analysis of the power relations is crucial before you begin, but it is sometimes necessary to take on this role in the short term with disempowered communities that have urgent needs. In the advocacy role practitioners may need to be catalysts for change, to change opinions or attitudes or actions or to mobilise resources. It may sound obvious, but advocacy requires that practitioners have the ability to understand the views of those they represent and the ability to accurately and assertively present them to powerbrokers. Inevitably, advocacy will cause some degree of instability so it is important to find allies and to develop media contacts (Ife 2002). Effective use of the media may be part of the advocacy role. Radio, television and print each require different skills. For television you need to be able to distil the message into a few seconds: word pictures, metaphors and analogies are helpful. Practitioners may need professional development in working with the media and other forms of advocacy. The media can be useful for lobbying elected officials. Practitioners may take on advocacy work as individuals or as members of an organisation. Working out which elected official you need to lobby is a skill in itself. A local politician with a particular portfolio may be the best. The larger the numbers involved, the more effective the lobbying and so working with other organisations is important. Face-to-face contact is also effective and writing a letter can only be seen to be effective advocacy if it initiates a response from the elected official (Wass 2000). There is a range of helpful resources for practitioners. Chapman and Lupton's book *The Fight for Public Health* (1994) is a good resource for public health media advocacy.

Social marketing

The diffusion of innovation theory has been discussed in this chapter in relation to change. As innovators and change agents, practitioners may need to formally market an idea on behalf of a group, organisation or community. Diffusion theory is used as an analytical tool in social marketing. Similar issues around empowerment arise in this role, as with advocacy. Further, there is a danger that individual behaviour change strategies may become victim-blaming devices, particularly for vulnerable groups that may not have the knowledge, skills and resources to make the desired change.

Social marketing has been used for many years in a diverse range of health improvement campaigns . . .

If we reflect on the theory as presented by AtKisson (1999) it is obvious that if everyone were an innovator or change agent we would not need social marketing strategies. Social marketing has been defined as:

> concepts and methods [that] borrow heavily from traditional marketing literature. However, social marketing is distinguished by its emphasis on so-called 'non-tangible' products—ideas, attitudes, lifestyle changes—as opposed to the more tangible products and services that are the focus of marketing in business, health-care, and non-profit service sectors. (Lefebvre & Flora, in McKenzie & Smeltzer 2001, p. 235)

Social marketing has been used for many years in a diverse range of health improvement campaigns such as immunisation, family planning, agricultural reforms and lifestyle changes to prevent cardiovascular disease, drug abuse and so on.

There are various social marketing planning frameworks: CDCynergy and SMART (social marketing assessment and response tool) are two models that fit the description of the essential characteristics of social marketing

(McKenzie & Smeltzer 2001). They both provide standard planning frameworks directed at developing programs with the aim of successfully persuading individuals to change their behaviour.

Baum (2002) reminds us of the limitations of social marketing in that the structural factors that prevent or restrict people's ability to change their lifestyle are often ignored. However, it is possible to couple social marketing with an advocacy role which in public health is issue and policy oriented. Advocacy is not primarily oriented at changing the knowledge, attitudes or behaviours of individuals, but rather the legislative, fiscal, physical and social environments in which individual change can take place (Chapman & Lupton 1994).

Activity 7.4
Writing a media release
http://www.allenandunwin.com/sustainhealth

7.3 Education for sustainability

In the end, we will conserve only what we love. We will love only what we understand . . . Baba Dioum

Public health in the 21st century will be characterised by an ecological approach to the environment . . .

While there is now general agreement on the continuing deterioration of the planet's natural resource cycles and on the need for a response that conforms to sustainable development principles, there is far less agreement on what our response should be in any particular place or profession. However, the Earth Charter (2000) supports the notion that education is one of the fundamental ways to transform society. Principle 14 states: Integrate into formal education and lifelong learning the knowledge, values and skills needed for a sustainable way of life. Further, part (a) states: Provide all, especially children and youth, with educational opportunities that empower them to contribute actively to sustainable development (p. 45).

Public health in the 21st century will be characterised by an ecological approach to the environment, an approach that was first legitimised in the Ottawa Charter for Health Promotion (Hancock 2000). Public health as a profession urgently needs to reconsider its role in maintaining the health of human populations, in the light of current state of the world environment reports. Parallel international events provide the teaching process with a clearly described and shared body of knowledge. These events include the outcomes of the major world meeting on sustainable development in Johannesburg in 2002, the United Nations Conference on Environment and Development in Brazil in 1992; the establishment of the worldwide community-based Earth Charter; the learning from the global programs of Healthy Cities and Local Agenda 21; and the agreement between the global agencies of the United Nations, the World Bank and World Resources Institute.

Conceptual framework for action

Becoming a learning society is a public and political process . . . it is about recreating our democracy within and as part of the 21st century world. (Duke, in Bradshaw 1999, p. 18)

The framework for learning and change presented in Chapter 1 is based on a combination of experiential and inquiry-based learning principles (Kolb et al. 1974). They argue that all learning is about change, and adult learning is best characterised as a form of personal inquiry into real world problems. This approach is well suited to responding to sustainability and health issues that require accepting the need for transformational change.

The transition learning model is another reference for practitioners involved in change facilitation at community or governance levels.

In *Transforming Lives, Transforming Communities* (1999) Bradshaw provides us with educational values, principles and a framework that can be used in education and in our roles as change agents in sustainability and health. The conceptual framework advocates the following eight lifelong learning goals:

- understand complex systems that interact unpredictably;
- identify and integrate existing and emerging personal, local, national and global perspectives;
- prosper with difference, paradox and multiple sets of realities;
- see and make connections between the past, the present and the future;
- encourage sustainability in relationships and the environment;
- engage in a process of change, privately and publicly, civically and occupationally, throughout life;
- extend learning styles and repertoires; and
- develop insights through questioning, through asking 'why?' and 'what if?' as well as 'what?' and 'how?' (Bradshaw 1999, p. 23)

These goals link our discussion in Chapter 6 with the discussion here in Chapter 7. Concepts that are common to all eight goals are multiplicity, connectedness, critical intelligence and transformation. These principles—

indicators of quality future education—work together interdependently whatever the topic, subject or discipline. Bradshaw asserts that in practice, learners and teachers assemble alternative perspectives, explanations and possibilities (multiplicity); together they then make connections between these and beyond these (connectedness). They ask questions about these (critical intelligence). All the while, learners and teachers consolidate by determining and taking thoughtful action that makes a difference personally, locally, nationally and/or globally (transformation).

The transition learning model is another reference for practitioners involved in change facilitation at community or governance levels. The model provides an integration of learning and teaching paradigms, with special attention to cultural dimensions. Personal attitudes are in a state of flux as people seek to minimise the cognitive dissonance between their attitudes toward a subject; for example, responsible natural resource management and pollution minimisation and their behaviour as in motor vehicle use for private purposes. The aim of this reconciliation process is to appear consistent to themselves. Dissonance tension can be quite high and is a motivation to maximise consonance. Attitudes are the outcome of the evaluation of decisions about people, events or objects where the cognition dimension establishes reference for beliefs or opinions as a value association and behaviour is the action intention. The constructionist theory of learning explains that people construct knowledge as opposed to merely collecting data and further, that in relation to the cognitive transformation processes, the information is altered or transformed after reflecting upon prior experience and previously held assumptions (James 2000, p. 13).

Skills in education are particularly important for change agents. Practitioners working for sustainability and health may be initially engaged in consciousness raising, which Friere (1972) used in teaching literacy in disempowered communities.

Learning communities

Kolb's ideas strongly influenced the field of action research and are now used as a framework for lifelong learning in a number of professions. The work gave rise to the idea of the learning organisation, an organisation that is continually expanding its capacity to create its future (Senge 1990).

Learning communities are groups that come together to share their knowledges and that integrate the perspectives of community, specialists,

Learning communities are groups that come together to share their knowledges and that integrate the perspectives of community, specialists, government and industry.

government and industry. Everyone is both a teacher and a learner. Fundamental to learning communities is respecting people's different knowledges. This is very different from the traditional Western 'didactic' lecture style, a 'top-down' instructional approach whereby acknowledged experts pass on their (assumed) superior knowledge to be absorbed by the 'empty vessels' waiting to be filled. Latin American educationalist Paulo Friere was a strong critic of this approach, arguing that it represents nothing more than the oppression of the majority by a privileged minority (Friere 1972). Friere's view of education as an essentially participatory process, an active partnership between teacher and learner and one that is truly transformational and pivotal to human development, fits well with the concept of the inter-generational and inter-cultural education that takes place in learning communities. The participatory learning approach involves respect for each other's learning, exchanging stories, listening to different groups and their values, and exploring open ways of learning. In this way learning communities can become empowered to identify their problems, critically assess their historical and social roots, envisage a healthier future for themselves and develop strategies to overcome barriers to sustainability (Wallerstein & Bernstein 1988). This is the cornerstone of empowerment.

In a global information era we need to construct a new and holistic knowledge that combines the lived experience of local community members with specialised knowledge from research, professions and industry, and an understanding of the strategic processes of politics and administration. We need to be savvy as well as holistic.

The section on Imagine Chicago gives an example of encouraging people's imagination and allowing the 'what if?' questions to be explored, goals and values to be made clear, and creative solutions to living more responsibly and sustainably sought. To work effectively, learning communities need to establish a culture which openly and boldly encourages the challenges to be explored in a constructive and non-adversarial way. Learning communities are essentially solution oriented and supportive of creative ideas. Their members respect and value the different knowledge constructs. They seek solutions that combine the lived experience of local community members, the specialist knowledge of professional experts, the strategic knowledge of government and the integrative knowledge of those whose role it is to work holistically across other groups (Brown et al. 2001).

Prior to putting the thinking into action, the teaching-learning process needs to move into designing action plans and reflecting on their

Prior to putting the thinking into action, the teaching-learning process needs to move into designing action plans and reflecting on their implications, effects and the principles of what should be done.

The cycle continues with the action being evaluated: what works, and if it has not worked what we can learn from the experience?

implications, effects and the principles of what should be done. Here the Earth Charter and Health Charter principles offer useful guidelines for action. The cycle continues with the action being evaluated: what works, and if it has not worked what we can learn from the experience? This may involve examining the barriers to change in view of what was tried, and requires a continuing commitment to the process.

In Chapter 6 we discussed the need to examine our values in acting for sustainability. If we are to act as change agents, we need to think about how all of us learn. The D4P4 model for learning and changing is covered in Chapter 1. Seven kinds of intelligence (Box 7.6) is another perspective on learning—one that is consistent with our general discussion, in particular about how individuals may make connections in their explorations.

Box 7.6 Seven kinds of intelligence

Linguistic People with high linguistic intelligence have a knack for language and learn best by saying, hearing and seeing words. They learn best through books, records, and tapes, being engaged in discussion and informal writing.

Spatial People with spatial intelligence usually learn visually and need to learn through images, pictures, metaphors and colours. Films, slides, diagrams, maps charts, art activities, visualisation exercises, contribution kits and vivid stories help them learn.

Bodily kinaesthetic People who excel in this area learn best by moving their bodies and working with their hands. Their learning activities need to be kinetic, dynamic and visceral; role playing, drama, creative movement, hands-on activities and sport are best.

Musical Some people learn best through rhythm and melody, by singing, tapping out or whistling.

Interpersonal People with interpersonal inclinations learn best by relating to and co-operating with others. Social games that emphasise concepts and skills or community projects are ideal.

Logical mathematical These people look for concepts, abstract patterns and relationships. Experiments, puzzles and exploring new ideas are best for them.

Intrapersonal These people learn best if left to learn for themselves.

Source: Gardner 1983

7.4 Research for sustainability

'Would you tell me, please, which way I ought to go from here?' said Alice. 'That depends a good deal on where you want to get to,' said the Cat. Lewis Carroll

Participatory approaches

Chapter 5 provides an in-depth discussion on monitoring and evaluation in sustainability and health. Here we outline a number of participatory approaches to research in the context of how change might occur. Participatory approaches have evolved, primarily since the 1960s, from several sources and traditions. Pretty et al. (1995) outline the following five as particularly important.

Activist participatory research: inspired by Paulo Friere and his work in education with disempowered communities. This approach aims to empower people by raising their awareness of their circumstances through dialogue. Its key contribution to the current approaches is the recognition that disempowered people can be creative and capable, and outsiders have a role as catalysts and facilitators in their empowerment.

There are a variety of terms for participatory approaches.

Agro-ecosystem analysis: developed by Gordon Conway and colleagues. This approach draws on systems and ecological thinking, combining analysis of systems (productivity, stability, sustainability, equity) with pattern analysis of space, time, flows and relationships, relative values and decisions. Among major contributions to current approaches are its use of transects, informal mapping and diagramming and the use of scoring and ranking to assess innovations.

Applied anthropology: through observation and conversation, 'development professionals' learn to appreciate the richness of rural people's lives.

Field research on farming systems: acknowledgement of the rationality of small and poor farmers on one hand and their activities as experimenters on the other provides an insight to researchers into the complexity of farming systems.

Rapid rural appraisal: this approach is a reaction to the limitations of questionnaires. In answering the question 'whose knowledge counts', it seeks to enable outsiders to gain insight and information in a cost-effective and timely manner.

Source: Chambers 1992, in Pretty 1995, p. 55

There are a variety of terms for participatory approaches. Apart from the terms outlined above, you may be aware of participatory action research, participatory rural appraisal and rapid catchment analysis, to name three. Whatever these are called, Pretty et al. (1995) outline some common principles: a defined methodology and systemic learning process; multiple perspectives; group learning process; context specific; facilitating experts and stakeholders; and leading to change. In short, all participants must be involved in the entire process. The main aim is to seek diversity, not to simplify complexity. A combination of research styles is needed to analyse complexity. Participatory approaches involve people from different disciplines and sectors and from inside and outside the community. These approaches are context specific and necessarily flexible. The role of the external 'expert' is to help others do their own research. This process will eventually lead to increased community capacity for participatory research and action, and therefore change. Education for sustainability and research for sustainability are both underpinned by the same participatory processes.

Public health practitioners can no longer afford to work in isolation from other professions . . .

Public health practitioners can no longer afford to work in isolation from other professions, from government agencies or indeed from the communities whose health and wellbeing are at stake. We must learn how to work co-operatively and collaboratively with other stakeholders. This means opening channels of communication, and respecting and valuing the knowledge constructs that provide a holistic and systemic view of an increasingly complex array of 21st century issues of public health and ecological sustainability.

Conclusion

Throughout this book we have talked about worldwide change through, for example, the Earth Charter, Agenda 21 and Healthy Cities. This chapter has been about change and the possibilities available to public health practitioners to embrace innovation and to become change agents. Our task is to increase awareness that human activity is affecting human health. We have major tasks ahead of us if we are to control population, develop a new economic paradigm, reduce consumption, reduce the economic gap between rich and poor, develop sustainable agricultural practices, control pollution, apply new technology for renewable energy resources and conserve natural resources. We cannot hope to achieve any of these without changing the way we live. As innovators and change agents we can work at the international, national, provincial or local level. Whatever the level, change needs to occur. As practitioners we need to remember that from little things big things grow (Kelly & Carmody 1991).

References

AtKisson, A. 1999, *Believing Cassandra: An optimist looks at a pessimist's world*, Scribe Publications Pty Ltd, Melbourne

Balaton Group, http://www.unh.edu/ipssr/Balaton.html [14 February 2004]

Baum, F. 2002, *The New Public Health,* Oxford University Press, South Melbourne

Beilharz, L. 2002, *Building Community: The shared action experience*, Solutions Press, Bendigo

Bradshaw, D. 1999, *Transforming Lives, Transforming Communities: A conceptual framework for further education*, Adult, Community and Further Education Board, Victoria, Melbourne

Brown, V.A., Nicholson, R., Stephenson, P., Bennett, K.J. and Smith, J. 2001, *Grass Roots and Common Ground: Guidelines for community-based environmental health action*, Regional Integrated Monitoring Centre, University of Western Sydney, Richmond, New South Wales

Browne, B. and Jain, S. 2002, *Imagine Chicago: Ten years of imagination in action*, http://www.imaginechicago.org. or http://imaginechicago.org/possibility_publication.html [11 February 2004]

Burrows, B.C., Mayne, A.J. and Newbury, P. 1991, *Into the 21st Century: A handbook for a sustainable future*, Adamantine Press, Twickenham

Carson, R. 1962, *Silent Spring*, Fawcett Publications, Greenwich, Connecticut

CDCynergy, http://www.cdc.gov/communication/cdcynergy.htm [11 February 2004]

Chapman, S. and Lupton, D. 1994, *The Fight for Public Health: Principles and practice of media advocacy*, BMJ, London

Costanza, R. and Jorgensen, S. eds 2002, *Understanding and Solving Environmental Problems in the 21st Century: Toward a new, integrated hard problem science*, Elsevier, Oxford

Earth Charter Commission 2000, *The Earth Charter Initiative Handbook*, Earth Charter Commission, New York

Friere, P. 1972, *Pedagogy of the Oppressed*, Penguin, London

Gardner, H. 1983, *Frames of Mind: The theory of multiple intelligences*, Basic Books, New York

Giddens, A. 1984, *The Constitution of Society: Outline of the theory of structuration*, University of California Press, Berkeley

Green, L. and Kreuter, M. 1999, *Health Promotion Planning: An educational and ecological approach*, Mayfield Publishing Company, Mountain View, California

Hancock, T. 2000, 'Healthy Communities Must Also Be Sustainable Communities', *Public Health Reports*, vol. 115, pp. 151-6

Heron, J. 1999, *The Complete Facilitators Handbook*, Kogan Page Ltd, London

Ife, J. 2002, *Community Development: Community-based alternatives in an age of globalisation*, Pearson Education, Sydney

James, R. 2000, *The Transitional Learning Model: A handbook for training design*, Vocational and Education and Training Publications, Perth

Kelly, P. and Carmody, K. 1991, 'From Little Things Big Things Grow' [CD], *Comedy,* Mushroom/Larrikin, Sydney

Kolb, D.A., Rubin, I.M. and McIntyre, J.M. 1974, *Organisational Psychology: An experiential approach*, Prentice Hall, New Jersey

McKenzie, J.F. and Smeltzer, J.L. 2001, *Planning Implementing and Evaluating Health Promotion Programs*, Allyn and Bacon, Boston

McPhillips, K. ed 2002, *Local Heroes: Australian crusades from the environmental frontline*, Pluto Press, Annandale, New South Wales

Meadows, D.H., Meadows, D.L., Randers, J. and Behrens, W.W. 1972, *The Limits to Growth: A report for the club of Rome's project on the predicament of mankind*, Potomac Associates, London

Nicholson, R., Stephenson, P., Brown, V.A. and Mitchell, K. eds 2001, *Common Ground and Common Sense: Community-based environmental health planning*, Commonwealth of Australia, Canberra

O'Brien, E. 2002, 'The Lead Group: Responding to the problem of lead contamination' in *Local Heroes: Australian crusades from the environmental frontline*, ed. K. McPhillips, Pluto Press, Sydney

Pretty, J., Guijt, I., Thompson, J. and Scoones, I. eds 1995, *Participatory Learning and Action: A trainer's guide*, IIED Participatory Methodology Series, International Institute for Environment and Development, London

Rapport, D. 2001, 'Pessimism of the Intellect and Optimism of the Will', *Ecosystem Health*, vol. 7, no. 4, pp. 187-91

Rogers, E.M. 1995, *Diffusion of Innovations*, The Free Press, New York

Senge, P.M. 1990, *The Fifth Discipline: The art and practice of the learning organisation*, Doubleday, London

Townsend, M. 1998, *Making Things Greener: Motivations and influences in the greening of manufacturing*, Ashgate Publishing Limited, Aldershot

Wallerstein, N. 1992, 'Powerlessness, Empowerment, and Health: Implications for Health Promotion Programs', *American Journal of Public Health*, January/February, vol. 6, no. 3, pp. 197-205

Wallerstein, N. and Bernstein, E. 1988, 'Empowerment Education: Friere's ideas adapted to health education', *Health Education Quarterly*, vol. 15, no. 4, pp. 379-94

Wass, A. 2000, *Promoting Health: The primary health care approach*, Harcourt Saunders, Sydney

Wheeler, K.A. and Perraca Bijur, A. eds 2000, *Education for a Sustainable Future: A paradigm of hope for the 21st century*, Innovations in Science Education and Technology, Kluwer Academic/Plenum Publishers, New York

Yassi, A., Kjellstrom, T., Kok, T. and Guidotti, T. 2001, *Basic Environmental Health*, Oxford University Press, New York

MANAGING chapter eight

Public health leadership and management for sustainability

Rae Walker, Jan Ritchie and Michael Sparks

Summary

The nature of the problems outlined in previous chapters and the costs of failing to move toward sustainability make it imperative that the transition is initiated across society. This chapter puts the case that the key to global ecological integrity is integrated action among all the sectors of our social fabric, which means recognising that we need to be working in a new paradigm since this requires a social revolution. This chapter argues for public health practitioners to become ready to provide leadership in the management of human systems for sustainability, taking the management role that meets the requirements of this serious situation. Sections cover analysing issues at multiple levels, managing complex systems (hierarchical, network and market forms) and identification of drivers for public health leadership in sustainability for health.

Chapter 8 Managing

Public health leadership and management for sustainability

Rae Walker, Jan Ritchie and Michael Sparks

Key words

Management for sustainability, leadership, adaptive management, drivers for transition and change, levels of action, analysis of human systems

Learning outcomes

From this chapter, public health practitioners and students will:

- gain knowledge about the management of human systems that support the sustainability of natural systems and human health;
- be ready to provide leadership in the management of human systems for ecological sustainability;
- be able to examine issues to be managed in their social and ecological context;
- analyse human systems and be able to identify appropriate approaches to management;
- recognise that management for sustainability means working in a new paradigm.

Outline

8.1 The challenge to public health of managing for sustainability

8.2 Analysing issues at multiple levels

8.3 Managing complex systems: three organisational forms

8.4 Managing hierarchical or formal organisations for sustainability

8.5 Managing networks and communities for sustainability

8.6 Managing markets for sustainability

8.7 Leadership and drivers for sustainability: the role of public health

Learning activities

8.1 Building a tower

Reading

Carley M. and Christie I. 2000, *Innovative Management for Sustainable Development*, Earthscan, London

Ministry of Forests, GoBC, Canada 2000, *An Introductory Guide to Adaptive Management: For project leaders and participants,* http://www.for.gov.bc.ca/HCP/AMHOME/INTROGD/Toc.htm

8.1 The challenge to public health of managing for sustainability

As elucidated throughout this book, the issues being raised in attempting to achieve global ecological integrity require new understanding, and new frameworks for action. The entirety of this different manner of operating requires us to recognise we are entering a new phase of life on this planet that history will record as being guided by the principles of a whole new paradigm. The newness is invigorating but the challenges are immense. Obstacles abound at every step, with progress being obstructed by both active confrontation from vested interests and passive inertia from apathetic individuals. To coordinate, consolidate, integrate and synthesise innovative activity for sustainability ends requires exceptional courage and above average energy. This is indeed a tall order, but without overriding guidance at higher levels, actions that are unco-ordinated are likely to be relatively fruitless. Thus this final chapter suggests a range of relevant and meaningful management and leadership concepts based on the principles discussed in previous pages.

As elucidated throughout this book, the issues being raised in attempting to achieve global ecological integrity require new understanding, and new frameworks for action.

By this stage we have introduced our readers to an overview of what we feel is the public health problem and how we can address it; we have outlined the concern we feel at the lack of involvement of public health practitioners in the area of sustainability; we have revisited seminal documents and frameworks and introduced newer ones that clarify the issues needing to be understood; we have determined the fact that we work within different knowledge cultures and that there is a need to follow the rules of dialogue in order to communicate between these different cultures; we have discussed the importance of scoping the problems and evaluating the solutions; and we have explained ways of acting and innovating to achieve our goals. Everything we have covered so far reflects our belief that things must change. This chapter provides some ideas of managing for change at personal, local, national and above all global levels, building on the different paradigmatic principles already presented.

People can choose between ecological life-support system maintenance or degradation. This choice has identifiable and in many cases measurable effects on public health:

> *If a society opts for social institutions, technologies and conservationist behaviours that sustain the natural resource base—the life-supporting*

ecosystems—then the long term health of that population will be enhanced. In contrast, erosion of natural resources will cause economic difficulties and regional conflicts and will eventually harm the health of even distant wealthy populations. (McMichael 2002, p. 93)

The ways social systems operate need to change if life-support systems are to be maintained. Human health is threatened, as is all life, so social and organisational change that supports the maintenance of ecological integrity, at multiple levels of social systems, must become 'core business' for public health. Public health managers and the organisations in which they work have, in their own context, a responsibility to lead change in our social systems toward the systems that support ecological integrity and human health.

Public health practice is well placed to make this change. The philosophical ideals of public health in recent decades—the New Public Health principles—are well documented (see Chapter 1 and Baum 2002) and depict adherents of these ideals as having an enlightened view of the knowledges covered in Chapter 4. In this ideal, lay perceptions and community opinions are valued alongside the views of public health researchers. Political and economic perspectives are key in decision-making, determining priority actions and appropriate interventions.

Understanding the contribution of factors in the social and physical environment of individuals to their health has allowed a strong focus in public health practice on the environmental determinants of health. The call to public health action exhorts practitioners to work in ways that empower people to make choices over how they would like to be healthier. Including global ecological integrity as an essential determinant of human health becomes a commonsense move for those with these values, and the consequent need to manage and lead others in addressing this integrity becomes obvious.

The broad categories of actions required of managers who work toward sustainability and health include:

- increased efficiency of resource use and decreased waste production;
- management practices that improve the resilience of natural resource systems;
- dealing cautiously with risk and irreversibility;
- integration of social and environmental considerations into economic decision-making, including proper valuing of environmental resources; and

The ways social systems operate need to change if life-support systems are to be maintained.

- community involvement in decisions. (Department of Environment, Sport and Territories 1992)

From the point of view of immediate relevance to public health practice, these actions would probably be best approached in reverse. Public health has extensive management experience in sponsoring community development programs for health (Baum 2002). However, this book adds an overriding principle to management for sustainability that we feel has not been considered adequately to date. The most important aspect of managing in this context is bringing together the various knowledge cultures held by relevant stakeholders—cultures which are described so clearly in Chapter 4. Unless we acknowledge that here we are moving into previously unvisited territory in harnessing these viewpoints to move forward together for change, we will continue to be ineffective in attempting to achieve our goals.

Public health has extensive management experience in sponsoring community development programs for health.

Thus the overall task we set ourselves in this chapter is to review the latest in the management literature so that those attempting to be innovative and creative managers for sustainability can draw on what they feel will best arm them to achieve success.

8.2 Analysing issues at multiple levels

If choices that meet current needs without compromising environmental integrity are to be realistic, the options need to be placed in their social and ecological contexts. Soskolne and Bertollini (1999) argue that three domains of integrity are important: the domains of the individual, the social and the ecological (p. 8). They argue that these domains are related to each other and that disharmony in their relationships can be damaging for the overall system. It is possible to solve a problem at a local or individual level in a way that creates negative effects at social and/or ecological levels. For example, spraying DDT for malaria control can reduce the immediate hazard posed by mosquitoes but has also created wider effects in human populations (Soskolne & Bertollini 1999). The 'good choices' are those that do not create unwanted effects in any of the domains (Figure 8.1). The individual domain consists of individuals and the groups in which they live, work and play: families, work groups or recreational groups. The social domain is made up of culture, economy, social class and social institutions such as government. The ecological domain consists of ecological and biophysical systems. As also indicated in the Mandala of Health described in Chapter 1, we cannot make good choices without this wider awareness.

Figure 8.1 Management domains

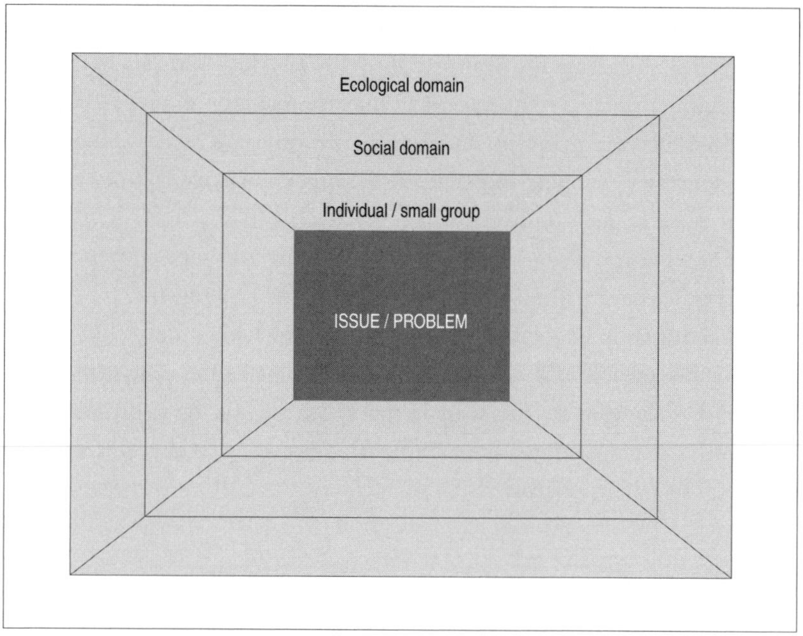

8.3 Managing complex systems: three organisational forms

In order to achieve progress towards ecological sustainability we need to organise elements within our complex social systems in new ways. We can consider this to be a process of co-ordinating existing resources for sustainability purposes. In complex social systems three models of co-ordination can be used to characterise and analyse the ways in which any human management system is co-ordinated, from a large global consortium such as the pharmaceutical giants, to state departments of health or a school food outlet (Frances et al. 1991). These models are comparable to the public policy discourses of market, state and community respectively (Adams & Hess 2001). Adler (2001) argues, from a slightly different perspective, that there are three ideal types of organisational form: markets, hierarchies or formal organisations, and networks. Powell (1990) describes the view of some economists that the three organisational forms are best conceived as governance structures. The key idea is that there are three major and very different ways of organising social activity, each operative at any scale (Figure 8.2).

Figure 8.2 Three organisational forms for sustainability management

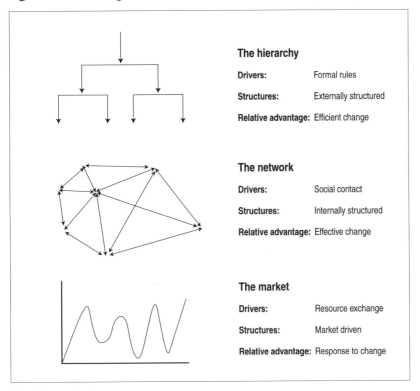

It is common for markets, hierarchies and networks to contribute to the co-ordination of activities in a complex social system, but in different ways (Skelcher et al. 1996). In any real life setting the organisational forms (or models of co-ordination) co-exist but with unequal status. For example, in formal organisations such as government departments and hospital administrations, the hierarchical form of co-ordination is dominant. There are markets and networks in trading resources and informal co-operative systems, but these are subordinate to the hierarchy. In communities, networks are dominant, with hierarchies and markets still present but subordinate to the collective informal knowledge of individual histories and capacities. In commerce and industry, markets are dominant, with administrative hierarchies and informal networks subordinate to resources trading.

Each of the models can be used to co-ordinate activities and events that otherwise appear unrelated. They are used in leadership and management to make sense out of an apparently chaotic system, in a way that all the participants in the system can understand. By co-ordinating otherwise disparate activities, coherence, morale and efficiency can be advanced in a social system (Frances et al. 1991; O'Toole 1997). Each model uses a characteristic approach to achieving social co-ordination and each can appear in diverse forms. Markets co-ordinate through the 'invisible hand' of a price system in market exchange, for example, through subsidies for crucial medications and school food outlets. Hierarchies work in the same organisations through authoritative administrative systems that consciously organise linkages between component parts. Networks co-ordinate through social, political and economic relationships that cross the boundaries of established organisational units (Frances et al. 1991). Through Activity 8.1, the public health leader and manager will find an understanding of the three organisational forms.

Activity 8.1
Building a tower

Aim: this learning activity endeavours to give participants an opportunity to experience leadership behaviour across a range of organisational modes. Groups will build a tower from supplied materials.

Why do we do it?

This chapter takes the reader through three very different organisational forms requiring therefore three very different managing processes.

Where and with whom do we do it?

Ideally three groups are needed for this activity, each with at least six members. It is best for the groups to be in the same room, which should be big enough for each group to work independently but in view of the others. Usually one and a half hours are devoted to this activity.

How do we do it?

As well as placing members in three groups, it is necessary to appoint an observer for each group and two judges overall.

The observers need a briefing sheet asking them to document the following:
* How the group organised for work.

- How decisions were made: through selection of alternatives? Through consensus? Through railroading?
- Whether participation was even or there was domination of a few?
- Missing task and maintenance functions?
- How the group members reacted to winning or losing.

The groups need instructions:

- One group is told it is working in a formal hierarchical organisation with a strong leader, two deputies and three followers; the second that it is in a network where everyone is expected to give an equal contribution; and the third group is operating in a market system where it is paid according to output, so the bigger each member's personal contribution the better.
- Each group is given a box of Lego blocks of the same number and shapes.
- Each is to build its tower to be judged on height, strength, beauty and inventiveness.
- Each will have one hour to build its tower.
- The winning group judged by the two judges will receive an award.

How do we review the activity?

At the end of the hour the judges make judgment based on the set criteria and present the award (a piece of fruit?). Then groups meet with their observers to discuss the exercise. Observers report back on the process they observed and general discussion follows on the value of the activity.

The social systems that affect ecological sustainability are complex. The management of organisations and complex systems to enhance sustainability and human health requires understanding of and skill in the appropriate harnessing of each organisational form. If public health is to attain leadership in managing for sustainability, an understanding of these different organisational forms is essential.

An illustration of the ways the three organisational forms intersect in a complex enterprise is provided by studies of urban regeneration partnerships in Britain (Lowndes & Skelcher 1998). Urban regeneration partnerships are created out of local collaborations for urban renewal that at times are transformed into formal structures to undertake major projects. Urban renewal is a major factor in modern city administration and offers one of the greatest contributions to advancing both sustainability and health; the opportunities to rebuild or retrofit according to energy-efficient, resource-conserving principles are immense. The dominant organisational form in these partnerships is the network, but the partnership has a life cycle in which different organisational forms become important at different times in relation to particular partnership tasks.

Box 8.1 Three organisational forms co-existing in a complex system

Stage of development	Organisational form
Pre-partnership collaboration	Networks already exist linking individuals and organisations for co-operative joint action
Formalisation	Hierarchical structures established to manage a large-scale project overseen by a board of management with decisions implemented by staff. Network membership status becomes scattered.
Program delivery	Market processes of tendering and contracting are used for some aspects of work. These sit alongside network relationships used for other tasks.
Partnership conclusion	Network structures used to manage local activity when the formal project has concluded.

Source: After Lowndes and Skelcher 1998

A key skill required of managers in the complex systems of society is the ability to identify the particular organisational form(s) required for a task and to use the appropriate management strategies that can achieve the desired goals.

8.4 Managing hierarchical or formal organisations for sustainability

This section expands on the characteristics of the formal or hierarchical organisation. Public health personnel will be most familiar with this organisational form through their experiences of international, national, regional and local level governance for health.

Box 8.2 Ideal type characteristics of a bureaucracy

Key features	hierarchy or bureaucracy
Normative basis	employment relationship
Means of communication	routines
Methods of conflict resolution	administrative fiat, supervision
Degree of flexibility	low
Amount of commitment between parties	medium to high
Tone or climate	formal, bureaucratic
Actor preferences or choices	dependent

Source: After Powell 1990, p. 300

All large formal organisations, whether public, charitable or private, manifest qualities of a bureaucracy. The classical exponent of the theory of bureaucracy was Max Weber:

> *Bureaucracy, for Weber, was a mode of organisation. The concept of organisation was such that it subsumed such differing substantive entities as the state, the political party, the church or sect or firm. The defining characteristic of an organisation was the presence of a leader and an administrative staff. These persons were ordered into specific types of social relationship.* (Clegg 1990, p. 33)

The activities undertaken by managers are typically described in functional terms. For example, the acronym POSDCORB has been used to represent the key management functions of planning, organising, staffing, directing, co-ordinating, reporting and budgeting (Gulick & Urwick 1973, in Legge & Stanton 2002). Authority is a key to exercising power in a bureaucracy and can be based on the charisma of a leader, tradition or legal principles. The latter source of authority is typical of the modern state and government structures (Clegg 1990).

Order and the co-ordination of work in a bureaucracy are maintained through convention, social and legal rules that shape the behaviour of members and underpin the authority of the people who fill positions in the hierarchical structure of the organisation. Bureaucracy is, in principle, an objective and rule-directed structure in which business is supposed to be conducted by technical experts without reference to persons (Clegg 1990).

Formal organisations or bureaucracies are more complex and manifest more nuances than Weber described. For example, the formal hierarchical structure of a bureaucracy is accompanied by an informal network structure through which some business is unofficially transacted. Nevertheless, bureaucracies are characterised by hierarchical structures in which order is maintained through authority. Business is supposedly conducted in technically competent ways, in response to commands from above and according to the rules and conventions of the organisation.

A vast literature on management in bureaucracies has been produced and is readily available in bookstores and libraries. The next section discusses approaches and techniques for managing in bureaucracies that are used to advance a sustainability agenda. These are adaptive management, governance, benchmarking and the development of corporate environmental performance indicators.

Adaptive management

Adaptive management represents a variety of management approaches that incorporate an action learning cycle.

Adaptive management represents a variety of management approaches that incorporate an action learning cycle consisting of: problem assessment, program design, implementation, monitoring, evaluation and program adjustment or redesign for another cycle (Ministry of Forests 2000; Norton & Steinemann 2001). It has been widely used for community-based environmental management or ecosystem management (Norton & Steinemann 2001). Adaptive management systems are being used in Canada to improve forest management, in the United States for water management in the Everglades, for management of fish stocks and many other purposes (Ministry of Forests 2000). Adaptive management is:

> *a formal, systematic, and rigorous approach to learning from the outcomes of management actions, accommodating change and improving management. It involves synthesising existing knowledge, exploring alternative actions and making explicit forecasts about their outcomes. Management actions and monitoring programs are carefully designed to generate reliable feedback and clarify the reasons underlying outcomes. Actions and objectives are then adjusted based on this feedback and improved understanding. In addition, decisions, actions and outcomes are carefully documented and communicated to others, so that knowledge gained through experience is passed on, rather than being lost when individuals move or leave the organization.* (Ministry of Forests 2000)

Adaptive management is especially valuable when working in contexts containing many uncertainties. These uncertainties can arise from:

- the issue being addressed: we may know too little about it, for example, health effects of electromagnetic fields, indoor air quality, a culture of suspicion in communities;
- the principles underlying a program being unfamiliar: the program implementation may be uncertain, for example, use of co-management (a collaborative management process) of public health and environmental projects in local communities; or
- the system being managed being complex: it may be too complex to understand fully and the precautionary principle must be exercised, for example, climate change and its public health effects.

Norton and Steinemann (2001) argue that adaptive management is characterised by three core principles:

1. Experimentalism: adaptive management is a consciously experimental approach to managing in a dynamic and surprising system. Hypotheses are formed at the problem assessment stage, interventions designed and evaluated in order to learn how to manage better, and management systems re-designed.
2. Multi-scalar analysis: ecosystems are complex and dynamic, and the effects of changes in them can appear over long periods of time and in diverse locations. Ecosystems are understood as functioning at different scales of magnitude and over extended periods of time, and these are taken into account in management decisions and processes.
3. Place sensitivity: places have a physical component made up of local subsystems and ecological conditions. Places also have a social component consisting of local communities, their relationship to their environment, values and history. Implementation of programs needs to accommodate the characteristics of the place in which they are implemented.

Adaptive management has evolved in more formal organisations, although it has potential for being an effective way of working in networks and markets.

Adaptive management is especially valuable when working in contexts containing many uncertainties.

Governance

To attain a greater understanding of the issues in managing for sustainability it is useful to undertake an analysis of the term 'governance', exploring its meaning in relation to this purpose. Governance means directing and controlling an organisation (Blandford & Smyth 2002) or a social system; it is used to refer to the role of governments in establishing and

Governments have the capacity, through their policies and the institutional arrangements they create, to shape the activities that take place across society.

implementing policies that shape activity in governmental jurisdiction or through collaboration across jurisdictions (Yencken 2002). It is also used to refer to the responsibilities of boards of management in relation to organisational performance, operations and compliance with laws and standards (Blandford & Smyth 2002). Because environmental systems have connections from local to global scales, governance for sustainability and health needs to be considered at multiple interacting levels. For example, Local Agenda 21 is an international agreement that for full implementation requires support at national and state or provincial government levels in order for local governments across a country to have maximum effect on environmental systems through local action.

Governments have the capacity, through their policies and the institutional arrangements they create, to shape the activities that take place across society. Yencken (2002) argues that governmental governance arrangements for sustainability need to achieve four things:

1. Every level of government needs to respond to environmental problems appropriately:
   - to the size of the problem and the magnitude of the response needed to make a difference;
   - to the forces creating the problem;
   - to the prevailing socio-economic systems needing to change;
   - in ways that achieve environmental, economic, social and cultural sustainability 'conjointly'; and
   - with acknowledgement that environmental problems emerge slowly and are frequently of uncertain dimensions.
2. Governments need to participate in international arrangements that strive to address the global nature of many environmental issues.
3. Strong inter-governmental arrangements are required to address national issues.
4. Governments at all levels need to view environmental policy as an adaptive learning process that achieves incremental improvements as initiatives appropriate to the problem evolve.

Government has at its disposal a number of mechanisms and powers that enable it to act for environmental sustainability. These include the capacity to:

- fund specific initiatives;
- organise initiatives across the whole of government;
- legislate on matters such as environmental standards;
- establish monitoring systems for environmental indicators; and
- require environmental auditing.

Government has the capacity to establish social environments, standards and requirements to which organisational management must respond.

Corporate governance, according to Blandford and Smyth (2002), refers to the ways boards of management organise and control:

- the productive work of the organisation;
- responses to external pressures; and
- modes of operation.

Other authors such as Kanter (1984) suggest senior management is also responsible for corporate governance. Corporate governance for sustainability and public health is about shifting the productive work and operations of the organisation towards those that are more environmentally sensitive and ecologically sustainable. Dias-Sardinha and Reijnders (2001) argue that there are six key strategic areas for action by organisations:

- compliance with relevant regulations and with voluntary codes of conduct in regard to environmental issues;
- pollution prevention;
- eco-efficiency;
- eco-innovation;
- eco-ethics or the use of environment-relevant norms to guide organisational decision-making and activities; and
- ecological sustainability of production and modes of operation.

Environmentally sensitive and ecologically sustainable corporate governance is crucial to bring about wide-scale changes required to secure public health in a stressed environment. An example of a corporate plan that includes sustainable development can be found at the 'Shell Canada' website (Shell Canada 2004) where the whole organisation has reformed to make the above strategic areas for action predominant in their operational plans. An example of a framework and strategies for action on environmental sustainability in formal organisations can be found in the *New Environmental Strategy for the National Health Service* (National Health Service Estates 2002).

Government has at its disposal a number of mechanisms and powers that enable it to act for environmental sustainability.

Benchmarking

Benchmarking is another process of relevance to managing for sustainability. There are many definitions of benchmarking, however, the one that captures most important elements of the concept describes it as: 'The process of continuously measuring and comparing one's business processes against comparable processes in leading organisations to obtain information that will help the organisation identify and implement improvements' (Anderson & Pettersen 1996). Benchmarking is essentially about reviewing the important aspects of an organisation, comparison with similar organisations, identification of reasons for differences, and identification of changes that might result in improvements. A key issue is the identification of the important aspects of the organisation that should be reviewed.

A key issue is the identification of the important aspects of the organisation that should be reviewed.

Environmental benchmarking is about applying the principles of benchmarking to the environmental performance of an organisation. There are three aspects of an organisation that might be benchmarked: first, its performance through the comparison of performance indicators (for example, achieving water quality targets); second, its processes (such as planning) for the protection of native vegetation; third, the strategic and planning choices made by the organisation and whether they are comparable with those of the best organisations in the field (for example, choices of environmental priorities). At a local government level the following might be the focus of an environmental benchmarking process:

- state of the environment, for example, air and water quality, noise pollution;
- resource management, for example, waste reduction;
- costs of environmental protection, for example, waste management costs;
- consumer satisfaction with environmental services;
- efficiency and effectiveness of enforcement of environmental rules and regulations;
- monitoring and performance measurement methods;
- environmental management systems; and
- policies for influencing the drivers of pollution. (Bolli & Emtairah 2001, p. 32)

Bolli and Emtairah (2001) have written a comprehensive handbook on environmental benchmarking for local government produced by the

European Environment Agency. It could be adapted for use by most organisations with public health interests.

Corporate environmental performance indicators

There are substantial debates around the definition of appropriate environmental performance indicators—the other process of importance to formal organisations for managing for sustainability. It is worth noting of course that the development of indicators is pertinent (but not a central issue) for other organisational forms as well. While the overall development of indicators for all parties to sustainability and health—communities, experts and organisations—is addressed in Chapter 5, organisations have a special responsibility in monitoring for their clients and their shareholders (or taxpayers in the case of many government activities). There is great variation between organisations, industries and governments as to the indicators developed, valued and used. Further, there are inconsistencies between environmental legislation and some of the emerging systems of environmental indicators. The World Resources Institute suggests a four-part system of in-organisation indicators based upon the notion of resource inputs and outputs of a firm:

- materials used—quantities and types of inputs;
- energy consumption—quantities and types of energy used or produced;
- non-product output—waste, treatment or waste disposal;
- pollutant releases—quantities and types of pollutants released to air, water and soil/landfill. (World Resources Institute 2002a)

Other environmental management systems use different sets of indicators. ISO 14000 is an international set of standards for environmental management systems. Like other International Standards Organisation (ISO) programs, ISO 14000 is a quality accreditation process focused on environmental management. It requires reporting against three inter-related types of indicators:

- operational indicators, which measure environmental stressors such as consumption of non-renewable resources like fuel or forest products;
- management indicators, which measure efforts to reduce environmental effects such as efforts to increase energy efficiency or training of staff in relation to environmental matters; and
- environment condition indicators, which measure aspects of environmental quality such as concentrations of pollutants. (World Resources Institute 2002b)

There are substantial debates around the definition of appropriate environmental performance indicators ...

Another environmental management system is environmental accounting. This contains two main strands: environmentally differentiated traditional accounting and ecological accounting (Karvonen 2000). Environmentally differentiated traditional accounting identifies and reports separately the costs of environmental issues such as taxes, permits and so on for the purpose of controlling and influencing them (Karvonen 2000). Ecological accounting is best represented by the concept of eco-balance, where a structured method is harnessed for reporting the physical flows of materials and energy of an organisation in a specific period. An eco-balance contains three elements: an analysis of inventories reporting all flows of materials and energy; the potential environmental impacts of these flows; and valuation of them in relation to each other (Karvonen 2000). The aspiration to adequately value ecological systems poses substantial challenges for economic theory and practice (Limburg et al. 2002). It requires a shift from valuation principles such as willingness to pay or willingness to accept, to principles such as the cost of human action related to the risk that the action will destabilise, or irrevocably alter, the life-support system (Limburg et al. 2002). The risk-avoidance principle is analogous to an insurance premium that is paid to protect against environmental destabilisation. The debate about appropriate valuation of the environment is continuing.

Another environmental management system is environmental accounting.

8.5 Managing networks and communities for sustainability

Although public health practitioners will be most familiar with hierarchical organisations, increasingly the roles of non-government organisations and community networks in the public health field have come to be valued. This section explores the characteristics of this organisational form and its value in complementing the formal type.

Box 8.3 Ideal type characteristics of a network

Key features	Network
Normative basis	complementary strengths
Means of communication	relationships

Methods of conflict resolution	norm of reciprocity, reputation concerns
Degree of flexibility	medium
Amount of commitment between parties	medium to high
Tone or climate	open-ended, mutual benefit
Actor preferences or choices	interdependent

Source: after Powell 1990, p. 300

The inability of command and control bureaucracies working on their own or vertically with international bureaucracies to deal with complex environment and development problems is a major concern worldwide (Carley & Christie 2000, p. 175). These words reflect the complexities of using networks for environmental management. Carley and Christie are not arguing that traditional bureaucracies should be replaced; they are good at many tasks (Carley & Christie 2000). Rather, they argue that ecological sustainability demands innovation in the ways social systems operate and that innovation can be accomplished most readily through networks known as 'action networks' that link government, business, non-government and community organisations in partnership. Action networks focus on the goal of ecological sustainability, which is viewed in a holistic frame, but are flexible and reflexive in the processes by which they work (Carley & Christie 2000). There are many examples of action networks being used for ecological sustainability and health, including:

- land use planning—using networks including community groups, environmental organisations, local government, industry and health organisations; and
- waste minimisation in hospitals—using networks of hospitals, purchasing organisations and environmental organisations.

Action networks are very different from traditional bureaucracies and need to be understood and managed in quite different ways. Mandell (1994, p. 100) argues that:

the use of management and co-ordination techniques based on theories borrowed from the literature on organisation theory or market theory cannot be applied wholesale. In fact, the concept of management, in terms of co-

ordination and control, is distinctly different from what is discussed in this literature.

Action networks are very different from traditional bureaucracies and need to be understood and managed in quite different ways.

In action network structures the key idea is the network itself: the trans-organisational arena in which action is triggered (Mandell 1994). Mandell calls such networks 'program structures', meaning that the network itself is a particular structure for the implementation of joint action. Program structures

> *are conceptualised as being separate from the organisations that may be represented in the program structure. Although public programs may be initiated through the efforts of people in individual organisations, when people come together to implement these programs, their perception is that they are operating in a distinct institutional arrangement. People are still committed to the interests of the individual organisations they represent, but they are also committed to the idea of a collaborative program to achieve action not achieved through individual effort. This commitment . . . is a mindset or way of thinking that recognises the legitimacy of the program structures as a distinct institutional arrangement and influences the actions and activities considered acceptable or appropriate in this context.* (Mandell 1994, p. 104)

Conceptualising action networks as distinct institutional arrangements allows us to consider the knowledge, norms and values, work rules and patterns of behaviour appropriate for the network (Mandell 1994).

Techniques for managing action networks, and the issues that need to be addressed, are different from those used in hierarchies or markets (O'Toole 1997). Network management techniques may be counter-intuitive for individuals skilled in managing in other models. For example, action networks do not have a 'head' with authority to make decisions on behalf of the partners, or the capacity to issue credible instructions to them. Instead, processes of consultation and consensus building are required to consolidate what is shared between partners to establish or reinforce the common ground on which they will jointly act.

Defining characteristics of action networks

Rummery (2002) argues that the evidence from studies of health and welfare partnerships (action networks) in Britain indicates that there are two critical and defining characteristics of these structures: interdependence and trust. Reciprocal interdependence (Thompson 1967) is what makes the formation of action networks necessary (Rummery 2002). Reciprocal interdependence means that the outcome of one organisation's work is an input to another and vice versa; each organisation is linked to the other(s) in reciprocal feedback loops. This relationship is the reason an action network is appropriate if organisations are to solve problems that matter to them, but it is also a key influence on the behaviour of participants in the action network.

The key players most frequently acknowledging ecological interdependence and participating in action networks are:

- governments at all levels;
- community organisations including public health, conservation and development interests;
- private sector interests including landholders, companies and industry associations; and
- scientific and research institutions. (Williams 2002, p. 3)

Trust that member organisations will 'deliver on jointly held objectives' . . .

For effective management of most ecological issues the action networks involving natural resources, industry and community interests need to be regional in scale, though some issues may be more appropriately addressed on larger or smaller scales (Williams 2002). The scale of the action network—whether it be local, regional or national—is a function of the scale of the interdependencies.

Trust that member organisations will 'deliver on jointly held objectives' is a feature of action networks around which adaptation and flexibility of the structure hinge (Rummery 2002); in the absence of trust, joint work is inhibited. There are many definitions of trust. A useful definition is that used by Zaheer et al. (1998, p. 143):

> *The expectation that an actor (1) can be relied on to fulfil obligations, (2) will behave in a predictable manner, and (3) will act and negotiate fairly when the possibility for opportunism in present.*

Trust diminishes the need for organisations to protect themselves against predatory behaviour and is also a source of efficiency in joint work (Adam and Walker 2001). Doubts about the trustworthiness of others in a network diminishes the willingness of participants to co-operate (Huggins 2000, p. 33). Adler (2001, p. 218) argues that trust has four dimensions: sources, mechanisms, objects and bases.

Each dimension has a number of components. The source of trust dimension has three: repeated interaction, calculation of interest and shared norms and values. Typically, a trust-based relationship would have its origins in at least one of these components, but in some instances relationships of apparent trust may be formed in which people act in trusting ways but hedge against the risk of betrayal (Huggins 2000). This has been termed 'swift trust' and is based on competent and faithful enactment of clear roles and their associated duties rather than the more established sources of trust (Huggins 2000, p. 34).

Trust diminishes the need for organisations to protect themselves against predatory behaviour and is also a source of efficiency in joint work.

The mechanisms for the deciding to trust dimension also has three components: personal contact, reputation and institutional context. While trust is influenced by individual relationships, it is also influenced by the institutional arrangements in organisations that define the social roles of members. Roles are institutionally defined, though there is some capacity for individuals to perform their assigned role in preferred ways. In the end, however, an individual is constrained by the organisational environment.

The objects of trust dimension has three components: individuals, organisations and systems. Relationships of trust may be with any or all of these levels. It is possible to trust individuals but not the individual's organisation or the system of which it is a part. Similarly, it is possible to trust the system but not the organisation and/or individual, and so on. If the object we consider trusting manifests certain qualities—the bases of trust—we are more likely to bestow trust upon it.

The bases of trust dimension includes multiple components such as consistency of behaviour, personal and role competence, loyalty, goodwill, confidentiality, honesty and integrity (Adam & Walker 2001). The bases of trust are the features of those objects in which we feel trust (Adler 2001), and features of relationships that can be managed (Limerick & Cunnington 1993). An individual, organisation or system can increase the likelihood of being trusted by manifesting the qualities in which we feel trust—the bases of trust.

Managing networks

As noted, many public health practitioners are most familiar with management work in formal hierarchical (bureaucratic) organisations; for example, the public service, local government or large health care organisations. Experience gained in these contexts may not provide useful guidance for the management of action networks. O'Toole (1997, p. 47) argues that in networks:

Standard nostrums of public administration probably do not apply. Managers in networked settings do not supervise most of those on whom their own performance relies, monitoring channels are typically diffuse and unreliable, and common organisational culture exercises a limited and indirect influence.

If network management is so different, what are the ground rules? From O'Toole's (1997) perspective there are four 'rules of thumb' that help people new to the complexities of network management:

1. Power in networks is a function of a person's ability to organise support from partners for a particular course of action (Mandell 2001). The authority associated with management positions in formal organisations should not be assumed. Attempting to exercise authority in network structures can weaken an individual's influence.

2. An individual's own network of relationships, and the resources controlled by those network members, is an important source of influence. Among other things, these networks provide 'strategic intelligence' that supports understanding and action in complex contexts. Personal work-related networks need to be reviewed and systematically rebuilt from time to time.

3. Effective network managers look for opportunities to co-ordinate the work of the full set of participants in the action network. The opportunities may be found in widely shared values, goals or practices that form the common ground for joint action.

4. Shifting the members of the action network toward joint action that will achieve shared goals, and helping to build trust between participants, are typically valued activities.

If we move beyond 'rule of thumb' management strategies we find three key strategies in network management (Mandell 2001):

1. Influencing members to participate. This includes developing champions and sponsors for the network, reframing existing rules, procedures, norms and values of network actors to support joint action, and developing a shared purpose and vision for the network. It also involves monitoring and influencing network membership to sustain joint action and change network dynamics when appropriate.

2. Securing commitment to joint action. This is about exercising influence in the network to achieve co-operation and collaboration between people

If network management is so different, what are the ground rules?

and organisations that may not normally do this. It involves marshalling resources, building agreements, establishing systematic communication processes, mediating between participants, and developing strategies to achieve common objectives.

3. Creating an environment that supports productive interaction by increasing the benefits and reducing the costs of participation. The manager becomes a facilitator of network work, making the decisions and actions required easier to achieve than they would otherwise be. Walker (2000) refers to a collaboration tactician, a term she uses to describe people who are skilled in making network structures function and who enjoy the skills of successful network managers. Win-win negotiation skills are paramount, as is the presence of attitudes which value one's own organisation in relation to others.

8.6 Managing markets for sustainability

The third organisational form that must be considered in managing for sustainability is the market.

The third organisational form that must be considered in managing for sustainability is the market. Although there is frequent overlap between the three organisational forms, this form is probably least familiar to public health practitioners and is thus often regarded with suspicion. However, since global ecological integrity can only be achieved through including corporations and private industry in shared action, it is essential that the characteristics of markets be understood as clearly as those of formal and network organisations.

Box 8.4 Ideal type characteristics of a market

Key features	Market
Normative basis	contract, property rights
Means of communication	prices
Methods of conflict resolution	negotiating, resort to courts for enforcement of contracts
Degree of flexibility	high
Amount of commitment between parties	low
Tone or climate	precision and/or suspicion, trust
Actor preferences or choices	independent

Source: after Powell 1990, p. 300

A market is a system for exchanging specific goods and services in a non-personal way, often controlled through a contract enforceable in law. In economic theory markets are a spontaneous co-ordination mechanism that imparts rationality and consistency to the self-interested actions of individuals and firms (Powell 1990). Relationships between people or firms in a market transaction are in theory impersonal, non-co-operative, self-interested and unconstrained (Powell 1990)—in contrast with hierarchies and networks. When we talk of managing markets for sustainability and health we are typically referring to ways of influencing the activity of firms in a marketplace. Firms operating in a competitive market have key processes that must be undertaken (for example, auditing), and key values that underpin decision-making (for example, efficiency). Many of the techniques for managing markets for sustainability and health are attempts to put new content into key processes (for example, environmental auditing), and to attach new actions to key values such as eco-efficiency. In this part of the chapter some major strategies for working towards ecological sustainability and health in market contexts are discussed.

A market is a system for exchanging specific goods and services in a non-personal way, often controlled through a contract enforceable in law.

Managing markets for sustainability

The strategies described here are key approaches to influencing the behaviour of business organisations operating in a market environment. The descriptions are brief and uncritical, include business language and concepts, and links to resources that provide more information are provided. Such a brief discussion can do no more than introduce ideas that have currency in the business community itself.

Eco-efficiency

Eco-efficiency is defined as:

> *The delivery of competitively priced goods and services that satisfy human needs and bring quality of life, while progressively reducing ecological impacts and resource intensity throughout the life cycle to a level at least in line with the earth's carrying capacity.* (World Business Council for Sustainable Development 2000, p. 4)

Eco-efficiency is considered to be a business management philosophy that focuses on business opportunities that provide both environmental and economic benefits. It is about innovation and subsequent economic growth and competitiveness (World Business Council for Sustainable Development 2000).

From the perspective of the World Business Council for Sustainable Development (2000), eco-efficiency has four objectives and four opportunities. The objectives are to:

- reduce consumption of resources;
- reduce the impact on nature;
- increase product or service value; and
- implement an environmental management system.

The opportunities lie in:

- re-engineering processes to reduce the consumption of resources;
- co-operation with other companies to convert waste into products;
- redesigning products; and
- finding new ways of meeting consumer needs.

Eco-efficiency is considered to be a business management philosophy that focuses on business opportunities that provide both environmental and economic benefits.

Eco-efficiency is a framework in which sustainability can be pursued through business activity in a competitive market; however, it requires that the social environment of the market also changes in a way that creates economic benefits for companies working in the framework. For example, it requires government to change elements of the market environment it creates for business such as shifting taxes—currently on labour and profit—to resource use and pollution, and it requires consumers to value 'green products' and strengthen the demand for them (World Business Council for Sustainable Development 2000). Measurement of eco-efficiency is conceptualised as product or service value divided by environmental influence. Progress is achieved by providing more value per unit of environmental influence or unit of resource used (Verfaillie & Bidwell 2000). The World Business Council for Sustainable Development has produced indicators that can be used for decision-making, benchmarking and accountability (Verfaillie & Bidwell 2000).

Innovation

Innovation is viewed from a business perspective as the core process required to create a sustainable society: 'Our challenges in business are to create the major innovations necessary to enable a sustainable human existence and to ensure their acceptance by society' (Dormann & Holliday 2002, p. 9). This quotation captures a business perspective on the role of innovation in sustainable development. The role of business in innovation is to create products and services out of ideas and to deliver them to the marketplace in efficient ways. The innovation process is depicted by Dormann and Holliday (2002, p. 11) as moving further than is expected in the other organisational forms from 'idea' to 'research and development', 'product/service' and commercialisation of the latter.

New ideas, inputs and practices need to be incorporated into the process to ensure sustainability issues are addressed; these include economic, social and environmental ideas and issues. Dormann and Holliday (2002) argue that there are four major questions to be answered in regard to innovation in regard to sustainability:

- How can we ensure sustainability is part of the creative process?
- How can we ensure sustainability considerations are part of the management of development process?
- When and how can external viewpoints enrich the creative and development processes?
- What processes are most likely to leverage the value of our intellectual capital?

Innovation is viewed from a business perspective as the core process required to create a sustainable society.

Triple Bottom Line/single bottom line

Although the triple bottom line (TBL) has already been covered in previous chapters, it has relevance here so is briefly addressed again, this time from a management perspective. It is a way of measuring and reporting an organisation's performance against economic, social and environmental indicators. It has its origins in the business sector and is considered a way of shifting the focus of business activity away from economic performance only. Again, go to the website of Shell Canada (2004) to see how that corporation has moved from a bottom line purely based on economic indicators to now base its decisions on social and environmental factors as well.

Although the TBL is often represented by partially overlapping circles, with the area of overlap being the patch monitored and reported using TBL processes, more recently a nested model has been used. This model represents the economy as dependent on society, which is in turn dependent on the environment (Giddings et al. 2002). The latter is a more realistic if less focused depiction of the relationships, and has come to be known as the single bottom line (SBL). From a management perspective, this SBL provides probably the optimum framework for sustainability decision-making.

Competitive advantage

Virtually all corporate pollution is a sign of economic waste and the unproductive use of resources, and can be addressed by better technology or improved methods. Innovative corporate practices in the area of the environment, then, will often enhance internal competitiveness. Products that address environmental scarcities will also have enormous market potential. This means that companies should see environmental protection as an opportunity. (Porter 2002, p. 4)

Implicit in Porter's argument is the idea that the market provides incentives for sustainable practices. Companies can achieve competitive advantage in the marketplace by innovation in relation to the use of scarce resources, and by reducing the cost of resources through efficiency, waste minimisation and recycling. Exploiting a competitive advantage is a very important strategy for generating wealth in a market.

8.7 Leadership and drivers for sustainability: the role of public health

In the opening section of this chapter we made clear that we believe managing for sustainability means operating in a new paradigm. We stated our belief that this new approach should be viewed as core business for public health. Public health theory and practice must expand to include all aspects of this vigorously expanding area of knowledge and skills; however, from their recent experiences in the promotion of health and the prevention of disease, public health practitioners are in a position to take a lead in the required co-operative ventures that can only be attained through intersectoral, interdisciplinary and international collaboration.

The role of public health in tobacco control across the world is an example that augurs well as a model for public health leadership for sustainability (Chapman 2003). Australia, as one of the three leading countries in the world to succeed in reducing smoking rates across the whole population, is an interesting case study of harnessing and working with these three organisational forms. Initial efforts to reduce smoking-related morbidity and mortality focused on individuals changing their behaviour. Messages from hierarchical organisations emphasised an authoritative approach; however, it was soon recognised by public health personnel that exhorting individuals to 'do the right thing' and quit smoking for their better health was a lost cause, despite those working from the biomedical perspective continuing to uphold this approach. The recognition of the futility of this approach was achieved when community perceptions were tapped to reveal that the lack of obvious and immediate harm meant that death from lung cancer and other smoking-related conditions that were at risk of developing had little meaning to the vast majority of smokers. This recognition came from understanding networks and informal community groups. Tobacco control slowly moved to focus more on addressing the market issues involved, demonstrating that an understanding of the third organisational form was essential. Tobacco began to be viewed as a drug and the tobacco companies as the drug 'pushers'. Public health practitioners joined the fight to ban tobacco advertising, moving their focus from the demand (smokers themselves) to the supply (tobacco companies). Following this progress, active community groups worked to support non-smoking employees in using the law to protect their health through instigating smoke-free work environments. Australian government departments were the first to implement policies and practices reflecting this change in the law—again a return to focusing on hierarchical organisations, and their example has now been followed in many countries that seek to seriously address the problem. Analysis shows the effectiveness of the overall approach has been especially due to understanding the characteristics of all three organisational systems and using this knowledge to manage for the health of the public.

. . . we believe managing for sustainability means operating in a new paradigm.

The risk for public health is that despite the logic that practitioners in this arena could make very appropriate leaders, true leadership must inspire people to want to follow rather than be made to do so. Public health will lose dignity and respect if it arrogantly tries to place itself in a powerful leading position without demonstrating its potential to lead in a way that genuinely values global ecological integrity. Leadership is more than being in an authoritative position; effective leaders influence people through exhibiting such personal attributes as their values, ethics and skills in ways that attract the respect of others. Only once this respect is gained can the art and skill of guiding and directing for task accomplishment come into play. Thus the primary attributes needed for leadership are trustworthiness and ability to communicate a vision (Clark 1998).

Bolman and Deal (2003) offer some useful ideas in their recent publication *Reframing Organizations: Artistry, choice and leadership*. In the case of leadership for sustainability, the idea of reframing our perspectives is central to the task. The concepts of artistry and creativity fit well with the suggestions we are making here that these ideas are the foundations for a social revolution in our thinking and ultimately in our acting. It is relevant here to revisit the list in Chapter 1, Box 1.6, of the areas of knowledge and skills that public health practitioners should attain. Leadership is needed from the public health arena that facilitates the development of these knowledge and skill areas, not as an end in themselves but rather as a foundation for the new challenges. Feeling strong in our understanding of the basics will give courage to leaders and their followers who wish to move to new heights.

Public health will lose dignity and respect if it arrogantly tries to place itself in a powerful leading position without demonstrating its potential to lead in a way that genuinely values global ecological integrity.

Conclusion

In this chapter, we have restated our opinion that working towards sustainability and health will require a paradigm shift. Visionary and trustworthy leaders will be required to move society to new and constructive ways of dealing with these huge issues. We have built on previous chapters that clarified and exposed issues around sustainability and that provided a call to action. Managing and leading others to act requires a firm foundation of knowledge, but must depend on skills of implementation for optimum results to occur. Reading these words is one thing; acting and implementing is another. Co-ordinating and managing the extensive human and material resources involved in the quest for sustainability is the ultimate task.

Resources for leadership and management skills

An Introductory Guide to Adaptive Management. A web-based resource through which the principles of adaptive management of forests in Canada is encouraged. The emphasis is on the management process. Available at: http://www.for.gov.bc.ca/hfp/amhome/introgd.htm [22 January 2004]

Co-management of natural resources. A web-based resource in which the principles of network management are applied to stakeholder management of natural resources. Available at: http://nrm.massey.ac.nz/changelinks/cmnr.html [13 February 2004]

Eco-efficiency: creating more value with less impact. A discussion of the concept and principles of eco-efficiency prepared by the World Business Council for Sustainable Development. Available at: http://www.wbcsd.org [13 February 2004]

Bolli, A. and Emtairah, T. (2001) *Environmental Benchmarking for Local Authorities: From concept to practice*, European Environment Agency, Copenhagen. Available at: http://www.eea.eu.int [22 January 2004]

Innovation, Technology, Sustainability and Society. A report from the World Business Council for Sustainable Development on the role of innovation in creating sustainability. Available at: http://www.wbcsd.org [13 February 2004]

Measuring Eco-efficiency: a guide to reporting company performance. A discussion of appropriate indicators of eco-efficiency and systems for reporting prepared by the World Business Council for Sustainable Development. Available at: http://www.wbcsd.org [13 February 2004]

Partnership synergy. A web-based resource produced by the Centre for Advancement of Collaborative Strategies in Health. It includes a conceptual framework, research instruments for measuring synergy and dimensions of functioning and a partnership self-assessment tool. Available at: http://www.cacsh.org/ [13 February 2004]

Triple Bottom Line Toolkit. A resource kit produced by the City of Melbourne and the International Council for Local Environmental Initiatives for triple bottom line measurement and reporting in local government. Available at: http://www.melbourne.vic.gov.au [13 February 2004]

The World Resources Institute describes itself as a management institute for environment and business. Its website contains useful information in environmental performance indicators. Available at: http://www.wri.org [22 January 2004]

Managing and leading others to act requires a firm foundation of knowledge . . .

References

Adam, J. and Walker, R. 2001, 'Trust in Relationships between Primary Health Care Organisations', *Australian Journal of Primary Health Interchange*, vol. 7, pp. 56-60

Adams, D. and Hess, M. 2001, 'Community in Public Policy: Fad or foundation', *Australian Journal of Public Administration*, vol. 60, no. 2, pp. 13-23

Adler, P.S. 2001, 'Market, Hierarchy, and Trust: The knowledge economy and the future of capitalism', *Organisation Science*, vol. 12, pp. 215-34

Anderson, B. and Pettersen, P.G. 1996, *The Benchmarking Handbook: Step-by-step instructions*, Chapman and Hall, London

Baum, F. 2002, *The New Public Health*, Oxford University Press, South Melbourne

Blandford, J. and Smyth, T. 2002, 'From Risk Management to Clinical Governance', *Managing Health Services: Concepts and practice*, ed. M.G. Harris, MacLennan and Petty, Sydney

Bolli, A. and Emtairah, T. 2001, *Environmental Benchmarking for Local Authorities: From concept to practice*, European Environment Agency, Copenhagen, http://www.eea.eu.int [22 January 2004]

Bolman L. and Deal, T. 2003, *Reframing Organizations: Artistry, choice and leadership*, Wiley, New York

Carley, M. and Christie, I. 2000, *Innovative Management for Sustainable Development*, Earthscan, London

Chapman, S. 2003, *Tobacco and Health*, http://tobacco.health.usyd.edu.au/site/supersite/resources/docs/index.htm [2 May 2003]

Clark D. 1998, 'Concept of Leadership', *Big Dog's Leadership Page*, http://www.nwlink.com/~donclark/leader/leadcom.html [22 January 2004]

Clegg, S.R. 1990, *Modern Organisations: Organisation studies in the postmodern world*, Sage, London

Department of Environment, Sport and Territories 1992, *National Strategy for Ecologically Sustainable Development*, Australian Government Publishing Service, Canberra

Dias-Sardinha, I. and Reijnders, L. 2001, 'Environmental Performance Evaluation and Sustainability Performance Evaluation of Organisations: An evolutionary framework', *Eco-Management and Auditing*, vol. 8, no. 2, pp. 71-9

Dormann, J. and Holliday, C. 2002, *Innovation, Technology, Sustainability and Society*, World Business Council for Sustainable Development, Stevenage, United Kingdom

Frances, J., Levacic, R., Mitchell, J. and Thompson, G. 1991, 'Introduction', *Markets, Hierarchies and Networks: The co-ordination of social life*, eds G. Thompson, J. Frances, R. Levacic and J. Mitchell, Sage, London

Giddings, B., Hopwood, B. and O'Brien, G. 2002, 'Environment, Economy and Society: Fitting them together into sustainable development', *Sustainable Development*, vol. 10, no. 4, pp. 187-96

Huggins, R. 2000, *The Business of Networks: Inter-firm interaction, institutional policy and the Tec experiment*, Aldershot, Ashgate

Kanter, R.M. 1984, *The Changemasters: Corporate entrepreneurs at work*, Counterpoint, Boston

Karvonen, M.M. 2000, 'Environmental Accounting as a Tool for SMES in Environmentally Induced Economic Risk Analysis', *Eco-Management and Auditing*, vol. 7, no. 1, pp. 21-8

Legge, D. and Stanton, P. 2002, 'Learning Management (and Managing Your Own Learning)', *Managing Health Services: Concepts and practice*, ed. M.G. Harris, MacLennan and Petty, Sydney

Limburg, K.E., O'Neill, R.V., Costanza, R. and Farber, S. 2002, 'Complex Systems and Valuation', *Ecological Economics*, vol. 41, no. 3, pp. 409-20

Limerick, D. and Cunnington, B. 1993, *Managing the New Organisation: A blueprint for networks and strategic alliances*, Business and Professional Publishing, West Chatswood

Lowndes, V. and Skelcher, C. 1998, 'The Dynamics of Multi-Organisational Partnerships: An analysis of changing modes of governance', *Public Administration Review*, vol. 76, pp. 313-33

Mandell, M.P. 1994, 'Managing Interdependencies through Program Structures: A revised paradigm', *American Review of Public Administration*, vol. 24, no. 1, pp. 99-124

——2001, 'Collaboration through Network Structures for Community Building Efforts', *National Civic Review*, vol. 90, no. 3, pp. 279-87

Ministry of Forests, GoBC, Canada 2000, *An Introductory Guide to Adaptive Management: For project leaders and participants,* http://www.for.gov.bc.ca/HFP/AMHOME/INTROGD/Toc.htm [22 January 2004]

National Health Services Estates 2002, *New Environmental Strategy for the National Health Service*, Norwich, www.nhsestates.gov.uk/download/publications_guidance/envstrat.pdf [22 January 2004]

Norton, B.G. and Steinemann, A.C. 2001, 'Environmental Values and Adaptive Management', *Environmental Values*, vol. 10, pp. 473-506

O'Toole, L.J. 1997, 'Treating Networks Seriously: Practical and research based agendas in public administration', *Public Administration Review*, vol. 57, no. 1, pp. 45-52

Porter, M. 2002, 'Preface', *Tomorrow's Markets: Global trends and their implications for business*, World Resources Institute, World Business Council for Sustainable Development and United Nations Environment Program, New York

Powell, W.W. 1990, 'Neither Market nor Hierarchy: Network Forms of Organisation', *Research in Organisational Behavior*, vol. 12, pp. 295-336

Rummery, K. 2002, 'Towards a Theory of Welfare Partnerships', *Partnerships, New Labour and the Governance of Welfare*, eds C. Glendinning, M.A. Powell and K. Rummery, Policy Press, Bristol, United Kingdom

Shell Canada 2004, *Sustainable Development Policy*, http://66.46.147.14/code/values/dir_values.html [22 January 2004]

Skelcher, C., McCabe, A., Lowndes, V. and Nanton, P. 1996, *Community Networks in Urban Regeneration*, The Policy Press, Bristol

Soskolne, C.L. and Bertollini, R. 1999, *Global Ecological Integrity and 'Sustainable Development': Cornerstones of public health*, A Discussion Document, WHO European Centre for Environment and Health, Rome, http://www.euro.who.int/document/gch/ecorep5.pdf [22 January 2004]

Thompson, J.D. 1967, *Organizations in Action: Social science bases of administrative theory*, McGraw-Hill, New York

Verfaillie, H.A. and Bidwell, R. 2000, *Measuring Eco-Efficiency: A guide to reporting company performance*, World Business Council for Sustainable Development, Tockwith

Walker, R. 2000, *Collaboration and Alliances: A review for VicHealth*, Victorian Health Promotion Foundation, Melbourne

Williams, J. 2002, 'Roles, Responsibilities and Partnerships', *Ecological Management and Restoration*, vol. 3, no. 1, pp. 3-4

World Business Council for Sustainable Development 2000, *Eco-Efficiency: Creating more value with less impact*, World Business Council for Sustainable Development, Tockwith

World Resources Institute 2002a, *Corporate Epistemology: The way forward*, http://www.wri.org [30 September 2003]

——2002b, *In Search of Common Yardsticks*, http://www.wri.org [30 September 2003]

Yencken, D. 2002, 'Governance for Sustainability', *Australian Journal of Public Administration*, vol. 61, no. 2, pp. 78-89

Zaheer, A., McEvily, B. and Perrone, V. 1998, 'Does Trust Matter? Exploring the Effects of Inter-organisational and Interpersonal Trust on Performance', *Organisation Science*, vol. 9, no. 2, pp. 141-59

THE WAY FORWARD

Epilogue

The way forward

It has taken five editors, seven universities, ten international experts, thirty colleagues, twelve authors, ten trial courses and three years to develop this teaching text for incorporating sustainability into public health courses. This thorough consultative and collaborative process has meant that we, the editors, have been putting into practice the learning resources you will have found throughout this book. Looking forward from here, based on our learning during this process, we can say that:

- The personal and professional changes associated with working towards sustainability and health are not trivial. They involve taking part in social learning that goes beyond the usual teaching curriculum that services current expectations of public health. **Working together for sustainability and health means not only taking part in, but leading, major social change.**
- The changes to public health and environmental management are as significant as those that responded to the industrial revolution. We need to remember that current urban planning, local government services, public health services and civil engineering regimes, all now taken for granted as essential social structures, were all initiated at that time. **Working towards sustainability and health means being willing to stay open to similar ground-breaking initiatives, both from within and outside one's sector of action**.
- The collaborative processes and continuing learning spiral that provide the backbone of *Sustainability and Health* may seem complex on the first reading. Now that this learning resource has been trialled with your colleagues and fellow students, we hope you have found, as we have done, that it produces a synergy and a richer understanding of the topics than do more traditional teaching-learning processes. **Working together for sustainability and health is essentially a convivial, creative and productive process**.

We have presented the sustainability and health practitioner—whether in the public health professions, a student, or in some related occupation—with a challenging theoretical framework for moving decisions into action and a set of practical strategic tools for implementing that framework. Both the D4P4 decisions-into-action framework and the integrative tools are meant to be intensely practical and a core part of your own practice.

In our closing reflections, we return once more to the D4P4 framework, suggesting you apply it to your own use of the materials in this book.

As you began your course, your program or your project you needed a firm commitment to *what should be*, the principles of sustainable development, the broader principles of sustainability and the Earth Charter in order to give you a sense of direction in managing a program of change (Figure 1.3, Box 1).

From there, you went to the most reliable sources you could find on *what is* in relation to your chosen principles. Your descriptions of people and place will have included multiple and even contrasting perspectives, and been related to broad-based explanatory frameworks (Figure 1, Box 2).

Once you grounded the principles in the current realities of the literature, your occupation and your colleagues, you will have explored the creative potential for social learning and social change, reviewed fresh ideas from a range of researchers and futurists, and chosen those most appropriate to your situation in designing practical actions towards *what could be* (Figure 1.3). In applying the social learning and social change approach to your particular area in your particular field, you will have scoped the full context and potential of your program, and applied that to implementing and monitoring your and your collaborators' strategies and actions in order to discover *what can be* (Figure 1.3, Box 4).

From there you will have revisited *what should be*, re-examining first principles in the light of the learning from the evaluation to see whether you needed to re-interpret the principles in reflecting on what you have learnt. Thus, *Sustainability and Health: Supporting global ecological integrity in public health* represents a never-ending spiral of mutual learning as we all move a little toward the vast and difficult but essential goal.

Throughout this book we have proposed a new way of working in public health and related practice, giving guidelines for an inclusive, collaborative, systems-focused and future-oriented approach that includes personal responsibility for managing change. We have suggested that successful action to address sustainability and health requires as large a shift in thinking as did the moves of a century ago that led eventually to the elimination of cholera and tuberculosis as major scourges in Western populations, and to the eradication of smallpox completely. That action took us from isolating the disease carriers to recognising that it was the social context that needed to be changed. Personal hygiene and health controls in urban design were born from that change.

To achieve sustainability, the change is as great or greater; the scale is global, societies are multicultural and the adaptations required involve acute change in interactions between the social and physical worlds. Sustainability requires the linking of the social and physical worlds at personal, communal and global levels—a linkage that we have termed *global ecological integrity.* As we were developing our materials for this book, our global ecological integrity was unexpectedly jeopardised. A communicable disease that could well have been as equally serious a pandemic as those mentioned above erupted into a world that thought it had the capacity to control such infectious diseases. In January 2003, severe acute respiratory syndrome (SARS) reared its ugly head, emerging as a new and threatening public health problem that crossed environmental boundaries (World Health Organisation 2003). The occurrence of a new disease with a rapid global spread was just such an event that we, as authors of *Sustainability and Health,* were predicting and to which we had hoped to provide some responses.

A close examination of what happened with SARS, and why, offers a benchmark for comparison which we believe our readers might find interesting. Throughout this book we have emphasised a need for innovative and collaborative approaches to addressing sustainability. The SARS epidemic has given us an example of the very environment-related risks to health that this entire set of learning materials is intended to prevent. Yet there were already in existence a series of global and local responses that could easily be described as innovative and collaborative. Is it possible to find something that we can learn here that strengthens our resolve and ability to put the components of this book into action before, rather than after, the event?

From the start, SARS was problematic locally and globally, socially and environmentally, and professionally across a wide range of response areas. If we analyse SARS as a public health problem, we can see that it initially could not be clearly defined from previous experience of disease identification or transmission. However, its effects were immediate and tangible; they arose through human/environment interaction and were spread at an unprecedented rate through human/environment transmission.

Although the original infected population only affected some 8000 people, the very infection rate and the high case fatality rate of 15 per cent was of immense concern, both immediately and as a precedent for the future (World Health Organisation 2003). The knowledge bases for living, listening, grounding, knowing, scoping, acting, innovating and managing—covered in the eight chapters of this book—were called into play in new ways, closely related to those we have discussed here. Let us briefly analyse global performance in reacting to SARS according to the principles set out in the book.

In Chapter 1 we talked about *Living*. The existence of a public health threat from SARS was not apparent for three months, which allowed it time to reach 27 countries. Atypical pneumonia is not an uncommon diagnosis in a Third World country where elaborate technology is not available for differential diagnosis, but the cases appearing in developed countries where laboratory testing could occur, showed the disease did not fit a recognised and identifiable pattern. SARS spread globally as rapidly as it did due to this disparity in public health resources, high urban density and the ease with which humans have been able to move around the globe in recent decades, especially by air.

Clearly viewing disease from an ecological perspective helped identify and control the way the epidemic spread. If the perspective and skills offered here had been in place, it would have allowed sustainability and health practitioners to work towards prevention, rather than remediation, of the next global threat.

In Chapters 2 and 3 we spoke about *Listening* and *Grounding*. Even though it took a mere three months for SARS to move from a few instances of atypical pneumonia to a potential global threat, WHO took leadership in collaboration between mass media outlets and expert information channels—all vehicles which often act in isolation or competition—to work in a global partnership to proclaim the situation across the world. Even the choice of the simple four-letter abbreviation, SARS, has allowed easy discussion and demystification so the messages could reach all concerned. The worldwide information network allowed almost instantaneous dissemination when there was a will to inform and the technology was easily available and accessible. China was initially the exception, until the urgency of the issue eventually overcame early political censorship.

WHO broadcast daily bulletins on the Internet in clear lay person's languages to clarify the problem and to inform people worldwide on how they could protect themselves and prevent the spread to others. The clear information and the recognition of the widespread responsibilities of individuals, communities, specialist practitioners and governments allowed transfer of information to catch up with the rapid spread of the disease.

In Chapter 4 we discussed *Knowing*. It is interesting to view the SARS example from this perspective. The response to SARS among threatened societies was shared very obviously across the five knowledge cultures, as follows. Individuals reconsidered personal hygiene; communities sought to safeguard their members through such diverse actions as special SARS hospitals working to protect their healthcare workers and villages in China, keeping a sanitised area through replacing their village walls.

Specialists worked around the clock to result in the coronavirus involved being identified. The epidemiology of the patterns of incidence and prevalence gave us a clearer picture of the spread of SARS, and of the response through isolation and antibiotic regime that proved effective in reducing transmission. Private industry and governments not necessarily friendly to each other all collaborated freely. Strategists mounted policy and legislative campaigns to protect citizens, and openness and citizen responsibility emerged even in closed societies.

Most constructively, WHO co-ordinated an extraordinary global surveillance and research information system in collaboration with national governments and affected communities to come up with a co-ordinated, holist response that respects global ecological integrity beyond any one way of knowing or any one jurisdiction. It sent teams to work in every stricken country and region, co-ordinated specialisations for collaboration across borders and worked toward a shared understanding of the human condition in the new global context. If such teams had been in place before the event, monitoring prospective risks and responses, SARS may have been prevented altogether or stopped at source.

In Chapter 5 we spoke of *Scoping*. WHO's co-ordination of a surveillance and information system to result in a global response indicated the organisation saw SARS as a part of a complex system that could only be understood by working with complexity. WHO enlisted many experts and communities in working to build a nested understanding of those complex factors and how they related to each other.

However, what emerged here was the predictability of such an event in a world of changing climatic and environmental living conditions, rapid global transport and close urban proximity to others. In scoping we have suggested that negotiating a vision for global ecological integrity will continue to predict the potential for crises such as SARS but hopefully provide a cohesive way of acting to prevent the problems arising in the first place.

In Chapters 6 and 7 we introduced *Acting* and *Innovating*. The remarkable severity of the disease was the primary focus of the world's attention, and almost certainly gave a new signal to the world.

The global response was probably more remarkable in the skills it highlighted for the future. With SARS the call to collaboration between public health and other practitioners and the communities concerned was positively received because of the severity and immediacy of the problem. However, whereas SARS was visible, tangible and immediate and therefore something to which we needed to respond, sustainability is intangible, distant and barely visible, particularly to urban dwellers. SARS fitted our instinctive and patterned response, but sustainability is comparatively foreign and needs to harness new and old skills to a new future.

Our usual response to something foreign tends to be escape or denial. We realise we cannot gain by trying to escape from global ecological disintegrity, so we have been falling back on denying it to become comfortable again. This presents change agents with the challenge of problem definition that we must overcome if we are to harness enthusiasm for our cause. Solutions of this nature are hard to recommend through the written word. AtKisson's (1999) optimism is the best overall perspective we can offer to assume as an ongoing commitment. To build on this optimism, we have suggested searching for critical incidents, social change strategies and teachable moments where we can raise the profile of sustainability and global ecological integrity so it becomes relevant and meaningful for those to whom we are addressing the message.

In Chapter 8 we discussed *Managing and leadership*. In managing the SARS situation it appeared that strategists fell back on old habits. We saw evidence of enforced quarantine of infected people and reintroduction of border protection in the form of nurses at the airport who re-directed potential carriers of the virus to isolation facilities, thus preventing people bringing the disease into the country. This was expressed to our communities in terms of 'public health safety' and was hard to criticise as a management strategy because it is all we know, and has worked throughout the centuries. However, is enforced discipline the best way towards us as a society protecting ourselves, or is there another way? This is a question which needs to be considered in a context of participation and collaboration as key principles of working towards sustainability.

As the way forward from this book, we hope that readers will see their way clear to work towards sustainability in such a way that past understandings of infectious disease control can be built on to provide successful worldwide prevention of similar potential global threats. It is not necessary to reject the old, but it is essential to recognise the need to change earnestly. It is now up to public health practitioners to act as leaders and role models in embedding their efforts to enhance human health within an overall context of global ecological integrity.

The editors:

Valerie A. Brown
John Grootjans
Jan Ritchie
Mardie Townsend
Glenda Verrinder
February 2004

References

AtKisson, A. 1999, *Believing Cassandra: An optimist looks at a pessimist's world*, Chelsea Green Publishing, Vermont

World Health Organisation 2003, *Communicable Disease Surveillance and Response: SARS*, http://www.who.int/csr/sar [10 July 2003]

The editors

Emeritus Professor Valerie A. Brown AO, BSc, MEd, PhD

Director, Local Sustainability Project and Visiting Fellow, School of Resources, Environment and Society, Australian National University

Valerie is Vice-president, Australian National Biocentre, http://www.sustainability.org; member of ACT Sustainability Expert Reference Group and ACT Health Promotion Board; and sits on the editorial boards of the journals *Local Environment, Environmental Health* and *Ecosystem Health*. Previously Foundation Chair in Environmental Health at the University of Western Sydney Hawkesbury, Professor Valerie A. Brown has established research and post-graduate teaching programs on local sustainability in Australia, Malaysia and China and has contributed to national and international policies on public health and environmental sustainability. Valerie was appointed an Officer of the Order of Australia in 1999 for advocacy for sustainable development. Her publications include (alone and with others) *Landcare Languages* 1995; *Risks and Opportunities: Managing environmental conflict and change* 1995, *Managing for Local Sustainability* 1997; *Western Sydney Regional State-of-the-Environment Report 2000*; and *Towards Whole-of-Community Engagement: A toolkit for whole-of-community collaboration* 2003.

John Grootjans RN BAppSc GrdDipEd MAppSc PhD

Senior Lecturer, Charles Sturt University, Faculty of Nursing
Project Manager, Sustainability and Health Project, Griffith University

Dr John Grootjans has national and international experience in undertaking educational programs in the fields of sustainability and health, Aboriginal and Torres Strait Islander health, primary health care, public health, community development and remote area nursing. After beginning his nursing career in southern New South Wales in 1975, he became a nurse educator in the NSW College of Nursing before moving to the Northern Territory to work with Aboriginal people on community and health development in East Arnhem Land. He was a senior lecturer at Batchelor College 1990-97, acting as Head of School of Health Sciences and completing his PhD on the multiple issues for indigenous health worker education. He then took up a post as Lecturer in Primary Health Care at the University of Sydney. John managed the Commonwealth-funded Public Health Education and Research Program (PHERP) innovations project 2000-04. At the same time he developed and taught the first Australian post-graduate program in sustainability and health in Griffith University's School of Public Health. He has undertaken a range of research consultancies in community health development in the developing countries of the Pacific region, including East Timor.

Associate Professor Jan Ritchie BAppSc (Physiotherapy) MPH PhD

School of Public Health and Community Medicine, University of New South Wales

Jan has a Degree in Physiotherapy from the University of Sydney (USyd) and a Master of Health Personnel Education and PhD in Public Health from the University of New South Wales (UNSW). She is currently an Associate Professor in the School of Public Health and Community Medicine at UNSW, where she is Academic Program Advisor for Postgraduate Public Health Studies. She is very active in the national health promotion arena, being a long-standing Associate Director of the Australian Centre for Health Promotion, University of Sydney and currently holding the position of President of the Australian Health Promotion Association. She has worked extensively with the World Health Organization and the Australian Agency for International Development to promote the health of people in Pacific Island countries. Her primary research interest is community-based participatory research, attempting to better promote the health of patients, clients, consumers and community members.

Dr Mardie Townsend BSocSc PhD

Senior Lecturer, School of Health and Social Development, Deakin University

Mardie Townsend is a Senior Lecturer in the School of Health and Social Development at Deakin University, where she teaches on the links between 'people, health and place'. She is also course co-ordinator for the Bachelor of Health Sciences degree. In 1984, Mardie began her tertiary studies as a mature-aged student in the multidisciplinary Bachelor of Social Science (Socio-Environmental Assessment and Policy) course at RMIT. She completed a PhD in environmental sociology in 1996. Her research interests include the links between human health and contact with nature/ natural environments; social and health impact assessment; urban and rural health and wellbeing; and future trends in housing and neighbourhoods. In collaboration with Parks Victoria, the Lort Smith Animal Hospital and a range of other organisations, Mardie is leading research into the health benefits of contact with nature. Mardie also spent two years as a consultant in housing policy and practice in the United Kingdom and 10 years as a consultant in Australia, where her work involved strategic planning for community housing, community consultation and social impact assessment.

Glenda Verrinder RN Midwife GradDipHigher Ed MHealth Science

Lecturer, School of Public Health, La Trobe University, Bendigo

Glenda has been lecturing for seven years in public health theory and practice. Prior to that she spent 20 years working in community-based health care agencies in both urban and rural environments, and five years in acute health care settings. She has an ongoing relationship with community-based agencies and local government in the region. Her teaching, research and publications reflect her interests in public health in general and in particular primary health care, health promotion, ecological sustainability and health, environmental health and qualitative research. She sits on the editorial boards of Qualitative Health Research and Environmental Health, and is an active member of the Public Health Association of Australia and the Australian Environmental Health Educators' Forum.

Index

Aboriginal and Torres Strait Islander definition of
        health 143
Aborigines 74, 85, *see also* indigenous people
accountability, local/global 12
action groups
    environmental 59-60
    as settings for innovation 256-7
action in health and sustainability practice 102,
        Chapter 6
    acting collectively, *see* participation in decision making
    acting individually 235-9
    barriers to 246-8
    ethical guidelines/obligations 236-7
    planning, *see* planning in health and sustainability
        practice
    and systems thinking 201-12
action networks 291-4
    and trust dimension 293-4
adaptive management approaches 284-5
Adler, P.S. 278, 293
advocacy role 251, 252, 260-1
Agenda 21, *see* Local Agenda 21
agricultural production
    globalisation and 62
    monoculture 62
    see also food
aid to developing countries 53
air 206
    pollution 5, 10, 47, 48, 140-1, 186-7, 212, 214
Alma-Ata Declaration on Primary Health Care, USSR
        (1978) 84, 93-7, 99-100, 101, 143, 214
    key principles 93-4, 99-100, 143
Almås, R. 49
Aristotle 71
asbestos 5
AtKisson, A. xx, 15, 177, 233-5, 248-9
Australia
    Constitution of 85
    and international/UN conventions 91-2, 93
Australian Conservation Foundation 60
Australian Ecologically Sustainable Development
        Strategy 11
Australian National Public Health Strategy and
        Implementation Plan 11
Australian National State-of-the Environment Advisory
        Council 176

Balaton Group 177, 251, 259

Bates, G.M. 204
Bateson, W. 71
Baum, F. xx, 3, 18-19, 262
Bawden, R. 208
Believing Cassandra (A. AtKisson) xx, 248-9, 250
Bellagio principles 11
    guidelines for practical assessment of progress toward
        sustainable development 215-17
benchmarking, environmental 288-9
Berger, P.L. 143
Berry, T. 67
Bertollini, R. 19-20, 277
Bianchi, E.C. 66
Bierle, T. 227
biodiversity
    conservation of 12, 122
    depletion 8, 10
biomimicry 55
biophilia hypothesis 63-5
Birch, David 146, 147
Blandford, J. 287
Bohm, D. 150
Bolli, A. 288-9
Bolman, L. 301-2
Bradshaw, D. 263-4
Brower, David 67
Brown, Valerie A. 32, 146, 147
Browne, B. 253-5
bureaucracy, characteristics of 283-4, 291, *see also*
        hierarchies/formal organisations in managing
        sustainability

cancer 5, 166, 183
    lung 301
*Cannibals with Forks: The triple bottom line of
        21st century business* (J. Elkington) 56-7
capital, financial, physical and human 56-8
capitalism
    development of 49
    natural, *see* natural capital/capitalism
Capra, F. 3, 20, 71
Carley, M. 291
Carson, Rachel 30, 45, 107, 245
CDCynergy social marketing planning framework 261
change
    approaches to 233-5
    barriers to environmental 245, 246-8

climate 18-19, 239
global 1, 14, 45
sustainable 21-4
see also innovation/innovators; structural change
Chapman, S. 261
chemical pollutants 107-10
Chernobyl disaster 214
Chicago: 'Imagine Chicago' movement 253-5, 265
Christian perspective on spirituality and the Earth 67
Christie, I. 291
City Farm youth project 219-20
climate change 118-19
solutions 239
Club of Rome 14, 15
Coehlo, P. 67
Common Ground and Common Sense (R. Nicholson
    et al.) 153-4
communication skills 216, 232, 259, *see also* participation
    in decision-making
communities, learning 26-6
community
    -based action for health 152-4
    engagement in change 152-4, 258-9
    knowledge 138, 139, 140, 142, 143, 144, 147, 157,
        158
    life 121-2
    values 202
COMPASS monitoring system 177, 233
consciousness raising 251, 252-3
Constanza, Robert 146
Convention on Biological Diversity (1995) 204
Conway, Gordon 267
'cornucopian enchantment' perspective of
    sustainability 53
corporate environmental performance indicators 289-90
corporate governance for sustainability 287
Crimes (Torture) Act 1998 (Australia) 91-2
Curitiba, Brazil 234

D4P4 (decisions-into-practice) framework xiii, 2, 21-8,
        41, 83, 150, 156, 163, 167, 171, 180, 188, 308,
    see also decision-making
Dashboard (software) 177
DDT, use of 107, 277
Deal, T. 301-2
d'Eaubonne, Francois 68, 69
decision-making 12, 14
    framework/perspective 169-72, *see also* frameworks
    group, *see* participation in decision-making

indicators 176-7
knowledge cultures in 139, 141-3, 145-6, 148, 149
nominal group process 224-6
processes 226, *see also* D4P4; problem solving
scoping in: Chapter 5
sectors 170-2, *see also* knowledge
Declaration of Alma-Ata, *see* Alma-Ata Declaration on
        Primary Health Care
deductive and inductive problem solving 165, 166-9, 171
deity, the Earth as 66-7
depression, economic 52
deregulation, market 50, 51, 52
dialogue in a multiple knowledge learning community
        150-2
Dias-Sardinha, I. 287
discrimination, *see* Universal Declaration of Human
        Rights
disease
    and the environment 8, *see also* cancer
    infectious 4, 5, 211, 309-12
    see also health risk
dot.com bubble 52
DPSEEA framework for environmental health monitoring
        178, 179, 180, 181
Drengson, A. 210, 238

Earth as deity 66-7
Earth Charter (2000) 121-6, 169, 184, 262, 266, 268,
        308
Earth Summit, *see* United Nations Conference on
        Environment and Development
eco-efficiency
    definition of 297-8
    objectives and opportunities 298
eco-feminism 68-70
ecological
    economics 53-4
    integrity, *see* global ecological integrity
    issues, action networks on 291-4
    perspectives 45-7, 202
    system and human society 20-1, 45-7
Ecological Footprint Calculator software 224
ecology
    deep 60, 68, 238
    and human health 45-7
    and indigenous people 70-2
economics and sustainability 5,12, 40, 48-59
    capitalism and globalisation 49, *see also* globalisation
    ecological economics 53-4

economic liberalism 50-1
economic rationalism 50
Keynesianism 51-2
natural capitalism 54-6
single bottom line 58-9
'the cornucopian enchantment' perspective 53
triple bottom line 56-8, 145, *see also* triple bottom line principle
EcoSummit in Halifax, Nova Scotia (2000) 246-7
education for sustainability 262-6
conceptual framework for action 263-4
learning communities 264-6
types of intelligence 266
education, public health, *see* public health education
educational institutions facilitating sustainability 119-21
Elkington, J. 56-7, 236
empowerment strategies for change 252
Emtairah, T. 288-9
energy use 5, 9, 14, 245
see also oil
environment, natural: negative effects of the built environment on 212, 213, 214, *see also* pollution
environment and sustainability: Earth Charter (2000) 121-6, 169, 184, 262, 266, 268, 308
environmental health monitoring 177-8, 179, 180-7
indicators 176-7, 182
environmental issues
adaptive management of 284
benchmarking for 288-9
and change, *see* change
corporate performance indicators 289-90
and ecology, *see* ecological, ecology
frameworks (conferences and conventions) 106-21
health 3-10, 30-2
risk/health risk xx, 4, 47, 177-82, 185, 186-7, 247, *see also* disease; pollution
and scepticism 47-8
the systemic nature of 206-7
and waste management, *see* waste
see also environmentalism and sustainability
environmentalism and sustainability 40, 59-75
action groups/perspectives 59-60, 256-7
and feminism 68-70
human health and benefits of nature 63-5
indigenous people and the environment 70-2
and individual action 60-1, 62, 63
spirituality and the environment 65-7
and technologies to reduce consumption 63
equity 18, 85, 124, *see also* human rights; inequality

erosion, soil 75
ethical guidelines for practice 236-7

fair trade movement 62
family planning 53
Farman, Joe 111
feminism and sustainability 68-70
feminist ecology 66
fertiliser use 74
The Fight for Public Health (S. Chapman and D. Lupton) 261
fish stocks 74
Flannery, T.F. 70
food 207
consumption 62
crises, Third World 53
production 9, 62, 70-2
web problems 214
foreign aid to developing countries 53
forest
clearing 10
management 284
fossil fuels 15, *see also* energy use; oil
Foucault, M. 69, 149
Fourth World 83
frameworks
decision-making, *see* decision-making
environmental 106-21, 178, 179, 180-2
health-based 93-106
holistic 121-7
of knowledge: Chapter 4
social marketing 261-2
strategic 84-93
and tools 83-4
Friere, Paulo 265, 267
Frumkin, H. 65
futures wheels, 'no oil' 211-12, 213

Gaia hypothesis 45, 66
Gandhi, Indira 211
Gandhi, Mahatma 61
gas, natural 9
genetically modified crops/organisms 27, 122, 136-8, 140
genuine progress indicator (GPI) 59, 176
Giddens, A. 250
Gilding, P. 58-9
global ecological integrity xiv, xx, 1, 3, 8-10, 11, 19-20, 21, 122-4, 145, 309
global indicators of sustainability loss (1950-95) 9

Global Reporting Initiative (GRI) 57-8
global warming 8, 9, 10, 14, 27, 48, 245
globalisation 1, 2, 49
   ecological and human costs of 62-3
   positive collaborative action 209
   production cost cutting 62
governance, organisational 285-7
   corporate 287
governments and sustainability management 286-7
greenhouse gas emissions 9, 26, 48, 117-19
Greenpeace 60
'greenwashing' products 62-3
gross national product (GNP) 50
group action, *see* participation in decision-making
Gullone, E. 65

Hailes, J. 236
Hancock, T. 15, 16-18, 32, 42-3, 73, 144, 178, 209-10,
   212
Harremoës, P. 166
Harvard Negotiating Process 152
Hawken, Paul 54, 55, 56
HEADLAMP project, WHO 181
health
   - based frameworks (conferences/conventions) 84,
      93-106
   benefits of the natural environment 63-5
   community-based action for 152-4
   definitions of xv, 24-5, 143
   ecological perspective on 45-7
   and environmental issues 3-10, 30-2, 206-7
   risks, *see* health risk
   see also public health
Health and Environmental Analysis for Decision-making
   (WHO) 181
Health for All by the year 2000 strategy (WHO) 97-9,
   100, 266
health practice, *see* public health practice
health risk
   assessment 30, 166
   environmental xix, 4, 140-1, 177-8, 179, 205
   from SARS 309-12
   from smoking 300-1
   see also disease
Healthy Cities project (WHO) 16-17, 18, 214, 218-19,
   220, 263, 268
Heerwagen, J.H. 65
Heron, J. 258
hierarchies/formal organisations in managing
   sustainability 278, 279, 280, 281, 282-90

adaptive management 284-5
benchmarking 288-9
bureaucracies 283-7
corporate environmental performance indicators
   289-90
governance 285-7
Hippocrates of Kos 4
holistic frameworks
   Earth Charter 121-6
   knowledge, *see* knowledge
   perspective in assessing progress towards sustainabable
      development 215
Human Frontiers, Environments and Disease
   (T. McMichael) xx, *see also* McMichael A.J.
human relationship with the natural environment 63-7,
   209-10
human rights 85-93, 122, 124-5
   health 94
human society in the global ecological system 20-1, 45-7
human species, conditions for the physical survival of the
   15, 234-5

Ian Potter Foundation 258
Ife, J. 202, 251, 258
ignorance, knowledge and 144-5, 246
imagination as a social movement 253-4, 265
Imagine Chicago: Ten years of imagination in action
   (B. Browne and S. Jain) 253
'Imagine Chicago' movement 253-5, 265
indicators
   corporate environmental performance 289-90
   decision-making 176-7
   design websites 191-2
   environmental health monitoring 176-7, 182
   genuine progress (GPI) 59, 176
   of sustainability loss (1950-95) 9
indigenous people
   and the environment/food production 66-7, 70-2, 74
   the law/code of conduct 71-2
   life expectancy 93
indigenous sacred sites 74
indigenous spirituality 66-7
IndoPacific Conference on Environment and Health
   (2002) 146-7
industrial revolution 5, 149
inequality 86
   economic 50-1, 52
   health 94
   racial 49, 85

innovation/innovators: Chapter 7
  barriers to 246-8
  diffusion of 248-51
  from a business perspective 298-9, 300
  in education for sustainibility, *see* education for
    sustainability
  innovators defined 249
  and research for sustainability 267-8
  roles/perspectives of practitioners 251-62
  settings for 256-7
  structuration theory 250-1
  see also change; structural change
Inoue, Y. 210
Institute for Educational Studies 150
intelligence, types of 266, *see also* education for
  sustainability
Intergovernmental Agreement on the Environment
  (1992) 204
Intergovernmental Forum on Chemical Safety 107
International Association of Public Participation 227
International Conference on Health Promotion, Ottawa
  (1986) 100-6, *see also* Ottawa Charter for Health
  Promotion
International Conference on Primary Health Care, Alma-
  Ata, USSR (1978), *see* Alma-Ata Declaration on
  Primary Health Care
international conventions/treaties, *see* health-based
  frameworks; United Nations; Universal
  Declaration of Human Rights; *and by name* of
  conference/convention
International Council for Local Environmental Initiatives
  (ICLEI) 204-5, 209
International Labour Organisation 107
International Standards Organisation (ISO) programs
  289-90
International Union for Health Promotion and Education
  (IUHPE) 209
irrigation 9

Jain, S. 253-5
justice/social justice 84-5, 124-5, 251, 252
  perspective 202, *see also* human rights

Kahn, P.H. 64
Kant, E. 168, 169
Kanter, R.M. 287
Kellert, S.R. 64
Kelly, George 152
Keynes, John Maynard 51

Keynesianism 51-2
Kickbusch, I. 207, 210
Kidner, D.W. 209
kinship relations, indigenous 71-2
Kirschenmann, F. 204
knowledge
  constructions of: Chapter 4
  divided in public health 141-3
  holistic 134-6, 139, 140-1, 143, 144, 147, 148, 155,
    157, 158, 170, 172
  and ignorance 144-5
  individual 135, 136-9, 142, 143, 147, 158, 170, 172
  local/community 135, 138-9, 142, 143, 144, 147, 148,
    157, 158
  networking 154-5, 158
  and power 149
  re atmospheric lead 140-1, 186-7
  re genetic modification 137-8, 140
  re persistent organic pollutants (POPs) 145-5
  and rules for dialogue 150-1
  specialised/scientific 135, 138-9, 140, 142, 143, 144,
    147, 149, 157, 158, 170, 172
  strategic 135, 138-9, 142, 143, 144, 158, 172
  synthesis of, *see* synthesis of knowledges
  and whole-of-community action web 152-4
Kolb, D.A. 22, 23, 24, 167, 264
Kuhn, T.S. 139, 149
Kuznets, S. 50-1
Kyoto Protocol on Greenhouse Gases 9, 26, 48, 117-19

land use 207
  planning 291
  productive 9
Lawrence, G. 49
lead, atmospheric 140-1, 186-7, 260
LEAD Action News 260
learning communities 264-6
life expectancy 48
  indigenous 93
Light, A. 236
The Limits of Growth (Club of Rome) 14, 15
Limits to Growth (D.H. Meadows et al.) 245
listening and coordinating ideas: Chapter 2
Local Agenda 21   32, 84, 112, 215, 217-8, 219, 263,
  268, 286
Lomborg, B. 47-8
Lovelock, J. 45, 66
Lovins, A. and H. 54-5, 56
Lowe, I. 31, 32
Luckmann, T. 143
Lupton, D. 261

MacDonald, M. 13
McMichael, A.J. xx, 8, 32, 45-6, 84, 146, 147
McMurray, A. 93-4
McPhee, J. 67
management/leadership for sustainability: Chapter 8
    actions required by managers 276-7
    adaptive 284-5
    analysing issues 277-8
    behaviour 280-1
    benchmarking 288-9
    in bureaucracies 283-7, see also hierarchies/formal
        organisations in managing sustainability
    of complex systems 278-82
    corporate environmental performance indicators
        289-90
    and corporate governance 287
    domains 277-8
    environmental 284
    organisational forms, see hierarchies/formal
        organisations in managing sustainability; markets,
        managing; networks, managing
    resources for 302-3
    the role of public health 300-2
    in urban regeneration partnerships 281-2
Mandala of Health 15, 17, 42-3, 73, 144, 178
Mandell, M.P. 292
market deregulation 50, 51, 52
markets, managing 278, 279, 280, 281, 282, 296-300
    ideal type characteristics of a market 296-7
    innovation and business 298-9, 300
    markets defined 297
    and triple/single bottom line 299
Marxism 202
Meadows, Donella and Dennis 14
Men in Trees 219-20
Merchant, C. 69
Mill, John Stuart 236
monitoring environmental health 177-8, 179,
    180-3
    DPSEEA framework 178, 179, 180, 181
    PSR framework 181-2, 183
monitoring strategies 164, 165-9
    and deductive and inductive approaches 165, 166-9,
        171
monitoring sustainability and health programs: Chapter 5
Montreal Protocol on Substances that Deplete
        the Ozone Layer (1987) 110-11, 235, see also
        ozone depletion
Muir, John 63

National Environmental Health Strategy 152
National Health Service (Britain) 52
natural capital/capitalism 54-8
    strategies and principles 55-6
natural environment, negative effects of the built
        environment on 212, 213, 214
nature
    children and 64
    human relationship with (biophilia) 63-7, 209-10
    human separation from 70-1
networks, managing 278, 279, 280, 281, 282, 290-6,
        301
    action networks 291-4
    network characteristics 290-1
    rules/strategies 295-6
New International Economic Order 94
New Public Health principles 18-21, 32, 276
New Public Health, The (F. Baum) xx, 3, 18-19, 276
Nicholson, R. 153
nominal group process for planning 224-6
Norton, B.G. 285

O'Donoghue, Loitja 146
oil
    'no oil' futures wheel 213
    replacements 15
    use 9
organisational forms for management, see hierarchies/
        formal organisations in managing sustainability;
        markets, managing; networks, managing
Orians, G.H. 65
Ottawa Charter for Health Promotion 17, 100-6,
        215, 226, 262
Our Common Future (World Commission on
        Environment and Development) 145
ozone depletion 8, 9, 14, 117, 235, 345
    Montreal Protocol (1987) 110-11, 235

participation in decision-making 226-35
    approaches in 229, 267-8
    communication skills 232
    conflict management/resolution in 232-3
    consensus in 231
    constructs, collaboration and co-operation skills
        229-30
    decision-making processes 226
    democracy in 226-7
    evaluation techniques 230-1
    spectrum of 228

peace/tolerance 125-6
Perraca Bijur, A. 208, 255
perspectives
    action group 59-60, 256-7
    business 298-9, 300
    Christian 67
    'cornucopean enchantment' 53
    decision-making 169-72
    ecological 45-7, 202
    holistic (on sustainable development assessment) 215
    of practitioners of change 251-62
    public health theoretical: Chapter 2
    in systems thinking 201-8, *see also* knowledge,
        constructions of
pesticides 166, 205, 245, *see also* pollution
Pimentel, D. 8
planning in health and sustainability practice 212-26
    analysis 221
    appropriate technology in 223-4
    Bellagio Principles 215-17
    City Farm youth project 219-20
    essentials for 214-19
    Local Agenda 21 217-18
    models defining interractions 221-3
    research questions 221
    setting priorities 224-6
    WHO Healthy Cities project 218-19
plant species for medical use 10
pollution 4-5, 214
    chemical 107-10
    industrial 14, 368
    lead, atmospheric 140-1, 186-7, 260
    persistent organic pollutants (POPs) 107-10, 145-6, *see
        also* air, pollution; pesticides; soil; water
population: world 9, 14, 46, 53, 245
Porter, M. 300
poverty 46, 51, 58, 124, 211
    in Third World countries 53
Powell, W.W. 278-9
precautionary principle 18, 146, 166, 203-5
    defined 204
    implementing 205
Pretty, J. 267, 268
Prigogine, I. 20
problem solving
    deductive and inductive 166, 167-9, 171
    using models for analysis 247
production systems/models 55-6
PSR (pressure-state-response) framework 181-2, 183
public health, *see* health; New Public Health; public

health education; public health practice
public health education 14, 19, 20
    disciplinary areas in 29-30
    and global change 14
public health practice xix-xx, 2, 8
    criteria for practitioners 28-33
    defined xvi
    designing and monitoring programs: Chapter 5
    divided knowledges in 141-3
    and environmental issues 3-10, 30-2, *see also*
        environmental issues
    evidence-based 133-43
    history/phases 4-5, 19
    knowledges in, *see* knowledge
    management/leadership: Chapter 8
    new ideas for 18-21
    theoretical perspectives: Chapter 2
    and tobacco control 300-1

Racial Discrimination Act 1975, (Australia) 86, 91-2
Rapport, David 146, 247
Rees, W.E. 20, 32, 176
Reijnders, L. 287
research for sustainability 267-8
resource depletion, *see* air; food; oil; water
Rio Declaration on Environment and Development
        (1992) 112-17, *see also* United Nations
        Conference on Environment and Development
risk, dealing with 12
    health, *see* health risk
    environmental 177-82, 185, 186-7, 247
Rittel, H. 131
rivers 42-3, 72-5, *see also* water sources and waterways
Rocky Mountain Institute (2002) 55-6
Roosevelt, F.D. 52
Ross, H. 152
Rummery, K. 292
Rural City Farm project, *see* City Farm youth project

St Luke's Anglicare 258-9
SARS (severe acute respiratory syndrome) epidemic
        309-12
scepticism of environmental issues 47-8
science and sustainability 40, 41-8
    the classical approach 44-5
    human health and ecology 45-7
scoping sustainability: Chapter 5, *see also* monitoring
        sustainability and health programs;
    and brainstorming 190-1
    framework/perspective 169-73

and grounding 192-6
information sources 173-84
program stages 187-90
purpose/place in the research process 187-9
SWOT analysis in scoping process 189
sewerage 210-11
Sex Discrimination Act 1984, Australian 86, 91-2
Shell Canada 287, 299
shelter/physical environment 206-7
Silent Spring (R. Carson) 45, 107, 245
siltation of rivers 75
Simon, Julian 53
single bottom line (SBL) 58-9, 299
Skeptical Environmentalist, The (B. Lomborg) 47
slavery 49, 85
SMART (social marketing assessment and response tool)
    planning framework 261-2
Smith, Adam 50
Smithson, M. 160
smoking rates 300-1
Smuts, J.C. 135
Smyth, T. 287
social justice, *see* justice
soil degradation 10, 15
soil salination 214
Soskolne, C.L. 19-20, 21, 236
species, disappearing 9
spirituality and the environment 65-7
    indigenous 66-7
Steinemann, A.C. 285
Stockholm Convention on Persistent Organic
    Pollutants 107-10
structural change 33-4, 245-51
    advocacy 251, 252, 260-1
    barriers to 246-8
    capacity building for 251-62
    community engagement 152-4, 258-9
    consciousness raising 251, 252-3
    diffusion of innovation theory 248-51
    and empowerment 252
    and imagination as a social movement 253-5
    LEAD group 260
    networking strategy 259-60
    roles/perspectives of practitioners 251-62
    settings/groups for 256-7
    shared action for 258-9
    social animation for 258, 259
    for social justice 251, 252
    social marketing for 261-2

techniques for soft revolution 258
visioning for 255
sustainability xvi, 2
    in action 146-7
    community-based action for 152-4
    and constructions of knowledge, see knowledge
    corporate governance for 287
    defined xix
    designing and monitoring: Chapter 5
    and economics, see economics and sustainability;
    and environmentalism, see environmentalism and
        sustainability
    five strategies of 145
    frameworks (conventions and protocols): Chapter 3
    global indicators of loss of (1950-95) 9
    holistic frameworks (Earth Charter) 121-6
    indicators (single bottom line) 58-9
    management/leadership for: Chapter 8
    perspectives on 201-8, see also knowledge
    precautionary principle 203-5
    principles of xvi, xviii, 2, 11, 20-1, see also D4P4
        framework
    as public health practice 28-33
    reasons for 3
    research for 267-8
    and science 40, 43-8
    the stakeholders 155-6
    Talloires Declaration 119-21, 177
    three elements of 56-8, 144-5, 178, 179
sustainability and health
    definitions 11-18
    and environmental issues 3-10, *see also*
        environmental issues
    ideas/perspectives: Chapter 2
    and natural capitalism 55-6
sustainable development xvi, 2, 5, 11-18, 245
    and change 33-4, 245, *see also* change
    conditions for/implementation of 14-18, 234-5
    defined xvi, 11-18
    and new public health, *see* New Public Health
        principles
    principles 12, 13-14, 25
Sustainable Seattle city monitoring system 177, 233
Suzuki, D. 66
SWOT (strengths, weaknesses, opportunities, threats)
    analysis 189, 231
synthesis of knowledges 135-6, 143, 145, 146-8
    strategies for 149-52, 157
    tools for 152-6, 157

systems
  the futures wheel 211-12
  interconnectedness of 205-8, 209-10
  multiple perspectives 201-8
  the precautionary principle 203-5
  the sewerage principle 210-11
  and subsystems 205-6
  systems thinking 201-12
  the triple bottom line principle 203, *see also* triple
    bottom line principle
Szreter, Simon 52

Talloires Convention/Declaration 119-21, 177
technologies to reduce ecological impacts 63
theoretical perspectives of sustainability and health:
    Chapter 2
Third World countries 52, 53
Thoreau, Henry 61
tobacco control 300-1
Toulmin, S.E. 147
Townsend, M. 251
Transforming Lives, Transforming Communities
    (D. Bradshaw) 263-4
triple bottom line principle 56-8, 145, 179-80, 203, 205,
    208
  from a management perspective 299
trust dimension in action networks 293-4
The Turning Point (F. Capra) 3
Twine, R.T. 69

United Nations agencies 84-5, *see also by name*
United Nations Conference on Environment and
    Development (Earth Summit), Rio de Janeiro
    (1992) 13, 84, 112-17, 121, 145, 211, 217, 263,
    see also Earth Charter Local Agenda 21
United Nations conventions/conferences: Chapter 3
United Nations Development Program (UNDP) 59
United Nations Education Scientific and Culture
    Organisation (UNESCO) 84-5, 93, 97, 106, 121
United Nations Environment Program (UNEP) 106, 107,
    110, 111, 117
United Nations World Conference on Environment and
    Development (1986) 245
United States Environmental Protection Authority 107
United States Institute of Medicine, Research,
    Engineering and Science 13-14
Universal Declaration of Human Rights 85-91
universities facilitating sustainability (Talloires
    Declaration) 119-21, 177
UV radiation 5

Valdez Principles 177
values
  community 202
  ethical 24-5
  personal 201-3, 266
voluntary simplicity 60-2, 63
von Weizsäcker, Ernst 55

Wackernagel, M. 176
Walmer-Toews, David 146, 147
waste
  industrial 8
  managing/reducing 3, 5, 12, 15, 207
water 207
  depletion 14, 245
  pollution 8, 10, 47, 48, 74, 75, 177-8, 179, 184-5, 214
water sources and waterways 4, 8, 10, 75, 284, *see also*
    rivers
Weber, Max 283
welfare, public 50-1
welfare state 52, 53
Werner, D. 99
Wheeler, K.A. 208, 255
Wilderness Society 60
wildlife issues 60
Wilson, E.O. 63-4
windpower 9
women and the natural environment 68-70
World Bank 49, 51
World Commission on Environment and Development
    (1987) 8, 11, 145, 245
World Health Organisation (WHO) 8, 93, 97, 107, 310,
    310
  conferences/conventions 93-106
  definition of health 24-5, 143
  Health and Environmental Analysis for Decision-
    making, Linkage Analysis and Monitoring Project
    (HEADLAMP) 181
  Healthy Cities project 16-17, 18, 214, 218-19, 220,
    263, 268
  resolution WHA32.30 (Health for All by the year 2000
    strategy) 97-9, 100, 266

World Summit on Sustainable Development (2002) 26-7
World War II 51, 52, 85
World Wildlife Fund 60

Yencken, D. 286

Zaher, A. 293